Advances in Barrett's Esophagus

Editor

SACHIN WANI

GASTROINTESTINAL ENDOSCOPY
CLINICS OF NORTH AMERICA

www.giendo.theclinics.com

Consulting Editor
CHARLES J. LIGHTDALE

January 2021 • Volume 31 • Number 1

ELSEVIER

1600 John F. Kennedy Boulevard • Suite 1800 • Philadelphia, Pennsylvania, 19103-2899

http://www.theclinics.com

GASTROINTESTINAL ENDOSCOPY CLINICS OF NORTH AMERICA Volume 31, Number 1 January 2021 ISSN 1052-5157, ISBN-13: 978-0-323-79831-0

Editor: Kerry Holland

Developmental Editor: Donald Mumford

Gastrointestinal Endoscopy Clinics of North America (ISSN 1052-5157) is published quarterly by Elsevier Inc., 360 Park Avenue South, New York, NY 10010-1710. Months of issue are January, April, July, and October. Business and Editorial Offices: 1600 John F. Kennedy Blvd., Suite 1800, Philadelphia, PA, 19103-2899. Periodicals postage paid at New York, NY and additional mailing offices. Subscription prices are $363.00 per year for US individuals, $813.00 per year for US institutions, $100.00 per year for US and Canadian students/residents, $399.00 per year for Canadian individuals, $841.00 per year for Canadian institutions, $476.00 per year for international individuals, $841.00 per year for international institutions, and $245.00 per year for international students/residents. To receive student/resident rate, orders must be accompanied by name of affiliated institution, date of term, and the *signature* of program/residency coordinator on institution letterhead. Orders will be billed at individual rate until proof of status is received. Foreign air speed delivery is included in all *Clinics* subscription prices. All prices are subject to change without notice. **POSTMASTER:** Send address change to *Gastrointestinal Endoscopy Clinics of North America*, Elsevier Health Sciences Division, Subscription Customer Service, 3251 Riverport Lane, Maryland Heights, MO 63043. **Customer Service: 1-800-654-2452 (US). From outside the United States, call 1-314-447-8871. Fax: 1-314-447-8029. E-mail: JournalsCustomerService-usa@elsevier.com (for print support) or JournalsOnlineSupport-usa@elsevier.com (for online support)**.

Reprints. For copies of 100 or more, of articles in this publication, please contact the Commercial Reprints Department, Elsevier Inc., 360 Park Avenue South, New York, NY 10010-1710. Tel. 212-633-3874; Fax: 212-633-3820; E-mail: reprints@elsevier.com.

Gastrointestinal Endoscopy Clinics of North America is covered in *Excerpta Medica, MEDLINE/PubMed (Index Medicus), and MEDLINE/MEDLARS.*

Contributors

CONSULTING EDITOR

CHARLES J. LIGHTDALE, MD
Professor of Medicine, Division of Digestive and Liver Diseases, Columbia University, Medical Center, New York, New York, USA

EDITOR

SACHIN WANI, MD, FASGE, AGAF
Professor of Medicine, Associate Medical Director, Division of Gastroenterology and Hepatology, Medical Director, Esophageal and Gastric Center, University of Colorado Anschutz Medical Campus, Aurora, Colorado, USA

AUTHORS

JACQUES J.G.H.M. BERGMAN, MD, PhD
Department of Gastroenterology and Hepatology, Amsterdam University Medical Centers, University of Amsterdam, Amsterdam, the Netherlands

RAF BISSCHOPS, MD, PhD
Head of Endoscopy, Gastroenterology and Hepatology, University Hospital Leuven, Leuven, Belgium

MARCIA IRENE CANTO, MD, MHS
Gastroenterologist, Division of Gastroenterology and Hepatology, The Johns Hopkins Medical Institutions, Johns Hopkins Hospital, Baltimore, Maryland, USA

AMITABH CHAK, MD
University Hospitals Cleveland Medical Center, Case Western Reserve University School of Medicine, Cleveland, Ohio, USA

ASHWINEE CONDON, MD
Vatche and Tamar Manoukian Division of Digestive Diseases, David Geffen School of Medicine at UCLA, Los Angeles, California, USA

MICHAEL B. COOK, PhD
Senior Investigator, Division of Cancer Epidemiology and Genetics, National Cancer Institute, Rockville, Maryland, USA

WOUTER L. CURVERS, MD, PhD
Department of Gastroenterology and Hepatology, Catharina Hospital Eindhoven, Eindhoven, the Netherlands

ALBERT J. de GROOF, MD
Department of Gastroenterology and Hepatology, Amsterdam UMC, University of Amsterdam, Amsterdam, the Netherlands

PETER H.N. de WITH, PhD
Department of Electrical Engineering, VCA Group, Eindhoven University of Technology, Eindhoven, the Netherlands

HASHEM B. EL-SERAG, MD, MPH
Baylor College of Medicine Medical Center, McNair Campus (Clinic), Houston, Texas, USA

GARY W. FALK, MD, MS
Professor of Medicine, Division of Gastroenterology, University of Pennsylvania, Perelman School of Medicine, Philadelphia, Pennsylvania, USA

DOMENICO A. FARINA, MD
Department of Gastroenterology and Hepatology, Northwestern University, Chicago, Illinois, USA

REBECCA C. FITZGERALD, MD, FRCP, FMedSci
MRC Cancer Unit, Professor of Cancer Prevention, University of Cambridge, Honorary Consultant Gastroenterology, Cambridge University Hospitals NHS Foundation Trust, Director of Studies - Medical Science, Trinity College Cambridge, Cambridge, United Kingdom

CHARLOTTE N. FREDERIKS, MD
PhD Student, Department of Gastroenterology and Hepatology, University Medical Center Utrecht, Utrecht, the Netherlands

REHAN HAIDRY, BSc (Hons), MD, FRCP
Consultant Gastroenterologist, Department of Gastroenterology and Endoscopy, University College London Hospitals NHS Foundation Trust, London, United Kingdom

JOHN M. INADOMI, MD
Jon M. Huntsman Presidential Chair, Professor and Chair, Department of Internal Medicine, University of Utah School of Medicine, Salt Lake City, Utah, USA

PRASAD G. IYER, MD, MSc
Professor of Medicine, Division of Gastroenterology and Hepatology, Mayo Clinic, Rochester, Minnesota, USA

AMRIT K. KAMBOJ, MD
Instructor in Medicine, Division of Gastroenterology and Hepatology, Mayo Clinic, Rochester, Minnesota, USA

DAVID A. KATZKA, MD
Professor of Medicine, Division of Gastroenterology and Hepatology, Mayo Clinic, Rochester, Minnesota, USA

SRINADH KOMANDURI, MD, MS
Department of Gastroenterology and Hepatology, Northwestern University, Chicago, Illinois, USA

VANI J.A. KONDA, MD
Department of Gastroenterology and Hepatology, Baylor University Medical Center, Dallas, Texas, USA

PHILIPPE LECLERCQ, MD
Gastroenterology and Hepatology, University Hospital Leuven, Leuven, Belgium

MARTIN D. McCARTER, MD, FACS
Professor, Department of Surgery, Division of Surgical Oncology, University of Colorado Denver, Aurora, Colorado, USA

PAUL MOAYYEDI, MD, PhD, MPH
Paul Moayyedi Audrey Campbell Chair of Ulcerative Colitis Research, McMaster University, Hamilton, Ontario, Canada

V. RAMAN MUTHUSAMY, MD, MAS
Professor of Clinical Medicine, Medical Director of Endoscopy, UCLA Health System, Vatche and Tamar Manoukian Division of Digestive Diseases, David Geffen School of Medicine at UCLA, Los Angeles, California, USA

ESTHER A. NIEUWENHUIS, MD
Department of Gastroenterology and Hepatology, Amsterdam University Medical Centers, Amsterdam, the Netherlands

OLIVER PECH, MD, PhD
Department of Gastroenterology and Hepatology, Krankenhaus Barmherzige Brüder Regensburg, Regensburg, Germany

ROOS E. POUW, MD, PhD
Department of Gastroenterology and Hepatology, Amsterdam University Medical Centers, Amsterdam, the Netherlands

AKSHAY PRATAP, MD, MCh, FACS
Assistant Professor, Department of Surgery, University of Colorado, Aurora, Colorado, USA

KRISH RAGUNATH, MBBS, MD, DNB, MPhil, FRCP, FASGE
Professor of Medicine and Gastroenterology, Department of Gastroenterology, Curtin University Medical School, Royal Perth Hospital, Perth, Western Australia, Australia

JOEL H. RUBENSTEIN, MD, MSc
Research Scientist, Center for Clinical Management Research, Ann Arbor Veterans Affairs Medical Center, Professor of Medicine, Division of Gastroenterology, Department of Internal Medicine, University of Michigan Medical School, Rogel Cancer Center, University of Michigan, Ann Arbor, Michigan, USA

VINAY SEHGAL, MBChB, MRCP, PhD
Consultant Gastroenterologist, Department of Gastroenterology and Endoscopy, University College London Hospitals NHS Foundation Trust, London, United Kingdom

ANAMAY N. SHARMA, MD
University Hospitals Cleveland Medical Center, Case Western Reserve University School of Medicine, Cleveland, Ohio, USA

RHONDA F. SOUZA, MD
Division of Gastroenterology, Center for Esophageal Diseases, Baylor University Medical Center at Dallas, Center for Esophageal Research, Baylor Scott & White Research Institute, Dallas, Texas, USA

STUART JON SPECHLER, MD
Division of Gastroenterology, Center for Esophageal Diseases, Baylor University Medical Center at Dallas, Center for Esophageal Research, Baylor Scott & White Research Institute, Dallas, Texas, USA

MAARTEN R. STRUYVENBERG, MD
Department of Gastroenterology and Hepatology, Amsterdam UMC, University of Amsterdam, Amsterdam, the Netherlands

WEI KEITH TAN, MBChB
MRC Cancer Unit, University of Cambridge, Department of Gastroenterology, Addenbrookes Hospital, University of Cambridge, Cambridge, United Kingdom

AARON P. THRIFT, PhD
Assistant Professor, Section of Epidemiology and Population Sciences, Department of Medicine, Dan L Duncan Comprehensive Cancer Center, Baylor College of Medicine, Houston, Texas, USA

JOSEPH R. TRIGGS, MD, PhD
Assistant Professor of Clinical Medicine, Division of Gastroenterology, University of Pennsylvania, Perelman School of Medicine, Philadelphia, Pennsylvania, USA

FONS van der SOMMEN, PhD
Department of Electrical Engineering, VCA Group, Eindhoven University of Technology, Eindhoven, the Netherlands

THOMAS J. WATSON, MD, FACS
Professor, Department of Surgery, MedStar Georgetown University Hospital, Georgetown University School of Medicine, Washington, DC, USA

Bas L.A.M. WEUSTEN, MD, PHD
Gastroenterologist, Department of Gastroenterology and Hepatology, St. Antonius Hospital, Nieuwegein, the Netherlands; Gastroenterologist, Department of Gastroenterology and Hepatology, University Medical Center Utrecht, Utrecht, the Netherlands

Contents

Foreword: Barrett's Esophagus: Current Management and New Approaches xiii

Charles J. Lightdale

Preface: Advances and Opportunities in Barrett's Esophagus xv

Sachin Wani

Epidemiology of Barrett's Esophagus and Esophageal Adenocarcinoma: Implications for Screening and Surveillance 1

Michael B. Cook and Aaron P. Thrift

In the United States, the incidence of esophageal adenocarcinoma increased markedly since the 1970s with a recent stabilization. Despite evolving screening and surveillance strategies to diagnose, risk triage, and intervene in Barrett's esophagus patients to prevent esophageal adenocarcinoma, most cases present with advanced disease and poor resultant survival. Epidemiologic studies have identified the main risk factors for these conditions, including increasing age, male sex, white race, gastroesophageal reflux disease, abdominal obesity, cigarette smoking, and lack of infection with Helicobacter pylori. This review summarizes the current epidemiologic evidence with implications for screening and surveillance in Barrett's esophagus and esophageal adenocarcinoma.

Endoscopic Screening for Barrett's Esophagus and Esophageal Adenocarcinoma: Rationale, Candidates, and Challenges 27

Amrit K. Kamboj, David A. Katzka, and Prasad G. Iyer

Barrett's esophagus (BE) is the only known precursor to esophageal adenocarcinoma (EAC), a cancer with increasing incidence and poor survival. Risk of EAC in patients with BE is higher compared with the general population. Endoscopic screening for BE is performed to identify patients earlier in the metaplasia-dysplasia-carcinoma sequence from BE to EAC to enable eradication therapy. BE screening should be considered in individuals with multiple risk factors for BE and EAC. Challenges to BE screening include the absence of a cost-effective, widely applicable minimally invasive screening tool, gastroesophageal reflux disease centric screening recommendations, and limitations of current endoscopic surveillance practice.

Progress in Screening for Barrett's Esophagus: Beyond Standard Upper Endoscopy 43

Wei Keith Tan, Anamay N. Sharma, Amitabh Chak, and Rebecca C. Fitzgerald

Video content accompanies this article at http://www.giendo.theclinics.com.

The rapid increase in the incidence of esophageal adenocarcinoma in Western populations over the past 4 decades and its associated poor prognosis unless detected early has generated great interest in screening

for the precursor lesion Barrett's esophagus (BE). There have been significant developments in imaging-based modalities and esophageal cell-sampling devices coupled with biomarker assays. In this review, the authors discuss the rationale for screening for BE and the factors to consider for targeting the at-risk population. They also explore future avenues for research in this area.

Best Practices in Surveillance for Barrett's Esophagus **59**

Joseph R. Triggs and Gary W. Falk

Barrett's esophagus is the precursor lesion for esophageal adenocarcinoma. The goals of endoscopic surveillance are to detect dysplasia and early esophageal adenocarcinoma in order to improve patient outcomes. Despite the ongoing debate regarding the efficacy of surveillance, all current gastrointestinal societies recommend surveillance at this time. Optimal surveillance technique includes adequate inspection time, evaluation using high-definition white light and chromoendoscopy, appropriate documentation of the metaplastic segment using the Prague C & M criteria as well as the Paris classification should lesions be found, utilization of the Seattle biopsy protocol, and endoscopic resection of visible lesions.

Cost-Effectiveness of Screening, Surveillance, and Endoscopic Eradication Therapies for Managing the Burden of Esophageal Adenocarcinoma **77**

Joel H. Rubenstein and John M. Inadomi

The authors conducted a review of the literature of cost-effectiveness analyses regarding management of Barrett's esophagus, including screening, surveillance, and treatment strategies. Because of the presence of multiple systematic reviews on this topic, they chose to focus on more recent economic analyses, with an emphasis on comparative modeling because these analyses have been demonstrated to achieve greater validity and impact when there are multiple competing strategies that are clinically reasonable to pursue. The authors identified areas of consensus across studies regarding management strategies and also areas that require additional empirical data.

Advanced Imaging and Sampling in Barrett's Esophagus: Artificial Intelligence to the Rescue? **91**

Maarten R. Struyvenberg, Albert J. de Groof, Jacques J. Bergman, Fons van der Sommen, Peter H.N. de With, Vani J.A. Konda, and Wouter L. Curvers

Because the current Barrett's esophagus (BE) surveillance protocol suffers from sampling error of random biopsies and a high miss-rate of early neoplastic lesions, many new endoscopic imaging and sampling techniques have been developed. None of these techniques, however, have significantly increased the diagnostic yield of BE neoplasia. In fact, these techniques have led to an increase in the amount of visible information, yet endoscopists and pathologists inevitably suffer from variations in intra- and interobserver agreement. Artificial intelligence systems have the potential to overcome these endoscopist-dependent limitations.

Advances in Biomarkers for Risk Stratification in Barrett's Esophagus 105

Rhonda F. Souza and Stuart Jon Spechler

Dysplasia currently is the primary biomarker used to risk stratify patients with Barrett's esophagus, but dysplasia has a number of considerable limitations in this regard. Thus, investigators over the years have explored innumerable alternative molecular biomarkers for risk stratification in Barrett's esophagus. This report focuses only on those biomarkers that appear most promising based on the availability of multiple published studies corroborating good results, and on the commercial availability of the test. These promising biomarkers include p53 immunostaining, TissueCypher, BarreGEN, and wide-area transepithelial sampling with computer-assisted 3-dimensional analysis (WATS^{3D}).

Current Status of Chemoprevention in Barrett's Esophagus 117

Paul Moayyedi and Hashem B. El-Serag

Candidates for chemoprevention in Barrett's esophagus have long been suggested and there has been observational data to support many drugs, including statins, hormone replacement therapy, metformin, proton pump inhibitor therapy, and aspirin. Proton pump inhibitor therapy and aspirin are the most promising agents. Data suggest that aspirin and proton pump inhibitor therapy can decrease the risk of neoplastic progression in Barrett's esophagus. Further, the combination of aspirin and proton pump inhibitor therapy decrease all-cause mortality by approximately 33%. Future guideline groups need to evaluate the evidence rigorously, but the combination of proton pump inhibitor therapy and aspirin is promising.

Optimizing Outcomes with Radiofrequency Ablation of Barrett's Esophagus: Candidates, Efficacy and Durability 131

Philippe Leclercq and Raf Bisschops

The treatment of early Barrett's esophagus (BE) has undergone a paradigm shift from surgical subtotal esophagectomy to organ-saving endoluminal treatment. Over the past 15 years, several high-quality studies were conducted to assess safe oncological outcome of endoscopic resection of mucosal adenocarcinoma and high-grade dysplasia. It became clear that add-on ablative therapy with radiofrequency ablation (RFA) significantly reduces recurrence risk of neoplasia after resection. In this review, we highlight the most essential elements to optimize outcomes of RFA of BE, addressing the correct indication and patient selection in combination with the most efficient and safest treatment protocols to obtain long-term durability.

Updates in Cryotherapy for Barrett's Esophagus 155

Charlotte N. Frederiks, Marcia Irene Canto, and Bas L.A.M. Weusten

Cryotherapy is an ablation modality relying on freeze-thaw cycles to promote cell death through intracellular ice crystal formation, ischemia, and apoptosis. Currently, 2 different cryotherapy systems are available for esophageal use. The first is cryospray ablation, which involves repetitive applications of liquid nitrogen. The second system, cryoballoon ablation,

Measuring Quality in Barrett's Esophagus: Time to Embrace Quality Indicators **219**

Vinay Sehgal, Krish Ragunath, and Rehan Haidry

Endoscopic eradication therapy is a safe and effective therapy that has revolutionized the management of patients with Barrett's esophagus (BE)-related neoplasia. Despite this, there remains significant heterogeneity in clinical practice with consequent variation in patient outcomes. The aim of this article was to align consensus statements based on the best available evidence and expert opinion from the United States and United Kingdom to develop robust and measurable quality indicators that help to ensure patients with BE-related neoplasia receive the highest possible quality of care uniformly.

GASTROINTESTINAL ENDOSCOPY CLINICS OF NORTH AMERICA

FORTHCOMING ISSUES

April 2021
Video Capsule Endoscopy
David Cave, *Editor*

July 2021
Gastric Cancer
Chin Hur, *Editor*

October 2021
Optimizing Endoscopic Operations
John Vargo and Sunguk N. Jang, *Editors*

RECENT ISSUES

October 2020
Endoscopy in the Era of Antibiotic Resistant Bacteria
Jacques Van Dam, *Editor*

July 2020
Colorectal Cancer Screening
Douglas K. Rex, *Editor*

April 2020
Management of GERD: Looking with 2020 Vision
Kenneth J. Chang, *Editor*

RELATED CLINICS SERIES

Gastroenterology Clinics
(www.gastro.theclinics.com)
Clinics in Liver Disease
(www.liver.theclinics.com)

Foreword

Barrett's Esophagus: Current Management and New Approaches

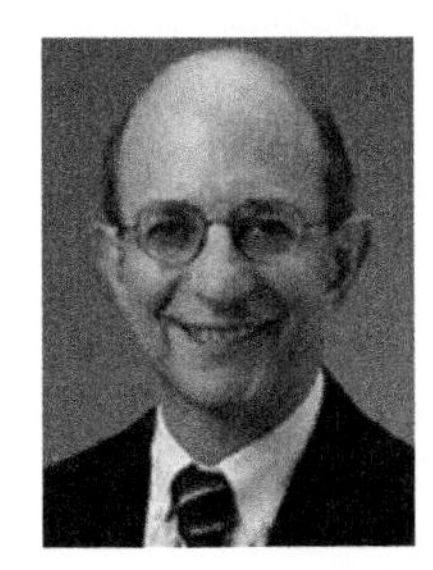

Charles J. Lightdale, MD
Consulting Editor

Barrett's esophagus stands as the primary indicator for an increased risk of esophageal adenocarcinoma. Endoscopic eradication of Barrett's esophagus with dysplasia has been clearly demonstrated in randomized controlled trials and multiple additional studies to markedly decrease the risk of developing adenocarcinoma of the esophagus. A paradigm shift in clinical practice and national and international guidelines has taken place with strong recommendations for endoscopic eradication therapy for early neoplasia in Barrett's esophagus, replacing esophagectomy in most patients. This battle is over, but the larger effort goes on to decrease mortality from the still accelerating incidence of esophageal adenocarcinoma. Most patients continue to present initially with highly lethal advanced cancer.

Dr Sachin Wani, a leader in the field, is the Editor for this issue of the *Gastrointestinal Endoscopy Clinics of North America* dedicated to Advances and Opportunities in Barrett's Esophagus. He has developed a thoughtful and comprehensive array of key topics in the current management of Barrett's esophagus and has assembled an extraordinary group of experts who present an authoritative state-of-the-art issue for practicing gastroenterologists, including new approaches to watch and possibly adopt.

Continued improvement in what we do and how we do it is a recurring theme in the articles relating to endoscopic therapy for dysplasia and early cancer in Barrett's esophagus. Major topics include the use of endoscopic mucosal resection and endoscopic submucosal dissection, optimized outcomes of radiofrequency ablation, and update on cryotherapy, a practical approach to refractory and recurrent Barrett's mucosa, and the role of surgical management of Barrett's-related neoplasia.

Gastrointest Endoscopy Clin N Am 31 (2021) xiii–xiv
https://doi.org/10.1016/j.giec.2020.09.008
1052-5157/21/© 2020 Published by Elsevier Inc.

There is a clear need for screening to identify patients with Barrett's esophagus, since most patients who have the condition are unaware of it. Articles are included on selective screening with endoscopy and with novel nonendoscopic methods. Of course, it is now evident that the overall risk of developing cancer in nondysplastic Barrett's esophagus is very low, in the range of 0.3% per patient-year. Thus, there must be huge improvements in risk stratification for patients with nondysplastic Barrett's esophagus. There are important articles on the latest epidemiology of Barrett's esophagus and esophageal adenocarcinoma, best practices and cost-effectiveness for screening and surveillance, advances in biomarkers for risk stratification, the use of advanced imaging and sampling in Barrett's, and the promise of endoscopic Artificial Intelligence to improve detection of subtle areas of dysplasia. Articles on the current status of chemoprevention and quality indicators in Barrett's management round out this terrific issue. Whether you are a card-carrying "Barrettologist" or a general gastroenterologist, you will not want to miss this splendid issue.

Charles J. Lightdale, MD
Department of Medicine
Columbia University Medical Center
161 Fort Washington Avenue
New York, NY 10032, USA

E-mail address:
CJL18@columbia.edu

Preface

Advances and Opportunities in Barrett's Esophagus

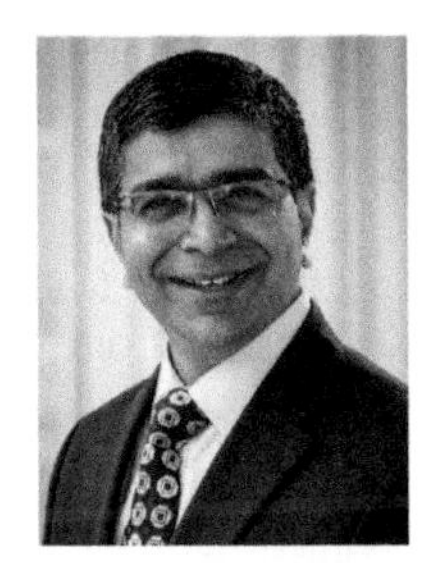

Sachin Wani, MD, FASGE, AGAF
Editor

The incidence of esophageal adenocarcinoma continues to increase in the Western population. While outcomes of patients with early esophageal adenocarcinoma has improved significantly, largely due to endoscopic eradication therapies and minimally invasive surgery, the 5-year survival rates for advanced cases remains dismal. Barrett's esophagus is the only precursor lesion for esophageal adenocarcinoma, and the last decade has seen significant improvements and innovations in this field. Some of the key advances include high-definition endoscopy, virtual chromoendoscopy, and endoscopic eradication therapies that have truly revolutionized our approach to detection and treatment of patients with Barrett's-related dysplasia and early esophageal adenocarcinoma. This approach has replaced the need for esophagectomy and allowed us to achieve outcomes comparable to surgery.

I am indebted to Dr Charlie Lightdale for this opportunity to guest edit this issue of *Gastrointestinal Endoscopy Clinics of North America* focused on Advances in Barrett's Esophagus. This issue provides a comprehensive state-of-the-art update in this field provided by experts in this field on topics ranging from epidemiology, screening, surveillance, endoscopic eradication therapy, and surgical management of Barrett's esophagus, and Barrett's-related neoplasia. We hope that this issue will serve as a valuable guide to clinicians and investigators. I am immensely grateful to all the authors who contributed to this issue despite their busy schedules.

This issue also highlights the new developments that have laid the foundation to address several challenges we have faced for several years. The development of newer minimally invasive sampling devices and progress in identifying the at-risk population have the highest potential to improve population-based screening and impact the epidemiology of esophageal adenocarcinoma in a meaningful way. The other areas that continue to remain problematic include the need for improved risk-stratification using clinical- and biomarker-based models and surveillance practices. The

Gastrointest Endoscopy Clin N Am 31 (2021) xv–xvi
https://doi.org/10.1016/j.giec.2020.09.007
1052-5157/21/© 2020 Published by Elsevier Inc.

establishment of quality indicators in screening, surveillance, and endoscopic eradication therapy as an infrastructure for continuous monitoring of quality has the potential to address variability in practices and population-based outcomes in Barrett's esophagus and esophageal adenocarcinoma.

Sachin Wani, MD, FASGE, AGAF
Professor of Medicine
Associate Medical Director
Division of Gastroenterology and
Hepatology Medical Director
Esophageal and Gastric Center
University of Colorado
Anschutz Medical Campus
1635 Aurora Court, Room 2.031
Auroa, CO 80045, USA

E-mail address:
sachin.wani@cuanschutz.edu

Epidemiology of Barrett's Esophagus and Esophageal Adenocarcinoma

Implications for Screening and Surveillance

Michael B. Cook, PhD[a,*], Aaron P. Thrift, PhD[b]

KEYWORDS

• History • Prevalence • Incidence • Survival • Biomarkers • Algorithms • Risk
• Genetics

KEY POINTS

- The causes of increasing incidence, male predominance, and racial differences of esophageal adenocarcinoma remain unknown.
- Primary risk factors of reflux, obesity, and cigarette smoking occur in only a subset of cases and are largely prevalent, providing weak discriminatory ability for screening and surveillance.
- Esophageal adenocarcinoma patients who have a prior diagnosis of Barrett's esophagus (<10% of all esophageal adenocarcinoma patients) have better outcomes compared with patients without a prior diagnosis of Barrett's esophagus.
- Biomarker studies in unselected Barrett's esophagus populations using whole esophageal sampling are warranted, and all biomarker studies should strive to be larger and have a strengthened statistical framework.
- Multiple prediction models have been derived for use in selecting high-risk patients for screening and surveillance; but require further validation and optimization before clinical application can be recommended.

HISTORY

Throughout the evolution of the definition of Barrett's esophagus (BE), the one thing that has remained constant is the identification of some form of columnar epithelium on histologic analysis. The first reporting of such a tissue found in the esophagus is attributed to Schmidt[1] in 1805. In the early part of the twenieth century, Stewart and

[a] Division of Cancer Epidemiology and Genetics, National Cancer Institute, 9609 Medical Center Drive, 6E430, Rockville, MD 20850, USA; [b] Section of Epidemiology and Population Sciences, Department of Medicine, and Dan L Duncan Comprehensive Cancer Center, Baylor College of Medicine, One Baylor Plaza, MS: BCM307, Room 621D, Houston, TX 77030, USA
* Corresponding author.
E-mail address: michael.cook@nih.gov

Gastrointest Endoscopy Clin N Am 31 (2021) 1–26
https://doi.org/10.1016/j.giec.2020.08.001
1052-5157/21/Published by Elsevier Inc.

Hartfall[2] and Lyall[3] noted that the presence of columnar epithelium in the esophagus—surrounding "ulcerations"—was an abnormality. Confusion and debate began to center on the origin of columnar epithelium in the esophagus and, in his famous treatise of 1950, Norman Rupert Barrett[4] proposed that a condition existed in which congenitally short esophagus resulted in the stomach being drawn up into the chest cavity—a type of hiatal hernia. However, even though the eponym of Barrett's was to stick, his initial theory of the origin of columnar epithelium was soon to be found incorrect. It was Allison and Johnstone[5] in 1953 who initially used the term "Barrett's ulcer" to refer to what was previously known as "peptic ulcer of the esophagus," reasoning that this would distinguish it from ulceration of esophageal squamous epithelium, which had been given the name "reflux esophagitis" by Barrett himself. Allison and Johnstone proposed that Barrett's ulcer was not due to a congenitally short esophagus with herniation of the stomach, but instead to a congenital gastric-lined esophagus. From scrupulous examination of specimens, they noted that there was no peritoneal covering, that the musculature was typically esophageal, islands of squamous epithelium existed within the columnar lining, and that oxyntic (parietal) cells were absent. This finding led them to propose that:

> *It appears better . . . . to refer to that congenital abnormality which from the outside looks like oesophagus and from the inside looks like stomach as 'oesophagus lined with gastric mucous membrane.'*

The association with reflux and hiatal hernia was spoken of, but they still considered BE to be wholly congenital, a view supported by embryologic studies of fetal development. Barrett[6] conceded his theory of congenitally short esophagus in 1957, now referring to this gastric-like lining as "lower esophagus lined by columnar epithelium," a term that in future publications was to be replaced by the eponym "Barrett's esophagus." He too still thought the condition to be of congenital origin, yet in 1957 he did acknowledge that an acquired pathogenesis may exist:

> *If the cardiac valve of a normal person were to become incompetent and if the lower oesophagus were, as a result, to be bathed for a long time by digestive gastric juice, the squamous epithelium could be eaten away and totally replaced by columnar cells.*

Thus, perhaps the eponym is merited. Two years later, in 1959, Moersch and colleagues[7] are credited with the first publication whereby the changes of the distal esophagus following reflux esophagitis are discussed without inferring a congenital origin, instead referring to "inflammatory metaplasia." Their study of 36 esophageal resections was the first convincing evidence that persistent gastroesophageal reflux disease (GERD) was central to the cause of columnar-lined esophagus. This perspective was strengthened in 1970 in a series of landmark canine experiments by Bremner and colleagues[8] in which they showed normal esophageal squamous repair in the absence of GERD but re-epithelialization with a columnar lining when GERD was induced.

What is now considered the defining feature of BE—goblet cells—were first noted by Bosher and Taylor[9] in 1951. Despite subsequent confirmatory observations,[5,10] the histology of BE continued to be debated for the next 20 years. In 1976, some clarity emerged from a study by Paull and colleagues[11] with descriptions of 3 types of metaplasia, including specialized columnar epithelium—which we now call intestinal metaplasia, synonymous with BE. Paull only hinted at the potential carcinogenic importance of intestinal metaplasia, and it was not until the early 1990s that intestinal metaplasia was generally accepted to be the most prevalent, distinctive epithelium, and highest in conferring risk of esophageal adenocarcinoma (EA).[12,13]

EPIDEMIOLOGY

Population Prevalence of Barrett's Esophagus

The population prevalence of BE is a crucial statistic upon which all primary and secondary prevention strategies are based, yet it remains largely unknown primarily because of the fact that many individuals with BE are asymptomatic.[14] The BE prevalence in selected populations—such as endoscopic or surgical series—is no substitute, and so there are few studies that provide an accurate estimate. The first reliable study, published in 1990, assessed the prevalence of long-segment BE in a large series of randomly selected subjects for autopsy and compared this with a prevalence from the endoscopy practice of the Mayo Clinic.[15] The finding of 4 BE cases was approximately 21 times of that which was expected (0.19), and this equated to an age- and sex-adjusted BE prevalence estimate of 376 per 100,000 population (0.376%). Other estimates of BE population prevalence come from randomly selected populations that underwent endoscopy. A Swedish study[16] of 1000 randomly selected volunteers detected a total of 16 cases of BE, five of which were classified as long-segment BE (≥2 cm), yielding population prevalences of 1.6% and 0.5%, respectively. An Italian study[17] of 1033 adults reported a BE population prevalence of 1.3% (0.2% for long segment and 1.1% for short segment). A computer simulation disease model has also been used to estimate the population prevalence of BE.[18] Aligning simulation models with EA rates from the US Surveillance, Epidemiology, and End Results (SEER) cancer registry data, the investigators estimated a BE population prevalence of 5.6%. Thus, in predominantly European ancestral populations, estimates for BE population prevalence range from 0.4% to 5.6%. Perhaps surprisingly, Asian countries may also have BE population prevalences in this range, despite the lower incidence of EA. A recent meta-analysis of 4 Asian-based studies indicated a BE population prevalence of 0.7%,[19] and a Taiwan-based study of 3385 subjects undergoing routine esophagogastroduodenoscopy examination as part of a health checkup provided a BE population prevalence of 2.6%.[20] The Taiwan study provided details of segment length, showing that most diagnoses were short-segment BE, a characteristic that has previously been described in other selected endoscopic series from Asian countries, and which is in accordance with the lower incidence of EA in Asian populations.

Incidence Trends of Barrett's Esophagus

Assessing incidence trends of BE is a near impossibility because of the large pool of asymptomatic, undiagnosed subjects that are estimated to exist in most populations. As such, the best estimates are derived from clinical data with the hope that these may mirror relative change of all BE cases, including those never diagnosed. Typically, the denominator in such studies is the number of endoscopies rather than the total population at risk.

In the United States, the first report of BE incidence was from the Mayo Clinic, which found a rate of 9.5 per 1000 endoscopies per annum that was stable over the period 1965 to 1986; the crude rate did dramatically increase but this was wholly accounted for by a similar increase in the number of endoscopies.[15] Two other US studies also presented evidence for no change in BE incidence through the 1990s, once adjusted for number of endoscopies.[21,22] However, a fourth US study did provide evidence for an increase.[23] The investigators found that endoscopy-suspected BE increased from 32.2 to 82.8 per 1000 endoscopies and histologically diagnosed BE from 6.7 to 27.6

per 1000 endoscopies during 1991 to 2000. More recent studies covering the mid-1990s through 2010 indicate that BE incidence has been stable and then may have declined.[24–26]

In contrast to those studies in the United States, most European studies have suggested an increase in BE incidence, including Scotland,[27] United Kingdom,[28] Switzerland,[29] the Netherlands,[30] Spain,[31] and Northern Ireland,[32] as has a study from Australia.[33] The most recent European study from the United Kingdom and the Netherlands provides evidence for a decrease and then stabilization of BE incidence.[34]

Statistics of BE incidence need to be interpreted with several caveats in mind: increasing enthusiasm and education about BE, especially short-segment BE, and changes in referral patterns have not been measured and therefore remain unadjusted for. It has been suggested that the increasing epidemiologic evidence of the strength of BE as a precursor to EA served to increase the awareness of this lesion.[27] It is unknown what effect this has had on referral practices; obviously more patients are being referred for endoscopy, but the relative influences of altered incidence of heartburn symptoms and increased awareness of sequelae complications, by both patient and provider, are unknown. Overall, it is likely the evidence supports increased BE incidence in Western Europe and Australia, while further evidence is needed to confirm or refute similar trends in the United States.

Incidence and Survival of Esophageal Adenocarcinoma

For the purpose of this review, the most recent data were analyzed from the SEER 9 registries[35] (covering approximately 10% of the US population) in which 21,358 cases of invasive EA (defined using *International Classification of Diseases for Oncology, Third Edition* site codes, C15.0–C15.9; and histologic codes, M8140–8575) were diagnosed between 1975 and 2017. The overall age-adjusted incidence rate for EA during 1975 to 2017 was 2.0 per 100,000 person-years. EA incidence rates increased from 0.4 per 100,000 person-years in 1975 to 2.8 per 100,000 person-years in 2017 (**Fig. 1**). EA incidence also varies by US state, with North American Association of Central Cancer Registries (NAACCR) data (SEER*Stat Database: NAACCR Incidence Data – CiNA Analytic File, 1995-2016, Public Use [which includes data from Centers for Disease Control and Prevention's National Program of Cancer Registries, Canadian Council of Cancer Registries Provincial and Territorial Registries, and the National Cancer Institute's SEER Registries], certified by the NAACCR as meeting high-quality incidence data standards for the specified time periods, submitted December 2018) showing highest rates predominantly in northern and northeastern states (**Fig. 2**). Although EA rates increased dramatically between the mid-1970s through 2000,[36] SEER 18 delay-adjusted data[37] show that the rate of increase has slowed in subsequent years and EA incidence has stabilized in the United States through 2017 (**Fig. 3**). Absolute rates of EA remain significantly higher among white men in the United States compared with women and non-whites; however, similar rates of change and secular trends have been observed in all subgroups of the US population. For EA cases in the SEER 18 registries,[38] median relative survival has increased from 10.5 months in 2000 to 13.1 months for persons diagnosed in 2016. Overall 5-year observed survival rates increased from 15.4% for patients diagnosed with EA in 2000 to 18.4% for patients diagnosed with EA in 2012. The greatest absolute improvement in survival trends occurred in EA patients diagnosed with localized disease, approximately 32% of patients diagnosed with localized EA in 2000 survived 5 years after their diagnosis, whereas the 5-year observed survival rate for patients diagnosed with localized EA in 2012 was 48% (**Fig. 4**). Less striking improvements in 5-year

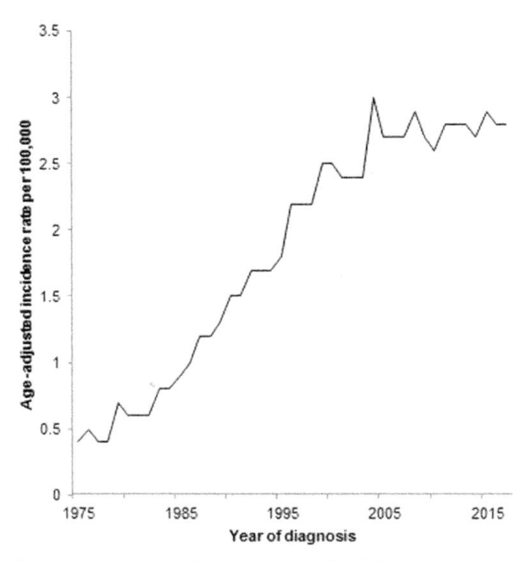

Fig. 1. Age-adjusted incidence rates of EA in the United States, 1975 to 2017. Rates are per 100,000 person-years. (Data source: Surveillance, Epidemiology, and End Results (SEER) 9 Registries.)

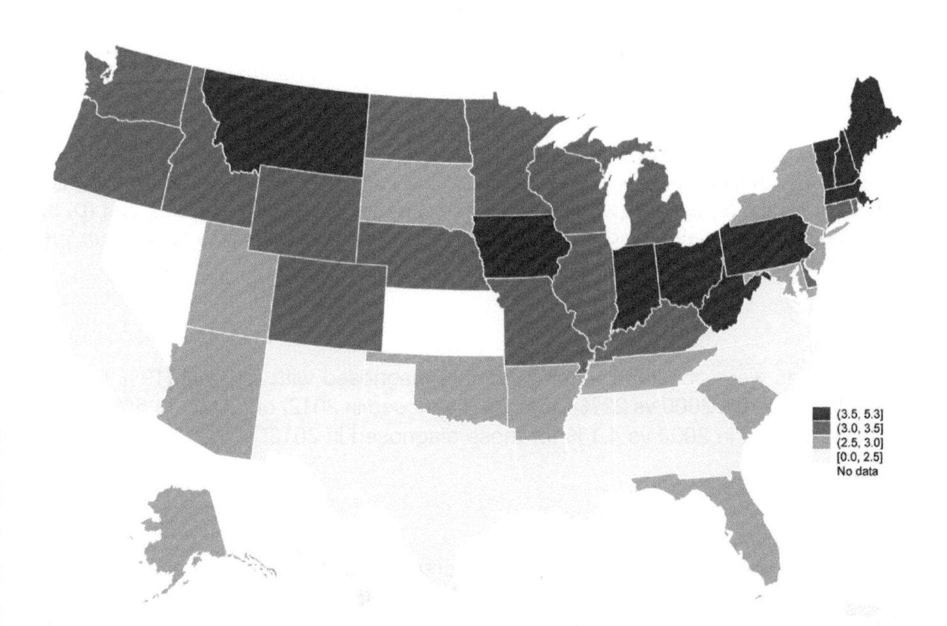

Fig. 2. Age-adjusted incidence rates of EA in the United States by state, 2012 to 2016. Rates are per 100,000 person-years. Darker blue hues denote higher incidence rate categories of EA. There were no data for the time period assessed for the states filled white. Alaska, Hawaii, and Puerto Rico have been repositioned for maximal resolution. (*Data from* North American Association of Central Cancer Registries (NAACCR) Incidence Data - CiNA Analytic File, 1995-2016.)

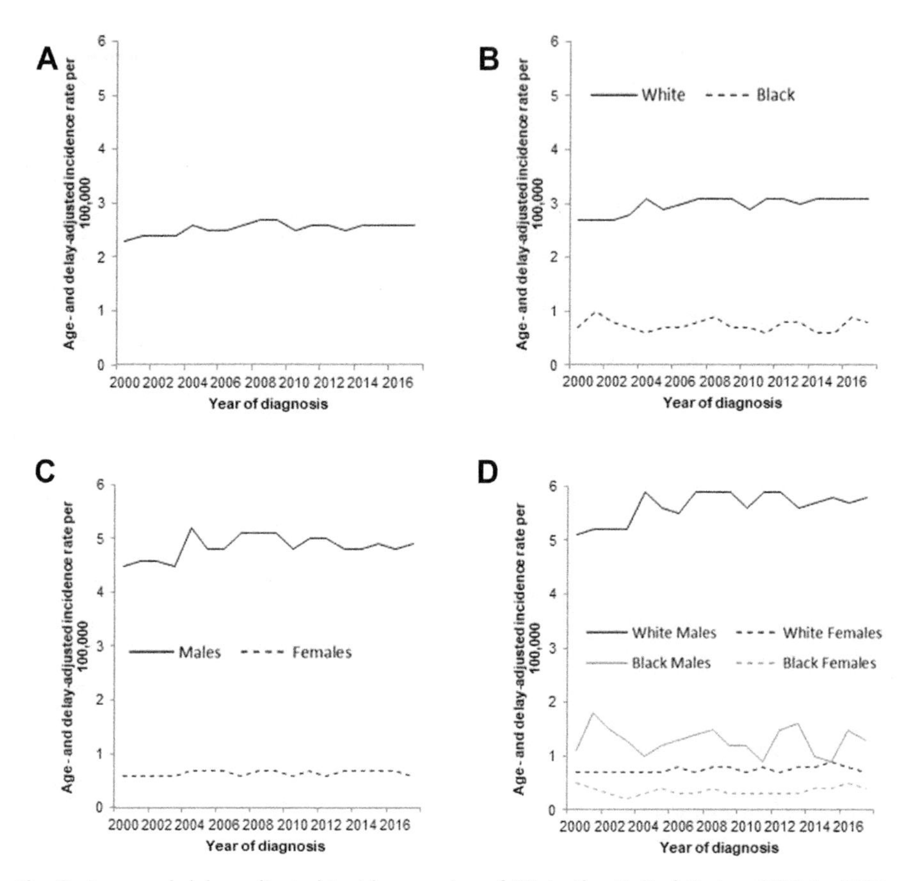

Fig. 3. Age- and delay-adjusted incidence rates of EA in the United States, 2000 to 2017. Rates are per 100,000 person-years. Age- and delay-adjusted incidence rates of EA are shown (*A*) for all; (*B*) by race (white and black); (*C*) by sex (males and females); and (*D*) by sex and race (white males, black males, white females and black females). (*Data from* Surveillance, Epidemiology, and End Results (SEER) 18 Registries.)

survival rates were observed among patients diagnosed with regional (19% for patients diagnosed in 2000 vs 22% for those diagnosed in 2012) or distant (2.5% for patients diagnosed in 2000 vs 4.1% for those diagnosed in 2012) stage EA.

NATURE OF THE PROBLEM

The central problems in primary prevention (screening) and secondary prevention (surveillance) of EA are the large undiagnosed BE population and the suboptimal ability to triage risk in the diagnosed BE population, respectively. The large undiagnosed BE population results in most EA cases presenting with late-stage disease and a resultant poor prognosis. In later discussion, the authors review the current epidemiologic evidence of risk factors, biomarkers, and algorithms that may be used to overcome this problem and identify a larger pool of subjects with BE. They then review the current evidence for triaging cancer risk in the diagnosed BE population, a difficulty that will

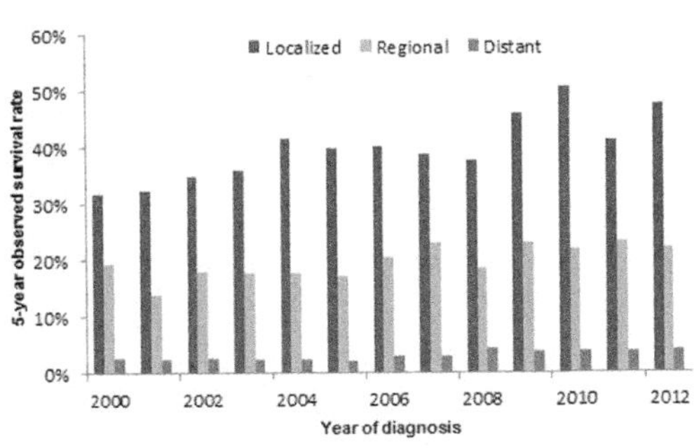

Fig. 4. Five-year survival rates for EA in the United States, 2000 to 2012, by stage at diagnosis (localized, regional, and distant stage). (*Data from* Surveillance, Epidemiology, and End Results (SEER) 18 Registries.)

be compounded should the primary prevention hurdle (population screening) be overcome.

CURRENT EVIDENCE

Population Screening for Barrett's Esophagus

There is a major caveat to this section. Most of the studies that are described have been conducted using selected BE populations, that is, patients who present with symptoms that merit endoscopic and histologic investigation. This caveat should not be glossed over, and it is an inherent limitation of studying a rare, largely asymptomatic condition that is expensive and difficult to diagnose.

Risk factors

Although clinical guidelines all recommend screening for BE, the screening population differs.[39–42] All guidelines, except those from the American Gastroenterological Association, condition screening for BE based on the presence of GERD symptoms (**Table 1**). Risk factors used to define high risk for purposes of screening generally include age $\geq$50 years, male sex, Caucasian race, GERD symptoms, smoking, and obesity. Here, the authors review the literature supporting these high-risk determinants as well as other potential risk factors for BE and EA.

Demographics

EA incidence increases with increasing age and is rare among persons aged less than 50 years. An intriguing and yet largely unexplained observation in EA is the striking sex disparity; across all countries, EA incidence rates in women remain significantly lower than those of men. The magnitude of the male predominance is greatest in the United States, where the male:female incidence rate ratio approaches 9:1.[43–45] EA is also more common in non-Hispanic whites than non-whites.[46] Likewise, BE is twice as common in men as in women and more common in non-Hispanic whites than other races/ethnicities.[47]

Environmental risk factors

Frequent GERD symptoms, cigarette smoking, and obesity are the main risk factors for EA and BE. Together, these 3 risk factors account for more than 70% of all cases of EA in Western populations[48,49] and are observed among most patients with BE.

Table 1
Barrett's esophagus screening guidelines for select gastroenterological societies

Society	Year	Screening Population
American College of Gastroenterology	2016	Men >5 y GERD, or with more than weekly symptoms + ≥2 risk factors: >50 y, central obesity (waist circumference >102 cm or waist-to-hip ratio >0.9), Caucasian, smoking, first-degree relative with BE or EA
British Society of Gastroenterology	2014	GERD with ≥3 risk factors: >50 y, Caucasian, male gender, obesity ± (+) family history
American Society for Gastrointestinal Endoscopy	2019	Individuals with a family history of EA or BE (high risk) OR GERD with ≥1 risk factors (moderate risk): >50 y, male gender, Caucasian, smoking, obesity
American Gastroenterological Association	2011	Multiple risk factors: >50 y, Caucasian, male gender, chronic GERD, hiatal hernia, obesity

In a pooled analysis of individual-level data from 5 case-control studies participating in the Barrett's and Esophageal Adenocarcinoma Consortium (BEACON; https://esocan.org/beacon/), there was a strong, dose-dependent relationship between frequency of GERD symptoms and EA risk. Compared with individuals with infrequent or no GERD symptoms, those with at least weekly and daily symptoms had 5-fold (odds ratio [OR] = 4.81, 95% confidence interval [CI]: 3.39–6.82) and 8-fold (OR = 7.96, 95% CI: 4.51–14.04) higher risk of EA, respectively.[50] For BE, individuals with frequent GERD symptoms occurring in early adulthood have especially high risk (first reported symptoms at age <30 years, OR = 15.1, 95% CI: 7.91–28.8).[51]

Cook and colleagues,[52] using pooled individual-level data from 10 case-control and 2 cohort studies in BEACON, found that ever smoking was associated 2-fold increased risk of EA (vs never smoking; OR = 1.96, 95% CI: 1.64–2.34) and showed that EA risk increased with increasing pack-years smoking history. Although EA risk among ever smokers appears to decline with increased years of smoking cessation, risk in former smokers does not return to the level observed for never smokers.[52,53] The evidence is less clear for BE. In the largest study to date, risk of BE was 1.7-fold as high among ever smokers as it was among never smokers (OR = 1.67, 95% CI: 1.04–2.67).[54] However, unlike for EA, BE risk does not increase with increasing cumulative exposure.

Compared with individuals with a normal body mass index (BMI <25.0 kg/m^2), individuals with BMI of 30.0 to 34.9 kg/m^2 and ≥40.0 kg/m^2 have 2-fold (OR = 2.39, 95% CI: 1.86–3.06) and 5-fold (OR = 4.76, 95% CI: 2.96–7.66) higher risk of EA, respectively.[55] Obesity in childhood and adolescence may also confer increased risk of EA independent of adult BMI.[56,57] Increasing evidence suggests that abdominal obesity confers greater risk for EA and BE than overall obesity.[58,59] A meta-analysis found more than 2-fold increased risk of EA associated with abdominal obesity (OR = 2.51, 95% CI: 1.54–4.06).[60] Likewise, abdominal obesity was associated with

2-fold higher risk of BE (OR = 1.98, 95% CI: 1.52–2.57).[60] These associations remained after controlling for BMI, whereas there were weak or no associations with BMI after controlling for abdominal obesity.

Alcohol consumption is not associated with increased risks of EA or BE.[61,62] The Continuous Update Project Report on diet, nutrition, and physical activity by the World Cancer Research Fund/American Institute for Cancer Research, which considers results from only cohort studies, reported that no dietary factors were judged to have strong evidence of an association with risk of EA and that there was limited suggestive evidence for an inverse relationship between physical activity and risk of EA.[63]

Helicobacter pylori is a gram-negative bacterium that infects half the world's human population and causes gastric cancer.[64] Conversely, *H pylori* infection is associated with lower risks of EA and BE. Two meta-analyses both reported more than 40% lower risk of EA for individuals infected with *H pylori* (in particular, those with the CagA-positive *H pylori* strain) compared with individuals uninfected with *H pylori*.[65,66] There is also strong evidence that *H pylori* infection is associated with lower risk of BE.[67,68]

Frequent users of aspirin and other nonsteroidal anti-inflammatory drugs (NSAIDs) have lower risk of EA. A pooled analysis of individual-level participant data in BEACON found that any use of aspirin or NSAIDs was associated with 30% lower risk of EA (OR = 0.68, 95% CI: 0.56–0.83).[69] Current users had an especially lower risk for EA (OR = 0.40, 95% CI: 0.24–0.97), and risk was shown to decrease linearly with both increased frequency and duration of use.[69] In contrast, a pooled analysis among BE studies in BEACON found no association between any NSAIDs and BE (OR = 1.00, 95% CI: 0.76–1.32).[70] Statins have also been shown to be associated with lower risks of EA and BE.[71,72]

Given the male predominance in BE and EA risk, studies have considered whether sex hormones might be involved. Case-control studies have found increased risk of EA associated with increased androgen:estrogen,[73] and increased risk of BE associated with higher levels of free testosterone and free dihydrotestosterone.[74,75] In a prospective study, prediagnostic concentrations of circulating dehydroepiandrosterone (highest quartile vs lowest quartile: OR = 0.28, 95% CI: 0.13–0.64), estradiol (highest quartile vs lowest quartile: OR = 0.55, 95% CI: 0.31–0.99), and free estradiol (highest quartile vs lowest quartile: OR = 0.56, 95% CI: 0.30–1.03) were associated with lower risk of a combined outcome of EA and gastric cardia adenocarcinoma.[76] In a second prospective study of EA, contrary to long-standing hypotheses,[77] higher circulating levels of testosterone were associated with lower risk for EA in men.[78] A recently published Mendelian randomization study found an association between genetically predicted levels of follicle-stimulating and luteinizing hormones and risk of BE and EA but no associations with other sex hormones, including dehydroepiandrosterone sulfate, testosterone, and estradiol.[79]

Genetic factors

Genome-wide association studies have identified and validated germline (inherited) loci associated with risk of EA and BE, including CRTC1, a transcription coactivator associated with increased cancerous activity, BARX1, a transcription factor that promotes esophageal differentiation, FOXF1, FOXP1, and TBX5, which encode transcription factors involved in esophageal development, and GDF7, which encodes a protein in the bone morphogenetic pathway that has been associated with BE.[80–83]

Algorithms

Early strategies to select patients for BE screening were based on only frequency and severity of GERD symptoms. However, because only around half of BE patients report symptoms of GERD,[16,17] symptoms alone discriminate poorly between persons with and without BE.[84–87] Several risk-stratification tools have since been developed that use demographic, lifestyle, and clinical information to discriminate between individuals at high and low risk for BE, with varying degrees of success with respect to discriminatory accuracy.[84,88,89] They also require further examination in external populations and prospectively before clinical implementation can be recommended.[90,91] Three recent validation efforts have shown that the Michigan Barrett's Esophagus pREdiction Tool, which incorporates GERD symptoms, age, waist-to-hip ratio, and pack-years of cigarette use to predict BE risk is robust and transportable to other populations.[87,92,93] However, the discriminatory ability of this tool (area under the receiver operating characteristic curve [AUC], ~0.70) is not at the level required for clinical application. To address this shortcoming, other factors, including blood-based biomarkers[85] and genetic information,[86,94] have been added to baseline models using demographic, lifestyle, and clinical factors, with modest success.

Precision Surveillance of Barrett's Esophagus

A similar caveat to that mentioned under Population Screening also applies to this section: all studies to have assessed preneoplastic (BE) tissues of EA cases have, by definition, been restricted to the BE subpopulation that is currently identified (symptom justifies endoscopic investigation). Rapid progressors, less symptomatic, and asymptomatic BE case populations—which comprise the majority as well as important, high-risk subsets of BE—are typically not identified and thus not studied. As such, evidence from studies of preneoplastic BE tissues may not be generalizable to the wider BE population, from which most EA cases derive. It is here that case-control (cross-sectional) studies of EA compared with BE controls may offer additional insights for putative risk prediction markers by studying unselected and complete EA populations.[95]

Risk factors

Risk factors for neoplastic progression in BE include age, sex, and cigarette smoking. Increasing age as a risk factor for neoplastic progression is inferred from cancer registry data, which show EA incidence of 1.0 per 100,000 person-years aged 40 to 49 years, 3.9 for ages 50 to 59, 9.3 for ages 60 to 69, 13.7 for ages 70 to 79, and 13.6 for 80+ years[37] and has empiric support as an independent predictor.[96–101] Male BE subjects have been shown to have 2 to 3 times higher risk of developing EA compared with female BE subjects,[102] which is not attenuated in multivariable models.[96–99,101,103] Cigarette smoking and pack-years have shown fairly consistent moderate associations with EA when compared with BE,[98,100,103–105] with a recent metaanalysis finding a 30% to 50% increased risk of ever smoking compared with never smoking.[96] Other lifestyle factors and demographics, such as GERD, excess adiposity, alcohol consumption, and race do not have good evidence for being risk factors for neoplastic progression in BE. GERD has consistently been inversely associated with EA when compared with BE.[95,105,106] In a study that conducted separate analyses of EA by prior diagnosis of BE, GERD was positively associated with the 13% of EA cases that had a prior diagnosis of BE,[95] yet inversely associated with the remaining 87% of EA cases that did not have a prior diagnosis of BE, when each were compared with a BE control group. A plausible interpretation is that most individuals diagnosed with EA do not have a recent history of severe GERD exposure.[107] With regards to excess adiposity, overweight at age 20 years (OR = 2.6, 95% CI: 1.2–5.5) and 10 years before questionnaire (OR = 1.8, 95% CI: 1.1–3.3) were associated with EA compared with BE controls in a hospital-based case-control study from the

Netherlands[105]; however, this observation does not have support from most other studies that have compared EA with BE.[96,98,100,104] In addition, abdominal obesity has been similarly null in relation to neoplastic progression in BE populations.[100,104] Studies of alcohol and neoplastic progression in BE have been null,[103,104,108] whereas race has been difficult to study because of the fact that most BE patients are of European ancestry.

Biomarkers

Endoscopic and histologic features Various endoscopic features have been associated with neoplastic progression in BE, including metaplastic segment length with studies showing a 17% to 19% increased risk per centimeter after multivariable adjustment.[96,109,110] Moreover, a recent pooled analysis of 10 studies showed annual rates of progression from nondysplastic BE to high-grade dysplasia or EA of 0.24% for short-segment BE (<3 cm) compared with 0.76% for long-segment BE (≥3 cm).[111] Other endoscopic features associated neoplastic progression in BE include esophageal contractility,[112] esophageal ulcer,[106,113] and nodularity.[113,114] The evidence for whether hiatal hernia is associated with neoplastic progression in BE is mixed with many studies finding no association,[97,106,109,115] although one of the largest case-control studies did report an OR of 1.2 per centimeter (95% CI: 1.0–1.4).[110] Esophageal stricture[106] and esophagitis[97,106] do not appear to be risk factors for neoplastic progression in BE.

The primary histologic feature associated with EA risk in BE is dysplasia. Diagnosis of high-grade dysplasia is often clinically treated as EA[42] because of the high risk of prevalent malignancy or subsequent progression. Low-grade dysplasia has a more contentious history as a marker of neoplastic risk because of low interobserver agreement and the possibility of true regression back to a nondysplastic state.[116] Larger specimen size[117] and simplified descriptive histologic criteria[118] appear to improve interobserver agreement, whereas expert confirmation[116] and persistence of low-grade dysplasia[119–121] are associated with higher risks of neoplastic progression. However, cancer risk still varies markedly between studies of low-grade dysplasia populations.[96,111,116,122] In the United States, this has resulted in low-grade dysplasia being used as a marker for either clinical intervention or increased surveillance, depending on patient-provider discussions.[116]

Molecular biomarkers Initial molecular biomarkers to stratify neoplastic risk in BE focused on using histochemistry to distinguish 3 subtypes of intestinal metaplasia.[123–125] Although subtype III was hypothesized to be a marker of disease progression,[126] further studies cast doubt on the specificity[127,128] and accuracy[129] of this biomarker. Despite this initial disappointment, further histochemical studies have provided more promising results. For example, in a nested case-control study of 29 cancer cases and up to 5 matched controls per case, diffuse/intense *TP53* staining in baseline BE biopsy was associated with an 11-fold increased risk of EA.[130] Prior smaller immunohistochemistry studies of low-grade dysplastic BE cases had suggested this association,[131–133] and subsequent studies and metaanalyses offered corroborating evidence.[134,135] This body of evidence led the British Society of Gastroenterology to recommend considering *TP53* immunohistochemistry as an adjunct diagnostic.[40,136]

A recent multiplexed immunofluorescence discovery and validation study of 14 markers implicated in BE progression or carcinogenesis more generally were tested in a multi-institutional case-control study comprising 79 progressors matched with 287 nonprogressors.[137] A 3-tier (low, intermediate, and high risk), 15-feature classifier based on 10 biomarkers (TP53, HER2, K20, COX2, CD68, HIF1a, p16INK4A, AMACR, CD45RO, and nuclear morphology) estimated a hazard ratio of 9.4 (95% CI: 4.6–19.2) when comparing high with low risk in the validation sample set, providing independent prognostic information. A subsequent external validation study estimated an OR of 4.7 (95% CI: 2.5–8.8) when comparing high- and low-risk groups within 58 progressors and 210 matched nonprogressors.[138] A prevalence-adjusted positive predictive value of 23% at 5 years[138] and evidence of cost-effectiveness[139] further emphasize the potential clinical value of this test. In a separate study, the investigators also found that this risk classifier could detect prevalent high-grade dysplasia/EA as a field effect in BE biopsies without dysplasia, indefinite for dysplasia or low-grade dysplasia,[140] with an OR of 46 (95% CI: 15–169) when comparing high- and low-risk groups. Therefore, this test may offer diagnostic as well as prognostic information that may be of particular value for BE patients in which intervention is not clearly indicated or desired.

Initial nucleic acid studies used flow cytometry to find that increased aneuploid and tetraploid cell fractions correlated with disease stage.[141,142] A cohort study[12] showed that 13 of 62 patients had increased G2/tetraploid cell fractions in baseline BE biopsies, nine of which subsequently progressed to high-grade dysplasia/EA. A later study of the Seattle Barrett's Esophagus Study cohort[143] reported increased baseline tetraploidy and aneuploidy had 5-year EA incidences of 56% and 43%, respectively, although most progressors had high-grade dysplasia at baseline. Many additional studies have been conducted in support of aneuploidy and tetraploidy as biomarkers of neoplastic progression,[144] albeit with evidence of publication bias and significant heterogeneity, the latter of which likely stems from variable BE study populations, technologies and assays, and thresholds of exposure.

A recent retrospective case-control study has shown that *TP53* mutations were more common (OR = 13.8, 95% CI: 3.2–61.0) in baseline BE biopsies of progressors (46%, 11/24) than nonprogressors (5%, 4/73) with significant associations also observed for *ARID1B*, *APC*, and *ERBB2*.[145] Importantly, Stachler and colleagues[146] noted that these mutations are early biomarkers that appear to precede aneuploidy in esophageal adenocarcinogenesis, which is in agreement with their prior cross-sectional study and forms the backbone of the current molecular model. Building on this model, a study using a high-resolution single-nucleotide polymorphism array has provided evidence that somatic copy number alterations of *CDKN2A/B* and *FHIT* were also predictive of neoplastic progression in nondysplastic baseline BE biopsy samples from 16 progressors and 42 nonprogressors.[147]

Other prospective studies have assessed multiple nucleic acid biomarkers in relation to neoplastic progression. One study based in the Seattle Barrett's Esophagus Study cohort found that 17p loss of heterozygosity (LOH), tetraploidy, aneuploidy, and 9p LOH estimated a relative risk of 38.7 (95% CI: 10.8–138.5) for EA diagnosis at 10 year of follow-up,[148] whereas another derived a 29 chromosomal feature model, which was reported to have an AUC of 0.94 for predicting EA risk.[149] Timmer and colleagues[150] conducted a similar nucleic acid analysis study, but restricted to a BE population without dysplasia, finding that *p16* loss, *MYC* gain, and aneusomy—when combined with age and BE circumferential segment length—identified a high-risk group with a hazard ratio of 8.7 (95% CI: 2.6–29.8) for neoplastic progression when compared with the low-risk group.

Other biomarkers of neoplastic progression in BE to have recently been assessed include methylation,[151,152] mutational load,[153,154] and cellular apoptosis susceptibility gene (CAS/CSE1L).[155] An in-depth discussion of these putative biomarkers is beyond the scope of this article but highlights the expansion of biomarkers being assessed in this field.

Finally, in addition to the prospective and retrospective studies described to have assessed preneoplastic (BE) tissues of EA cases, case-control (cross-sectional) studies comparing EA with BE are also of interest, as described at the outset of this section. Many of these discriminative markers are also in their infancy but include gene expression,[156] microRNA expression,[157–159] stromal lymphocytic phenotype,[160] neutrophil-lymphocyte ratio,[161] T-cell phenotype,[162,163] microbiome diversity,[164,165] and serum glycoproteins,[166] among others.

Algorithms

There are a limited number of algorithms for estimating risk of neoplastic progression in BE. One of the first was the Barrett's Esophagus Assessment of Risk score by Brown and colleagues[167] in 2018. This model estimated the risk of progressing from nondysplastic BE (N = 2591) to dysplasia (low/high grade) or EA (n = 133). Using 10-fold cross-validation, the model of age, sex, proton-pump inhibitor use, segment length, and history of esophageal candidiasis estimated an AUC of 0.76. Shortly thereafter, Parasa and colleagues[168] published their model—Progression in Barrett's Esophagus score, using a BE cohort of 2697 with 133 outcomes. This algorithm estimated risk of progressing from BE without dysplasia, indefinite for dysplasia, or with low-grade dysplasia to high-grade dysplasia or EA using 70% of the study population and included sex, smoking, segment length, and baseline-confirmed low-grade dysplasia resulting in an AUC of 0.76; the remaining 30% of the population demonstrated high model calibration. An external validation study, based in Northern Ireland and comprising 1198 BE patients with 54 progressors, estimated the AUC of this model as 0.70.[169] This external validation study is the only external validation study to date of any BE neoplastic progression model. A final model to be based on demographic/lifestyle/clinical factors was published by Holmberg and colleagues.[97] This nested case-control study based in the Swedish National Patient Registry compared BE without dysplasia, indefinite for dysplasia, or with low-grade dysplasia (n = 1089) with high-grade dysplasia or EA previously diagnosed with BE (n = 279). A final model of age, sex, and maximal segment length estimated an AUC of 0.71.

Recently, Hoefnagel and colleagues[170] developed a prediction model that combined molecular markers with demographic and clinical variables. This Dutch multicenter study included 334 nondysplastic BE patients, 32 of which progressed to high-grade dysplasia or EA. A model including age, BE circumferential length, and a clonicity score (based on fluorescence in situ hybridization probes for 20q13.2, c-MYC [8q24.12], and centromeres of chromosomes 7 and 17) estimated an AUC of 0.88.

Finally, Vaughan and colleagues[107] brought together an array of demographic, lifestyle, clinical, and molecular evidence to build an online risk calculator named IC-RISC (https://ic-risc.fredhutch.org/). This calculator emphasizes the importance of simplicity of use and communication of risk. The latter is especially important for providers and patients if professional guidelines are to advocate for personalized decisions in individuals with low-grade dysplasia.

CONTROVERSIES

A central controversy to the primary (screening) and secondary (surveillance) prevention strategies that underlie this review is whether BE is a necessary precursor of EA. Previous studies have reported that not all EA cases have concomitant BE.[171] A study using a rigorous biopsy protocol found that only 62% of EA patients had detectable BE,[172] while previous EA series have detected a BE prevalence range of 23% to 100%.[173–183] Sampling error as well as overgrowth and elimination by the expanding tumor are possible reasons for the variation of these estimates and the failure to observe BE in all EA subjects. The study of Chandrasoma and colleagues[181] found the prevalence of intestinal metaplasia decreased with increasing tumor size and stage, supporting the overgrowth/elimination theory. Meanwhile, Smith and colleagues[184] conducted a comprehensive retrospective and prospective review of clinical records and pathology specimens of 21 EA patients who underwent esophageal mucosal resection, finding evidence for intestinal metaplasia in all cases. Despite this, the controversy continues with a recent study going so far as to suggest that presence or absence of adjacent BE defines 2 distinct EA phenotypes[185]; a concept previously contemplated[180,186] but, overall, considered unlikely from the limited biological evidence that exists.[187–189]

FUTURE DIRECTIONS

Biomarkers for BE screening and risk triaging that have been discovered using biopsies will need to be validated in whole esophageal sampling specimens as well as total, unselected BE populations. A low-cost, single-timepoint specimen collection that can be used for sequential assessment of BE presence and neoplastic risk would be optimal. Algorithms that combine biomarkers and clinical parameters will need to be optimized and validated in external populations, and risk communication should be a central feature. If BE is determined to be an unnecessary precursor for EA, then population BE screening programs should collect information on other putative biomarkers of neoplastic progression gleaned from prospective and case-control studies.

Future BE biomarker studies could be strengthened in the following ways: state the a priori plan for building statistical models; consider interactions, transformations, and splines; refrain from categorizing predictors; use and report betas for risk models; use cross-validation and aim for external validation; use informed and a priori stated criteria for desired sensitivity and specificity; and assess model performance by incorporating population disease risk.

SUMMARY

Epidemiologic studies of demographic, clinical, and molecular biomarkers for BE screening and surveillance provide optimism for accurate risk prediction and precision surveillance. Movement toward larger-scale, collaborative studies—particularly focused on unselected BE populations without dysplasia, indefinite for dysplasia, or with low-grade dysplasia—is needed, as is further discovery and validation studies of biomarkers and algorithms. Cost-effective approaches for primary and secondary prevention of EA are within our grasp, but it is imperative that we conduct larger studies with a stronger and more clinically focused statistical framework.

CLINICS CARE POINTS

- Screening for Barrett's esophagus needs to go beyond patients reporting current symptoms of gastroesophageal reflux disease to include other established risk factors, such as smoking history and obesity.
- To date, no screening or surveillance algorithm has sufficient discriminatory accuracy or external validation to support clinical use.
- It is important to note that most evidence for cause and neoplastic progression is derived from selected Barrett's esophagus populations.

- Despite potential reverse-causation, case-control studies comparing esophageal adenocarcinoma with Barrett's esophagus may derive additional neoplastic predictors given the ability to characterize all patients with cancer with greater statistical power, as opposed to assessing a small subset of esophageal adenocarcinoma cases previously diagnosed with Barrett's esophagus.
- Biomarker studies must strive to use stronger statistical frameworks.
- Larger, collaborative studies—particularly those focused on Barrett's esophagus populations without dysplasia, indefinite for dysplasia, or with low-grade dysplasia—are needed to enhance biomarker discovery and validation efforts to increase the accuracy of predictive algorithms.

DISCLOSURE

None.

REFERENCES

1. Schmidt FA. De mammalium oesophage atque ventriculo. Halae: Batheana; 1805.
2. Stewart MJ, Hartfall SJ. Chronic peptic ulcer of the esophagus. J Pathol 1929; 32:9–14.
3. Lyall A. Chronic peptic ulcer of the oesophagus: a report of eight cases. Br J Surg 1937;24:534–47.
4. Barrett NR. Chronic peptic ulcer of the oesophagus and oesophagitis. Br J Surg 1950;38:175–82.
5. Allison PR, Johnstone AS. The oesophagus lined with gastric mucosa membrane. Thorax 1953;8:87–101.
6. Barrett NR. The lower esophagus lined by columnar epithelium. Surgery 1957; 41(6):881–94.
7. Moersch RN, Ellis FH, McDonald JR. Pathologic changes occurring in severe reflux esophagitis. Surg Gynecol Obstet 1959;108:476–84.
8. Bremner CG, Lynch VP, Ellis FH Jr. Barrett's esophagus: congenital or acquired? An experimental study of esophageal mucosal regeneration in the dog. Surgery 1970;68(1):209–16.
9. Bosher LH, Taylor FH. Heterotopic gastric mucosa in the esophagus with ulceration and stricture formation. J Thorac Surg 1951;21:306–12.
10. Morson BC, Belcher JR. Adenocarcinoma of the esophagus and ectopic gastric mucosa. Br J Surg 1952;6:127–30.
11. Paull A, Trier JS, Dalton MD, et al. The histologic spectrum of Barrett's esophagus. N Engl J Med 1976;295(9):476–80.
12. Reid BJ, Blount PL, Rubin CE, et al. Flow-cytometric and histological progression to malignancy in Barrett's esophagus: prospective endoscopic surveillance of a cohort. Gastroenterology 1992;102(4):1212–9.
13. Paraf F, Flejou JF, Pignon JP, et al. Surgical pathology of adenocarcinoma arising in Barrett's esophagus. Analysis of 67 cases. Am J Surg Pathol 1995; 19(2):183–91.
14. Shaheen N. Is there a "Barrett's iceberg? Gastroenterology 2002;123(2):636–9.
15. Cameron AJ, Zinsmeister AR, Ballard DJ, et al. Prevalence of columnar-lined (Barrett's) esophagus. Comparison of population-based clinical and autopsy findings. Gastroenterology 1990;99(4):918–22.

16. Ronkainen J, Aro P, Storskrubb T, et al. Prevalence of Barrett's esophagus in the general population: an endoscopic study. Gastroenterology 2005;129(6): 1825–31.
17. Zagari RM, Fuccio L, Wallander MA, et al. Gastro-oesophageal reflux symptoms, oesophagitis and Barrett's oesophagus in the general population: the Loiano-Monghidoro study. Gut 2008;57(10):1354–9.
18. Hayeck TJ, Kong CY, Spechler SJ, et al. The prevalence of Barrett's esophagus in the US: estimates from a simulation model confirmed by SEER data. Dis Esophagus 2010;23(6):451–7.
19. Qumseya BJ, Bukannan A, Gendy S, et al. Systematic review and meta-analysis of prevalence and risk factors for Barrett's esophagus. Gastrointest Endosc 2019;90(5):707–17.e1.
20. Chen YH, Yu HC, Lin KH, et al. Prevalence and risk factors for Barrett's esophagus in Taiwan. World J Gastroenterol 2019;25(25):3231–41.
21. Macdonald CE, Wicks AC, Playford RJ. Ten years' experience of screening patients with Barrett's oesophagus in a university teaching hospital. Gut 1997; 41(3):303–7.
22. Conio M, Cameron AJ, Romero Y, et al. Secular trends in the epidemiology and outcome of Barrett's oesophagus in Olmsted County, Minnesota. Gut 2001; 48(3):304–9.
23. Irani S, Parkman H, Krevsky B, et al. A decade (1991-2000) of increasing incidence of endoscopic and histologic Barrett's esophagus (BE) at a single academic medical center. Am J Gastroenterol 2003;98:S16.
24. Musana AK, Resnick JM, Torbey CF, et al. Barrett's esophagus: incidence and prevalence estimates in a rural Mid-Western population. Am J Gastroenterol 2008;103(3):516–24.
25. Yachimski P, Lee RA, Tramontano A, et al. Secular trends in patients diagnosed with Barrett's esophagus. Dig Dis Sci 2010;55(4):960–6.
26. Petrick JL, Nguyen T, Cook MB. Temporal trends of esophageal disorders by age in the Cerner Health Facts database. Ann Epidemiol 2016;26(2):151–4.e4.
27. Prach AT, MacDonald TA, Hopwood DA, et al. Increasing incidence of Barrett's oesophagus: education, enthusiasm, or epidemiology? Lancet 1997; 350(9082):933.
28. Watson A, Reed PI, Caygill CPJ, et al. Changing incidence of columnar-lined (Barrett's) oesophagus (CLO) in the UK. Gut 1999;44:W180.
29. Hurschler D, Borovicka J, Neuweiler J, et al. Increased detection rates of Barrett's oesophagus without rise in incidence of oesophageal adenocarcinoma. Swiss Med Wkly 2003;133(37–38):507–14.
30. van Soest EM, Dieleman JP, Siersema PD, et al. Increasing incidence of Barrett's oesophagus in the general population. Gut 2005;54(8):1062–6.
31. Alcedo J, Ferrandez A, Arenas J, et al. Trends in Barrett's esophagus diagnosis in Southern Europe: implications for surveillance. Dis Esophagus 2009;22(3): 239–48.
32. Coleman HG, Bhat S, Murray LJ, et al. Increasing incidence of Barrett's oesophagus: a population-based study. Eur J Epidemiol 2011;26(9):739–45.
33. Kendall BJ, Whiteman DC. Temporal changes in the endoscopic frequency of new cases of Barrett's esophagus in an Australian health region. Am J Gastroenterol 2006;101(6):1178–82.
34. Masclee GM, Coloma PM, de Wilde M, et al. Letter: incidence rates of Barrett's oesophagus and oesophageal adenocarcinoma in UK and the Netherlands - authors' reply. Aliment Pharmacol Ther 2014;40(4):404.

35. Surveillance Epidemiology and End Results (SEER) Program. (www.seer.cancer.gov) SEER*Stat Database: Incidence - SEER Research Data, 9 Registries, Nov 2019 Sub (1975-2017) - Linked To County Attributes - Time Dependent (1990-2017) Income/Rurality, 1969-2017 Counties, National Cancer Institute, DCCPS, Surveillance Research Program, released April 2020, based on the November 2019 submission.
36. Thrift AP, Whiteman DC. The incidence of esophageal adenocarcinoma continues to rise: analysis of period and birth cohort effects on recent trends. Ann Oncol 2012;23(12):3155–62.
37. Surveillance Epidemiology and End Results (SEER) Program. (www.seer.cancer.gov) SEER*Stat Database: Incidence - SEER 18 Regs Research Data + Hurricane Katrina Impacted Louisiana Cases with Delay-Adjustment, Malignant Only, Nov 2019 Sub (2000-2017) <Katrina/Rita Population Adjustment> - Linked To County Attributes - Total U.S., 1969-2018 Counties, National Cancer Institute, DCCPS, Surveillance Research Program, released April 2020, based on the November 2019 submission.
38. Surveillance Epidemiology and End Results (SEER) Program. (www.seer.cancer.gov) SEER*Stat Database: Incidence - SEER Research Data, 18 Registries, Nov 2019 Sub (2000-2017) - Linked To County Attributes - Time Dependent (1990-2017) Income/Rurality, 1969-2017 Counties, National Cancer Institute, DCCPS, Surveillance Research Program, released April 2020, based on the November 2019 submission.
39. Qumseya B, Sultan S, Bain P, et al. ASGE guideline on screening and surveillance of Barrett's esophagus. Gastrointest Endosc 2019;90(3):335–59.e2.
40. Fitzgerald RC, di Pietro M, Ragunath K, et al. British Society of Gastroenterology guidelines on the diagnosis and management of Barrett's oesophagus. Gut 2014;63(1):7–42.
41. Spechler SJ, Sharma P, Souza RF, et al. American Gastroenterological Association Technical Review on the management of Barrett's esophagus. Gastroenterology 2011;140(3):e18–52.
42. Shaheen NJ, Falk GW, Iyer PG, et al. ACG clinical guideline: diagnosis and management of Barrett's esophagus. Am J Gastroenterol 2016;111(1):30–51.
43. Xie SH, Lagergren J. A global assessment of the male predominance in esophageal adenocarcinoma. Oncotarget 2016;7(25):38876–83.
44. Xie SH, Lagergren J. The male predominance in esophageal adenocarcinoma. Clin Gastroenterol Hepatol 2016;14(3):338–47.e1.
45. Arnold M, Soerjomataram I, Ferlay J, et al. Global incidence of oesophageal cancer by histological subtype in 2012. Gut 2015;64(3):381–7.
46. Cook MB, Chow WH, Devesa SS. Oesophageal cancer incidence in the United States by race, sex, and histologic type, 1977-2005. Br J Cancer 2009;101(5):855–9.
47. Cook MB, Wild CP, Forman D. A systematic review and meta-analysis of the sex ratio for Barrett's esophagus, erosive reflux disease, and nonerosive reflux disease. Am J Epidemiol 2005;162(11):1050–61.
48. Engel LS, Chow WH, Vaughan TL, et al. Population attributable risks of esophageal and gastric cancers. J Natl Cancer Inst 2003;95(18):1404–13.
49. Olsen CM, Pandeya N, Green AC, et al, Australian Cancer Study. Population attributable fractions of adenocarcinoma of the esophagus and gastroesophageal junction. Am J Epidemiol 2011;174(5):582–90.
50. Cook MB, Corley DA, Murray LJ, et al. Gastroesophageal reflux in relation to adenocarcinomas of the esophagus: a pooled analysis from the Barrett's and

Esophageal Adenocarcinoma Consortium (BEACON). PLoS One 2014;9(7): e103508.

51. Thrift AP, Kramer JR, Qureshi Z, et al. Age at onset of GERD symptoms predicts risk of Barrett's esophagus. Am J Gastroenterol 2013;108(6):915–22.
52. Cook MB, Kamangar F, Whiteman DC, et al. Cigarette smoking and adenocarcinomas of the esophagus and esophagogastric junction: a pooled analysis from the International BEACON Consortium. J Natl Cancer Inst 2010;102(17): 1344–53.
53. Wang QL, Xie SH, Li WT, et al. Smoking cessation and risk of esophageal cancer by histological type: systematic review and meta-analysis. J Natl Cancer Inst 2017;109(12).
54. Cook MB, Shaheen NJ, Anderson LA, et al. Cigarette smoking increases risk of Barrett's esophagus: an analysis of the Barrett's and Esophageal Adenocarcinoma Consortium. Gastroenterology 2012;142(4):744–53.
55. Hoyo C, Cook MB, Kamangar F, et al. Body mass index in relation to oesophageal and oesophagogastric junction adenocarcinomas: a pooled analysis from the International BEACON Consortium. Int J Epidemiol 2012;41(6):1706–18.
56. Cook MB, Freedman ND, Gamborg M, et al. Childhood body mass index in relation to future risk of oesophageal adenocarcinoma. Br J Cancer 2015;112(3): 601–7.
57. Levi Z, Kark JD, Shamiss A, et al. Body mass index and socioeconomic status measured in adolescence, country of origin, and the incidence of gastroesophageal adenocarcinoma in a cohort of 1 million men. Cancer 2013;119(23): 4086–93.
58. Steffen A, Huerta J-M, Weiderpass E, et al. General and abdominal obesity and risk of esophageal and gastric adenocarcinoma in the European Prospective Investigation into Cancer and Nutrition. Int J Cancer 2015;137(3):646–57.
59. El-Serag HB, Hashmi A, Garcia J, et al. Visceral abdominal obesity measured by CT scan is associated with an increased risk of Barrett's oesophagus: a case-control study. Gut 2014;63(2):220–9.
60. Singh S, Sharma AN, Murad MH, et al. Central adiposity is associated with increased risk of esophageal inflammation, metaplasia, and adenocarcinoma: a systematic review and meta-analysis. Clin Gastroenterol Hepatol 2013; 11(11):1399–412.e7.
61. Freedman ND, Murray LJ, Kamangar F, et al. Alcohol intake and risk of oesophageal adenocarcinoma: a pooled analysis from the BEACON Consortium. Gut 2011;60(8):1029–37.
62. Thrift AP, Cook MB, Vaughan TL, et al. Alcohol and the risk of Barrett's esophagus: a pooled analysis from the International BEACON Consortium. Am J Gastroenterol 2014;109(10):1586–94.
63. World Cancer Research Fund/American Institute for Cancer Research. Continuous Update Project expert report 2018: Diet, nutrition, physical activity, and oesophageal cancer. 2018. Available at: dietandcancerreport.org. Accessed January 1, 2020.
64. Parsonnet J, Friedman GD, Vandersteen DP, et al. Helicobacter pylori infection and the risk of gastric carcinoma. N Engl J Med 1991;325(16):1127–31.
65. Nie S, Chen T, Yang X, et al. Association of Helicobacter pylori infection with esophageal adenocarcinoma and squamous cell carcinoma: a meta-analysis. Dis Esophagus 2014;27(7):645–53.

66. Xie FJ, Zhang YP, Zheng QQ, et al. Helicobacter pylori infection and esophageal cancer risk: an updated meta-analysis. World J Gastroenterol 2013;19(36): 6098–107.
67. Wang Z, Shaheen NJ, Whiteman DC, et al. Helicobacter pylori infection is associated with reduced risk of Barrett's esophagus: an analysis of the Barrett's and Esophageal Adenocarcinoma Consortium. Am J Gastroenterol 2018;113(8): 1148–55.
68. Eross B, Farkas N, Vincze A, et al. Helicobacter pylori infection reduces the risk of Barrett's esophagus: a meta-analysis and systematic review. Helicobacter 2018;23(4):e12504.
69. Liao LM, Vaughan TL, Corley DA, et al. Nonsteroidal anti-inflammatory drug use reduces risk of adenocarcinomas of the esophagus and esophagogastric junction in a pooled analysis. Gastroenterology 2012;142(3):442–52.e5 [quiz: e422–3].
70. Thrift AP, Anderson LA, Murray LJ, et al. Nonsteroidal anti-inflammatory drug use is not associated with reduced risk of Barrett's esophagus. Am J Gastroenterol 2016;111(11):1528–35.
71. Alexandre L, Clark AB, Bhutta HY, et al. Statin use is associated with reduced risk of histologic subtypes of esophageal cancer: a nested case-control analysis. Gastroenterology 2014;146(3):661–8.
72. Nguyen T, Khalaf N, Ramsey D, et al. Statin use is associated with a decreased risk of Barrett's esophagus. Gastroenterology 2014;147(2):314–23.
73. Petrick JL, Falk RT, Hyland PL, et al. Association between circulating levels of sex steroid hormones and esophageal adenocarcinoma in the FINBAR Study. PLoS One 2018;13(1):e0190325.
74. Cook MB, Wood S, Hyland PL, et al. Sex steroid hormones in relation to Barrett's esophagus: an analysis of the FINBAR Study. Andrology 2017;5(2):240–7.
75. Cook MB, Wood SN, Cash BD, et al. Association between circulating levels of sex steroid hormones and Barrett's esophagus in men: a case-control analysis. Clin Gastroenterol Hepatol 2015;13(4):673–82.
76. Petrick JL, Hyland PL, Caron P, et al. Associations between prediagnostic concentrations of circulating sex steroid hormones and esophageal/gastric cardia adenocarcinoma among men. J Natl Cancer Inst 2019;111(1):34–41.
77. Petrick JL, Cook MB. Do sex hormones underlie sex differences in cancer incidence? Testing the intuitive in esophageal adenocarcinoma. Am J Gastroenterol 2020;115(2):211–3.
78. Xie SH, Ness-Jensen E, Rabbani S, et al. Circulating sex hormone levels and risk of esophageal adenocarcinoma in a prospective study in men. Am J Gastroenterol 2020;115(2):216–23.
79. Xie SH, Fang R, Huang M, et al. Association between levels of hormones and risk of esophageal adenocarcinoma and Barrett's esophagus. Clin Gastroenterol Hepatol 2019. [Epub ahead of print].
80. Gharahkhani P, Fitzgerald RC, Vaughan TL, et al. Genome-wide association studies in oesophageal adenocarcinoma and Barrett's oesophagus: a large-scale meta-analysis. Lancet Oncol 2016;17(10):1363–73.
81. Becker J, May A, Gerges C, et al. Supportive evidence for FOXP1, BARX1, and FOXF1 as genetic risk loci for the development of esophageal adenocarcinoma. Cancer Med 2015;4(11):1700–4.
82. Palles C, Chegwidden L, Li X, et al. Polymorphisms near TBX5 and GDF7 are associated with increased risk for Barrett's esophagus. Gastroenterology 2015;148(2):367–78.

83. Su Z, Gay LJ, Strange A, et al. Common variants at the MHC locus and at chromosome 16q24.1 predispose to Barrett's esophagus. Nat Genet 2012;44(10): 1131–6.
84. Rubenstein JH, Morgenstern H, Appelman H, et al. Prediction of Barrett's esophagus among men. Am J Gastroenterol 2013;108(3):353–62.
85. Thrift AP, Garcia JM, El-Serag HB. A multibiomarker risk score helps predict risk for Barrett's esophagus. Clin Gastroenterol Hepatol 2014;12(8):1267–71.
86. Dong J, Buas MF, Gharahkhani P, et al. Determining risk of Barrett's esophagus and esophageal adenocarcinoma based on epidemiologic factors and genetic variants. Gastroenterology 2017;154(5):1273–81.e3.
87. Rubenstein JH, McConnell D, Waljee AK, et al. Validation and comparison of tools for selecting individuals to screen for Barrett's esophagus and early neoplasia. Gastroenterology 2020;158(8):2082–92.
88. Locke GR, Zinsmeister AR, Talley NJ. Can symptoms predict endoscopic findings in GERD? Gastrointest Endosc 2003;58(5):661–70.
89. Gerson LB, Edson R, Lavori PW, et al. Use of a simple symptom questionnaire to predict Barrett's esophagus in patients with symptoms of gastroesophageal reflux. Am J Gastroenterol 2001;96(7):2005–12.
90. Rubenstein JH, Thrift AP. Risk factors and populations at risk: selection of patients for screening for Barrett's oesophagus. Best Pract Res Clin Gastroenterol 2015;29(1):41–50.
91. Thrift AP, Kanwal F, El-Serag HB. Prediction models for gastrointestinal and liver diseases: too many developed, too few validated. Clin Gastroenterol Hepatol 2016;14(12):1678–80.
92. Thrift AP, Vaughan TL, Anderson LA, et al. External validation of the Michigan Barrett's Esophagus Prediction Tool. Clin Gastroenterol Hepatol 2017;15(7): 1124–6.
93. Ireland CJ, Thrift AP, Esterman A. Risk prediction models for Barrett's esophagus discriminate well and are generalizable in an external validation study. Dig Dis Sci 2020. [Epub ahead of print].
94. Kunzmann AT, Canadas Garre M, Thrift AP, et al. Information on genetic variants does not increase identification of individuals at risk of esophageal adenocarcinoma compared to clinical risk factors. Gastroenterology 2019;156(1):43–5.
95. Cook MB, Drahos J, Wood S, et al. Pathogenesis and progression of oesophageal adenocarcinoma varies by prior diagnosis of Barrett's oesophagus. Br J Cancer 2016;115(11):1383–90.
96. Krishnamoorthi R, Singh S, Ragunathan K, et al. Factors associated with progression of Barrett's esophagus: a systematic review and meta-analysis. Clin Gastroenterol Hepatol 2017;16(7):1046–55.e8.
97. Holmberg D, Ness-Jensen E, Mattsson F, et al. Clinical prediction model for tumor progression in Barrett's esophagus. Surg Endosc 2019;33(9):2901–8.
98. Cooper S, Menon S, Nightingale P, et al. Risk factors for the development of oesophageal adenocarcinoma in Barrett's oesophagus: a UK primary care retrospective nested case-control study. United Eur Gastroenterol J 2014;2(2):91–8.
99. de Jonge PJ, van Blankenstein M, Looman CW, et al. Risk of malignant progression in patients with Barrett's oesophagus: a Dutch Nationwide Cohort Study. Gut 2010;59(8):1030–6.
100. Kambhampati S, Tieu AH, Luber B, et al. Risk factors for progression of Barrett's esophagus to high grade dysplasia and esophageal adenocarcinoma. Sci Rep 2020;10(1):4899.

101. Bhat S, Coleman HG, Yousef F, et al. Risk of malignant progression in Barrett's esophagus patients: results from a large population-based study. J Natl Cancer Inst 2011;103(13):1049–57.
102. Cook MB, Coburn SB, Lam JR, et al. Cancer incidence and mortality risks in a large US Barrett's Oesophagus Cohort. Gut 2017;67(3):418–529.
103. Menke-Pluymers MB, Hop WC, Dees J, et al. Risk factors for the development of an adenocarcinoma in columnar-lined (Barrett) esophagus. The Rotterdam Esophageal Tumor Study Group. Cancer 1993;72(4):1155–8.
104. Hardikar S, Onstad L, Blount PL, et al. The role of tobacco, alcohol, and obesity in neoplastic progression to esophageal adenocarcinoma: a prospective study of Barrett's esophagus. PLoS One 2013;8(1):e52192.
105. de Jonge PJ, Steyerberg EW, Kuipers EJ, et al. Risk factors for the development of esophageal adenocarcinoma in Barrett's esophagus. Am J Gastroenterol 2006;101(7):1421–9.
106. Coleman HG, Bhat SK, Murray LJ, et al. Symptoms and endoscopic features at Barrett's esophagus diagnosis: implications for neoplastic progression risk. Am J Gastroenterol 2014;109(4):527–34.
107. Vaughan TL, Onstad L, Dai JY. Interactive decision support for esophageal adenocarcinoma screening and surveillance. BMC Gastroenterol 2019;19:109.
108. Lou Z, Xing H, Li D. Alcohol consumption and the neoplastic progression in Barrett's esophagus: a systematic review and meta-analysis. PLoS One 2014;9(10): e105612.
109. Pohl H, Wrobel K, Bojarski C, et al. Risk factors in the development of esophageal adenocarcinoma. Am J Gastroenterol 2013;108(2):200–7.
110. Avidan B, Sonnenberg A, Schnell TG, et al. Hiatal hernia size, Barrett's length, and severity of acid reflux are all risk factors for esophageal adenocarcinoma. Am J Gastroenterol 2002;97(8):1930–6.
111. Chandrasekar VT, Hamade N, Desai M, et al. Significantly lower annual rates of neoplastic progression in short- compared to long-segment non-dysplastic Barrett's esophagus: a systematic review and meta-analysis. Endoscopy 2019; 51(7):665–72.
112. Yadlapati R, Triggs J, Quader F, et al. Reduced esophageal contractility is associated with dysplasia progression in Barrett's esophagus: a multicenter cohort study. Dig Dis Sci 2020. [Epub ahead of print].
113. Alnasser S, Agnihotram R, Martel M, et al. Predictors of dysplastic and neoplastic progression of Barrett's esophagus. Can J Surg 2019;62(2):93–9.
114. Solanky D, Krishnamoorthi R, Crews N, et al. Barrett esophagus length, nodularity, and low-grade dysplasia are predictive of progression to esophageal adenocarcinoma. J Clin Gastroenterol 2019;53(5):361–5.
115. Krishnamoorthi R, Borah B, Heien H, et al. Rates and predictors of progression to esophageal carcinoma in a large population-based Barrett's esophagus cohort. Gastrointest Endosc 2016;84(1):40–6.e7.
116. Wani S, Rubenstein JH, Vieth M, et al. Diagnosis and management of low-grade dysplasia in Barrett's esophagus: expert review from the Clinical Practice Updates Committee of the American Gastroenterological Association. Gastroenterology 2016;151(5):822–35.
117. Wani S, Mathur SC, Curvers WL, et al. Greater interobserver agreement by endoscopic mucosal resection than biopsy samples in Barrett's dysplasia. Clin Gastroenterol Hepatol 2010;8(9):783–8.e2.

118. Ten Kate FJC, Nieboer D, Ten Kate FJW, et al. Improved progression prediction in Barrett's esophagus with low-grade dysplasia using specific histologic criteria. Am J Surg Pathol 2018;42(7):918–26.
119. Duits LC, van der Wel MJ, Cotton CC, et al. Patients with Barrett's esophagus and confirmed persistent low-grade dysplasia are at increased risk for progression to neoplasia. Gastroenterology 2017;152(5):993–1001.e1.
120. Kestens C, Offerhaus GJ, van Baal JW, et al. Patients with Barrett's esophagus and persistent low-grade dysplasia have an increased risk for high-grade dysplasia and cancer. Clin Gastroenterol Hepatol 2016;14(7):956–62.e1.
121. Song KY, Henn AJ, Gravely AA, et al. Persistent confirmed low-grade dysplasia in Barrett's esophagus is a risk factor for progression to high-grade dysplasia and adenocarcinoma in a US Veterans cohort. Dis Esophagus 2020;33(2): doz061.
122. O'Byrne LM, Witherspoon J, Verhage RJJ, et al. Barrett's Registry Collaboration of Academic Centers in Ireland reveals high progression rate of low-grade dysplasia and low risk from nondysplastic Barrett's esophagus: report of the RIBBON network. Dis Esophagus 2020. [Epub ahead of print].
123. Jass JR, Filipe MI. The mucin profiles of normal gastric mucosa, intestinal metaplasia and its variants and gastric carcinoma. Histochem J 1981;13(6):931–9.
124. Jass JR, Filipe MI. A variant of intestinal metaplasia associated with gastric carcinoma: a histochemical study. Histopathology 1979;3(3):191–9.
125. Jass JR. Role of intestinal metaplasia in the histogenesis of gastric carcinoma. J Clin Pathol 1980;33(9):801–10.
126. Peuchmaur M, Potet F, Goldfain D. Mucin histochemistry of the columnar epithelium of the oesophagus (Barrett's oesophagus): a prospective biopsy study. J Clin Pathol 1984;37(6):607–10.
127. Haggitt RC, Reid BJ, Rabinovitch PS, et al. Barrett's esophagus. Correlation between mucin histochemistry, flow cytometry, and histologic diagnosis for predicting increased cancer risk. Am J Pathol 1988;131(1):53–61.
128. Endo T, Tamaki K, Arimura Y, et al. Expression of sulfated carbohydrate chain and core peptides of mucin detected by monoclonal antibodies in Barrett's esophagus and esophageal adenocarcinoma. J Gastroenterol 1998;33(6): 811–5.
129. Smith JL, Dixon MF. Is subtyping of intestinal metaplasia in the upper gastrointestinal tract a worthwhile exercise? An evaluation of current mucin histochemical stains. Br J Biomed Sci 2003;60(4):180–6.
130. Murray L, Sedo A, Scott M, et al. TP53 and progression from Barrett's metaplasia to oesophageal adenocarcinoma in a UK population cohort. Gut 2006;55(10): 1390–7.
131. Weston AP, Banerjee SK, Sharma P, et al. p53 protein overexpression in low grade dysplasia (LGD) in Barrett's esophagus: immunohistochemical marker predictive of progression. Am J Gastroenterol 2001;96(5):1355–62.
132. Younes M, Ertan A, Lechago LV, et al. p53 Protein accumulation is a specific marker of malignant potential in Barrett's metaplasia. Dig Dis Sci 1997;42(4): 697–701.
133. Skacel M, Petras RE, Rybicki LA, et al. p53 expression in low grade dysplasia in Barrett's esophagus: correlation with interobserver agreement and disease progression. Am J Gastroenterol 2002;97(10):2508–13.
134. Snyder P, Dunbar K, Cipher DJ, et al. Aberrant p53 immunostaining in Barrett's esophagus predicts neoplastic progression: systematic review and meta-analyses. Dig Dis Sci 2019;64(5):1089–97.

135. Janmaat VT, van Olphen SH, Biermann KE, et al. Use of immunohistochemical biomarkers as independent predictor of neoplastic progression in Barrett's oesophagus surveillance: a systematic review and meta-analysis. PLoS One 2017;12(10):e0186305.
136. di Pietro M, Fitzgerald RC. Revised British Society of Gastroenterology recommendation on the diagnosis and management of Barrett's oesophagus with low-grade dysplasia. Gut 2017;67(2):392–3.
137. Critchley-Thorne RJ, Duits LC, Prichard JW, et al. A tissue systems pathology assay for high-risk Barrett's esophagus. Cancer Epidemiol Biomarkers Prev 2016;25(6):958–68.
138. Davison JM, Goldblum J, Grewal US, et al. Independent blinded validation of a tissue systems pathology test to predict progression in patients with Barrett's esophagus. Am J Gastroenterol 2020. https://doi.org/10.14309/ajg.0000000000000556.
139. Hao J, Critchley-Thorne R, Diehl DL, et al. A cost-effectiveness analysis of an adenocarcinoma risk prediction multi-biomarker assay for patients with Barrett's esophagus. Clinicoecon Outcomes Res 2019;11:623–35.
140. Critchley-Thorne RJ, Davison JM, Prichard JW, et al. A tissue systems pathology test detects abnormalities associated with prevalent high-grade dysplasia and esophageal cancer in Barrett's esophagus. Cancer Epidemiol Biomarkers Prev 2016;26(2):240–8.
141. Reid BJ, Haggitt RC, Rubin CE, et al. Barrett's esophagus. Correlation between flow cytometry and histology in detection of patients at risk for adenocarcinoma. Gastroenterology 1987;93(1):1–11.
142. Rabinovitch PS, Reid BJ, Haggitt RC, et al. Progression to cancer in Barrett's esophagus is associated with genomic instability. Lab Invest 1989;60(1):65–71.
143. Reid BJ, Levine DS, Longton G, et al. Predictors of progression to cancer in Barrett's esophagus: baseline histology and flow cytometry identify low- and high-risk patient subsets. Am J Gastroenterol 2000;95(7):1669–76.
144. Altaf K, Xiong JJ, la Iglesia D, et al. Meta-analysis of biomarkers predicting risk of malignant progression in Barrett's oesophagus. Br J Surg 2017;104(5):493–502.
145. Stachler MD, Camarda ND, Deitrick C, et al. Detection of mutations in Barrett's esophagus before progression to high-grade dysplasia or adenocarcinoma. Gastroenterology 2018;155(1):156–67.
146. Stachler MD, Taylor-Weiner A, Peng S, et al. Paired exome analysis of Barrett's esophagus and adenocarcinoma. Nat Genet 2015;47(9):1047–55.
147. Sepulveda JL, Komissarova EV, Kongkarnka S, et al. High-resolution genomic alterations in Barrett's metaplasia of patients who progress to esophageal dysplasia and adenocarcinoma. Int J Cancer 2019;145(10):2754–66.
148. Galipeau PC, Li X, Blount PL, et al. NSAIDs modulate CDKN2A, TP53, and DNA content risk for progression to esophageal adenocarcinoma. PLoS Med 2007;4(2):e67.
149. Li X, Paulson TG, Galipeau PC, et al. Assessment of esophageal adenocarcinoma risk using somatic chromosome alterations in longitudinal samples in Barrett's esophagus. Cancer Prev Res (Phila) 2015;8(9):845–56.
150. Timmer MR, Martinez P, Lau CT, et al. Derivation of genetic biomarkers for cancer risk stratification in Barrett's oesophagus: a prospective cohort study. Gut 2016;65(10):1602–10.

151. Nieto T, Tomlinson CL, Dretzke J, et al. A systematic review of epigenetic biomarkers in progression from non-dysplastic Barrett's oesophagus to oesophageal adenocarcinoma. BMJ Open 2018;8(6):e020427.
152. Dilworth MP, Nieto T, Stockton JD, et al. Whole genome methylation analysis of nondysplastic Barrett esophagus that progresses to invasive cancer. Ann Surg 2019;269(3):479–85.
153. Eluri S, Brugge WR, Daglilar ES, et al. The presence of genetic mutations at key loci predicts progression to esophageal adenocarcinoma in Barrett's esophagus. Am J Gastroenterol 2015;110(6):828–34.
154. Eluri S, Klaver E, Duits LC, et al. Validation of a biomarker panel in Barrett's esophagus to predict progression to esophageal adenocarcinoma. Dis Esophagus 2018;31(11).
155. Jiang K, Neill K, Cowden D, et al. Expression of CAS/CSE1L, the cellular apoptosis susceptibility protein, correlates with neoplastic progression in Barrett's esophagus. Appl Immunohistochem Mol Morphol 2018;26(8):552–6.
156. Varghese S, Newton R, Ross-Innes CS, et al. Analysis of dysplasia in patients with Barrett's esophagus based on expression pattern of 90 genes. Gastroenterology 2015;149(6):1511–8.e5.
157. Drahos J, Schwameis K, Orzolek LD, et al. MicroRNA profiles of Barrett's esophagus and esophageal adenocarcinoma: differences in glandular non-native epithelium. Cancer Epidemiol Biomarkers Prev 2016;25(3):429–37.
158. Revilla-Nuin B, Parrilla P, Lozano JJ, et al. Predictive value of microRNAs in the progression of Barrett esophagus to adenocarcinoma in a long-term follow-up study. Ann Surg 2013;257(5):886–93.
159. Wu X, Ajani JA, Gu J, et al. MicroRNA expression signatures during malignant progression from Barrett's esophagus to esophageal adenocarcinoma. Cancer Prev Res (Phila) 2013;6(3):196–205.
160. Porter RJ, Murray GI, Brice DP, et al. Novel biomarkers for risk stratification of Barrett's oesophagus associated neoplastic progression-epithelial HMGB1 expression and stromal lymphocytic phenotype. Br J Cancer 2020;122(4):545–54.
161. Campos VJ, Mazzini GS, Juchem JF, et al. Neutrophil-lymphocyte ratio as a marker of progression from non-dysplastic Barrett's esophagus to esophageal adenocarcinoma: a cross-sectional retrospective study. J Gastrointest Surg 2020;24(1):8–18.
162. Kavanagh ME, Conroy MJ, Clarke NE, et al. Impact of the inflammatory microenvironment on T-cell phenotype in the progression from reflux oesophagitis to Barrett oesophagus and oesophageal adenocarcinoma. Cancer Lett 2016;370(1):117–24.
163. Kavanagh ME, Conroy MJ, Clarke NE, et al. Altered T cell migratory capacity in the progression from Barrett oesophagus to oesophageal adenocarcinoma. Cancer Microenviron 2019;12(1):57–66.
164. Snider EJ, Compres G, Freedberg DE, et al. Alterations to the esophageal microbiome associated with progression from Barrett's esophagus to esophageal adenocarcinoma. Cancer Epidemiol Biomarkers Prev 2019;28(10):1687–93.
165. Elliott DRF, Walker AW, O'Donovan M, et al. A non-endoscopic device to sample the oesophageal microbiota: a case-control study. Lancet Gastroenterol Hepatol 2017;2(1):32–42.
166. Shah AK, Cao KA, Choi E, et al. Serum glycoprotein biomarker discovery and qualification pipeline reveals novel diagnostic biomarker candidates for esophageal adenocarcinoma. Mol Cell Proteomics 2015;14(11):3023–39.

167. Brown CS, Lapin B, Goldstein JL, et al. Predicting progression in Barrett's esophagus: development and validation of the Barrett's Esophagus Assessment of Risk Score (BEAR Score). Ann Surg 2018;267(4):716–20.
168. Parasa S, Vennalaganti S, Gaddam S, et al. Development and validation of a model to determine risk of progression of Barrett's esophagus to neoplasia. Gastroenterology 2018;154(5):1282–9.e2.
169. Kunzmann AT, Thrift AP, Johnston BT, et al. External validation of a model to determine risk of progression of Barrett's oesophagus to neoplasia. Aliment Pharmacol Ther 2019;49(10):1274–81.
170. Hoefnagel SJM, Mostafavi N, Timmer MR, et al. A genomic biomarker-based model for cancer risk stratification of non-dysplastic Barrett's esophagus patients after extended follow up; results from Dutch surveillance cohorts. PLoS One 2020;15(4):e0231419.
171. Tan MC, Mansour N, White DL, et al. Systematic review with meta-analysis: prevalence of prior and concurrent Barrett's oesophagus in oesophageal adenocarcinoma patients. Aliment Pharmacol Ther 2020;52(1):20–36.
172. Lagergren J, Bergstrom R, Lindgren A, et al. Symptomatic gastroesophageal reflux as a risk factor for esophageal adenocarcinoma. N Engl J Med 1999; 340(11):825–31.
173. Duhaylongsod FG, Wolfe WG. Barrett's esophagus and adenocarcinoma of the esophagus and gastroesophageal junction. J Thorac Cardiovasc Surg 1991; 102(1):36–41.
174. Haggitt RC, Tryzelaar J, Ellis FH, et al. Adenocarcinoma complicating columnar epithelium-lined (Barrett's) esophagus. Am J Clin Pathol 1978;70(1):1–5.
175. Hamilton SR, Smith RR, Cameron JL. Prevalence and characteristics of Barrett esophagus in patients with adenocarcinoma of the esophagus or esophagogastric junction. Hum Pathol 1988;19(8):942–8.
176. Streitz JM Jr, Ellis FH Jr, Gibb SP, et al. Adenocarcinoma in Barrett's esophagus. A clinicopathologic study of 65 cases. Ann Surg 1991;213(2):122–5.
177. Cameron AJ, Lomboy CT, Pera M, et al. Adenocarcinoma of the esophagogastric junction and Barrett's esophagus. Gastroenterology 1995;109(5):1541–6.
178. Clark GW, Smyrk TC, Burdiles P, et al. Is Barrett's metaplasia the source of adenocarcinomas of the cardia? Arch Surg 1994;129(6):609–14.
179. Li H, Walsh TN, Hennessy TP. Carcinoma arising in Barrett's esophagus. Surg Gynecol Obstet 1992;175(2):167–72.
180. Sabel MS, Pastore K, Toon H, et al. Adenocarcinoma of the esophagus with and without Barrett mucosa. Arch Surg 2000;135(7):831–5.
181. Chandrasoma P, Wickramasinghe K, Ma Y, et al. Is intestinal metaplasia a necessary precursor lesion for adenocarcinomas of the distal esophagus, gastroesophageal junction and gastric cardia? Dis Esophagus 2007;20(1): 36–41.
182. Takubo K, Aida J, Naomoto Y, et al. Cardiac rather than intestinal-type background in endoscopic resection specimens of minute Barrett adenocarcinoma. Hum Pathol 2009;40(1):65–74.
183. Aida J, Vieth M, Shepherd NA, et al. Is carcinoma in columnar-lined esophagus always located adjacent to intestinal metaplasia?: a histopathologic assessment. Am J Surg Pathol 2015;39(2):188–96.
184. Smith J, Garcia A, Zhang R, et al. Intestinal metaplasia is present in most if not all patients who have undergone endoscopic mucosal resection for esophageal adenocarcinoma. Am J Surg Pathol 2016;40(4):537–43.

185. Sawas T, Killcoyne S, Iyer PG, et al. Identification of prognostic phenotypes of esophageal adenocarcinoma in 2 independent cohorts. Gastroenterology 2018;155(6):1720–8.e4.
186. Johansson J, Johnsson F, Walther B, et al. Adenocarcinoma in the distal esophagus with and without Barrett esophagus: differences in symptoms and survival rates. Arch Surg 1996;131(7):708–13.
187. von Rahden BHA, Kircher S, Lazariotou M, et al. LgR5 expression and cancer stem cell hypothesis: clue to define the true origin of esophageal adenocarcinomas with and without Barrett's esophagus? J Exp Clin Cancer Res 2011; 30:11.
188. Mendes de Almeida JC, Chaves P, Pereira AD, et al. Is Barrett's esophagus the precursor of most adenocarcinomas of the esophagus and cardia? A biochemical study. Ann Surg 1997;226(6):725–33 [discussion: 733–5].
189. Engel U, McCombs R, Stranahan P, et al. Decrease in Le(x) expression in esophageal adenocarcinomas arising in Barrett's epithelium. Cancer Epidemiol Biomarkers Prev 1997;6(4):245–8.

Endoscopic Screening for Barrett's Esophagus and Esophageal Adenocarcinoma

Rationale, Candidates, and Challenges

Amrit K. Kamboj, MD, David A. Katzka, MD,
Prasad G. Iyer, MD, MSc*

KEYWORDS

- Barrett's esophagus • Screening • Esophageal adenocarcinoma
- Gastroesophageal reflux disease • Surveillance

KEY POINTS

- Only 7% of the approximately 10,000 esophageal adenocarcinomas diagnosed annually in the United States are detected through current screening and surveillance practices. This likely reflects the low proportion (33%) of prevalent Barrett's esophagus (BE) in the community that is currently in the surveillance pool.
- Screening for BE should be considered in those with multiple risk factors, including age greater than 50 years, male sex, chronic gastroesophageal reflux disease, white race, central obesity, smoking use, first-degree relative with BE or esophageal adenocarcinoma, and presence of hiatal hernia. Screening is not recommended in the general population.
- The greater the number of risk factors present, the higher the prevalence of BE.
- If initial evaluation is negative for BE, repeat evaluation for BE detection is not indicated given low yield, unless new clinical symptoms develop.

THE RATIONALE FOR BARRETT'S ESOPHAGUS SCREENING

There are approximately 18,440 new cases of esophageal cancer and 16,170 deaths from esophageal cancer annually.[1] Esophageal cancer has 2 histologic subtypes, adenocarcinoma and squamous cell carcinoma, and accounts for 1% of all cancers diagnosed in the United States.[1] Over the past 3 to 4 decades, there has been an

---

Funding: Funded in part by NCI R01 grant CA241164 (to P.G. Iyer).
Conflicts: A.K. Kamboj: None. D.A. Katzka: Education: Takeda. P.G. Iyer: Research funding from Exact Sciences, Pentax Medical, Medtronic, Nine Point Medical; Consulting: Medtronic, Symple Surgical.
Division of Gastroenterology and Hepatology, Mayo Clinic, 200 First Street SW, Rochester, Minnesota 55905, USA
* Corresponding author.
E-mail address: iyer.prasad@mayo.edu

Gastrointest Endoscopy Clin N Am 31 (2021) 27–41
https://doi.org/10.1016/j.giec.2020.08.002
giendo.theclinics.com

exponential increase in the incidence of esophageal adenocarcinoma (EAC), which now constitutes most cases of esophageal cancer diagnosed in the West.[2,3] There was a 463% increase in the incidence of EAC in Americans in 2000 to 2004 as compared with 1975 to 1979.[4] There is a marked male predominance for EAC with a male-to-female ratio of 9:1.[5,6] Known risk factors for EAC include Barrett's esophagus (BE), gastroesophageal reflux disease (GERD), male sex, white race, central obesity, and tobacco use.[7–9]

Despite advancements in its diagnosis and earlier recognition, EAC is associated with a poor 5-year survival rate of 10% to 20%.[10,11] The mortal threat of this disease results from 2 key mechanisms. The first is the propensity for metastasis at the earliest of stages owing to tumor access to lymphatic drainage in the esophageal submucosa. The second reason is the paucity of symptoms until advanced stages are reached. This combination almost always ensures a poor prognosis unless screening and surveillance are implemented from a preneoplastic state, that is, BE.

BE is the sole known precursor to the development of EAC and is characterized by metaplastic changes whereby the normal squamous epithelium of the distal esophagus is replaced by specialized columnar epithelium with intestinal metaplasia (IM).[7,12] BE is thought to progress to EAC in a stepwise manner, transitioning from nondysplastic BE (NDBE) to low-grade dysplasia (LGD) to high-grade dysplasia (HGD) to EAC. The risk of EAC in patients with BE is 30- to 125-fold greater than that in the general population.[13,14] The prevalence of BE in the general population is approximately 1% to 2% but may be as high as 5% to 15% in those with chronic GERD.[15–17]

Screening for BE currently includes patients with risk factors for the disease undergoing an endoscopic evaluation with esophagoduodenoscopy (EGD) or transnasal endoscopy (TNE). Esophageal biopsies are performed if the endoscopic appearance of the distal esophagus is consistent with BE with the presence of at least 1 cm of columnar-appearing metaplasia in the tubular esophagus. Given that the progression from BE to EAC is through a metaplasia-dysplasia-carcinoma sequence as described above, screening for BE is performed with the rationale that if patients can be identified at the time of metaplasia alone, they can be placed on endoscopic surveillance to enable the detection of dysplasia (low grade or high grade) or carcinoma (at an earlier stage).[18,19]

Over the past decade, randomized controlled trials and several prospective and retrospective cohort studies have shown that endoscopic eradication therapy (consisting of endoscopic resection of visible lesions followed by endoscopic ablation) can reduce progression to EAC by eliminating dysplasia and IM.[20–23] More recently, chemoprevention trials suggest that patients with NDBE may have prolonged time to all-cause mortality, EAC, and HGD when treated with high-dose proton pump inhibitors (PPIs) and/or aspirin.[24,25] If early-stage EAC (T1a EAC) is diagnosed during surveillance, it can be successfully treated endoscopically with excellent long-term survival (in distinction to potentially poor outcomes with surgery and chemoradiation in the treatment of more advanced EAC diagnosed after the onset of symptoms).[26,27]

Patients with EAC and prior history of known BE (presumably undergoing surveillance) are more likely to be detected with earlier-stage disease and receive endoscopic or surgical treatment compared with those with EAC and no prior known history of BE (not diagnosed in a surveillance program). A metaanalysis demonstrated that regular surveillance was associated with lower EAC-related and all-cause mortality (relative risk 0.60, hazard ratio 0.75).[28] In addition, this study showed that surveillance-detected EAC is diagnosed at earlier stages than EAC diagnosed outside of surveillance. Moreover, because there are no specific signs or symptoms associated with BE, it can only be detected via screening those with risk factors. The presence of alarm symptoms, such as dysphagia, odynophagia, and unintentional weight loss, often signal complications, such as a stricture or locally advanced EAC.

RISK FACTORS FOR BARRETT'S ESOPHAGUS AND ESOPHAGEAL ADENOCARCINOMA

Given that the metaplastic mucosa that occurs with BE is thought to occur uniformly in the presence of chronic GERD, it only stands to reason that GERD is often considered to be the primary risk factor for BE. Chronic GERD is strongly associated with BE with a summary odds ratio (OR) of 2.90 (95% confidence interval [CI], 1.86–4.54).[29] GERD symptoms increase the odds of long-segment BE by almost 5-fold (OR 4.92; 95% CI, 2.01–12.0) but may not have a significant association with short-segment BE (OR 1.15; 95% CI, 0.76–1.73) as shown in a systematic review and metaanalysis.[29] In patients with recurrent symptoms of GERD, the OR of EAC was 7.7 (95% CI, 5.3–11.4) compared with those without GERD symptoms.[30] The more frequent, prolonged, and severe the symptoms of GERD, the greater the risk of BE and EAC.[30–32] However, given that the overall prevalence of EAC is low and that 50% of the population experiences GERD symptoms on a monthly basis and 20% on a weekly basis, routine endoscopic screening of patients with GERD symptoms and no other risk factors is not supported.[31] The prevalence of BE in patients with GERD alone is estimated to be 3%.[33] In the setting of GERD plus another risk factor, the prevalence of BE increases to 12.2%.[33]

Age greater than 50 years is another strong risk factor for BE.[33–36] The prevalence of BE in the Western population older than the age of 50 years is 6.1%.[33] In individuals older than the age of 65 years, the prevalence of BE is approximately 16.7%.[37] The association of age and BE appears to be less prominent in the non-Western population, where the prevalence of BE in those older than the age of 50 years is about 1%.[38] Unless multiple other risk factors are present, screening is not recommended in those younger than 50 years even when GERD symptoms are present; for example, a man aged 35 years with GERD symptoms has a risk of EAC of 1 in 100,000.[39]

A substantial portion of first-degree relatives of individuals with BE have either short-segment or long-segment BE, suggesting that there may be a familial susceptibility to developing BE and EAC in a subset of the population.[40] After adjusting for other risk factors, family history was independently associated with BE or EAC with an OR of 12.23 (95% CI, 3.34–44.76).[41] There may be a greater than 2-fold risk of BE in first-degree relatives compared with those without a family history of BE and EAC.[42] Although 1 study suggested that close to 30% of first-degree relatives of patients with BE with HGD or EAC may have BE, the overall pooled prevalence of BE in this population is estimated at 23.4%.[33,43] It is estimated that 7% of cases of BE and EAC may be familial: these should be suspected in patients with younger age of onset of reflux symptoms and familial diagnosis of EAC or BE.[44] In contrast, in another study, there was no statistical difference in the risk of BE in a family member of a patient with BE with reflux symptoms compared with controls with reflux. However, these family members were more likely to experience reflux symptoms compared with controls theoretically increasing their risk for erosive esophagitis (EE) or BE compared with the general population.[45]

Central obesity is independently associated with BE and EAC.[46,47] BE may be present in 2% to 6% of patients with obesity undergoing EGD[48,49] with a pooled prevalence of 1.9%.[33] For every 1-kg/m^2 increase in the body mass index (BMI), the risk of EAC and BE increases by 16% and 12%, respectively.[46] Waist circumference is a better predictor of BE risk compared with BMI.[50]

Men are significantly more likely to have BE compared with women.[37,51,52] The prevalence of BE in men approaches 6.8%.[33] The incidence of EAC in women with GERD is extremely low and comparable to the risk of breast cancer in men.[39] The length of the BE segment was also found to be greater in men compared with women in 1 study.[53] Women are also less likely to have prevalent HGD or EAC compared with men (OR 0.52; 95% CI, 0.31–0.88).[53] Given the very low incidence of EAC in women, routine screening for BE is not recommended for this group unless multiple other risk factors are present.

White race is also a risk factor for BE.[52,54] Whites account for greater than 90% of all cases of BE.[55] The white-to-African American ratio for EAC is about 3:1.[56] The prevalence of BE in whites is approximately 6.1% and significantly higher compared with Hispanics (1.7%) and African Americans (1.6%).[54]

Tobacco use increases the risk of BE and EAC by about 2-fold.[57] There is a strong dose association between pack-years of cigarettes consumed and BE/EAC risk.[57] Compared with current smokers, those who quit smoking had lower risk of EAC after adjusting for pack-years.[57]

Most patients with BE have a hiatal hernia.[58] More than 95% of patients with BE have a hernia that is 2 cm in size or longer.[58] The hernia length and hiatal opening width in patients with BE were 3.95 cm and 3.52 cm, respectively, and both were significantly greater compared with controls with or without esophagitis.[58]

The risk factors shown to be associated with BE are summarized in **Table 1**. Multiple studies have demonstrated that the greater the number of risk factors present, the higher the chances of BE being present.[33,34] For each risk factor, the prevalence of BE increases by 1.2%.[33] When 3 or more risk factors were present, the odds of EE or BE were 3.7 times higher compared with those with 2 risk factors or less.[34] Moreover, when 5 or more risk factors were present, the odds of EE or BE were 5.7 times higher.[34]

Various risk scores and models exist that predict the risk of BE in an individual. The Michigan Barrett's Esophagus pREdiction Tool (M-BERET) is a model that incorporates GERD, age, abdominal obesity, and cigarette use and has been shown to more accurately classify the presence of BE compared with a model based on GERD alone (area under the curve [AUC] 0.72 vs 0.61, respectively).[65] The M-BERET has been externally validated in 4 independent datasets and maintains reasonable accuracy in discriminating patients with BE from population-based

Table 1
Risk factors associated with Barrett's esophagus

Risk Factor	Odds Ratio (95% CI)
Chronic gastroesophageal reflux disease	2.90 (1.86–4.54)[29]
Age >50 y	1.60 (1.1–2.4)[59]
Family history of Barrett's esophagus or esophageal adenocarcinoma	12.23 (3.34–44.76)[41]
Central obesity	1.98 (1.52–2.57)[60]
Male sex	Male/female sex ratio: 1.96/1 (1.77, 2.17/1)[61]
White race	3.95 (3.07–5.08)[62]
Tobacco use	1.42 (1.15–1.76)[63]
Hiatal hernia	3.94 (3.02–5.13)[64]

controls.[66] In addition, a risk prediction model for BE that combined a multibiomarker score (based on serum levels of interleukin [IL] 12p70, IL-6, IL-8, IL-10, and leptin) with demographic and clinical features had greater accuracy than with using GERD alone.[67] Although these risk scores and models may help identify high-risk patients and improve population screening, they are not routinely used in clinical practice given that the thresholds at which confirmatory testing is to be performed are not yet defined. These thresholds are likely dependent on the costs and performance characteristics of screening and confirmatory tests.

SELECTING CANDIDATES FOR BARRETT'S ESOPHAGUS SCREENING

National societies have independently published guidelines to select candidates for BE screening (**Box 1**).[19,38,68–70] The identification of screening criteria for these guidelines relies for the most part on demographic and clinical characteristics found commonly in patients with BE. In general, all societies do not recommend screening in the general population.[19,38,68–70] Instead, they recommend that BE screening should be considered in high-risk individuals. Moreover, before considering screening, the projected lifespan and comorbidities of the patient should be considered. Patients should be counseled that screening may detect BE, which could be followed by surveillance and/or dysplasia that could require endoscopic therapy. If BE is not found on the initial endoscopy, subsequent evaluation is not recommended given the low (<2%) yield of BE on repeat evaluation.[19] However, if the initial EGD shows moderate or severe esophagitis (Los Angeles Classification B, C, or D), high-dose PPI should be prescribed and repeat endoscopy should be performed after 8 to 12 weeks of treatment to evaluate for the development of BE (which can be present in 12%–15% of cases).[19]

GUIDELINES FROM NATIONAL SOCIETIES

The American College of Gastroenterology recommends that screening for BE may be considered in men with chronic (>5 years) and/or frequent (weekly or more) symptoms of GERD and two or more of the following risk factors for BE or EAC: age greater than 50 years, white race, presence of central obesity (waist circumference >102 cm or waist-hip ratio >0.9), current or past history of smoking, and a confirmed family history of BE or EAC in a first-degree relative.[19] Screening for BE in women is not recommended given the substantially lower risk of EAC in women with chronic GERD symptoms

Box 1
Summary of guidelines for Barrett's esophagus screening from gastroenterology and endoscopy societies

1. Screening for BE in the general population is not recommended.
2. Screening for BE should be considered in those with chronic reflux and multiple risk factors, including age greater than 50 years, male sex, white race, central obesity, smoking use, first-degree relative with BE or esophageal adenocarcinoma, and presence of hiatal hernia.
3. Screening for BE should generally not be performed in women with chronic GERD or men younger than 50 years with chronic GERD but may be considered in these individuals if multiple other risk factors are also present.

Data from Recommendations based on BE screening guidelines from ACG (2016), ASGE (2019), AGA (2016), ACP (2012), BSG (2014), and ESGE (2020).

compared with men. However, screening in women may be considered in select cases when multiple risk factors are present.[19]

The American Gastroenterological Association (AGA) suggests screening for BE in patients with multiple risk factors for EAC, including age 50 years or older, male sex, white race, chronic GERD, hiatal hernia, elevated BMI, and intraabdominal distribution of body fat.[68]

The American Society of Gastrointestinal Endoscopy recommends a screening strategy that identifies individuals at risk for EAC.[38] At-risk populations include those with a family history of BE and EAC (high risk) or patients with GERD and at least 1 other risk factor for EAC (moderate risk).[38] These other risk factors include age greater than 50 years, obesity/central adiposity, history of smoking, or male gender.[38]

The American College of Physicians suggests upper endoscopy be performed in men older than 50 years with chronic GERD symptoms (greater than 5 years) and additional risk factors, such as nocturnal reflux symptoms, hiatal hernia, elevated BMI, tobacco use, and intraabdominal distribution of fat.[69]

The British Society of Gastroenterology recommends endoscopic screening for BE in patients with chronic GERD symptoms and multiple risk factors (at least three of the following: age 50 years or older, white race, male sex, and obesity).[70] However, they suggest that the threshold of multiple risk factors should be lowered in the presence of family history, including at least 1 first-degree relative with BE or EAC.[70]

The European Society of Gastrointestinal Endoscopy suggests that endoscopic screening for BE should only be considered in high-risk individuals: that is, in those with long-standing GERD symptoms (ie, >5 years) and multiple risk factors (age ≥50 years, white race, male sex, obesity, or first-degree relative with BE or EAC).[71]

CHALLENGES WITH BARRETT'S ESOPHAGUS SCREENING

There are several challenges to screening for BE. The main goal of screening is earlier detection of dysplasia or EAC to enable improved outcomes. EAC is a cancer with a low incidence at the population level, which makes it difficult to detect. The global incidence rate of EAC worldwide is 0.7 per 100,000 person-years.[7] In the United States, 17,650 new cases of esophageal cancer were diagnosed in 2019 with EAC accounting for about 60% of the cases.[72,73] Despite recommendations for BE screening and surveillance, most cases (93%) of EAC are prevalent because they continue to be diagnosed after the onset of alarm symptoms, which are more indicative of advanced disease (**Fig. 1**).[73] In contrast, the low rate of progression from BE to EAC (annual risk of 0.12%–0.5%) questions the cost-effectiveness and impact of surveillance for incident neoplasia.[15,74] Furthermore, data suggest it is likely due to this low absolute rate of progression that most patients with BE die of non-EAC related causes, such as ischemic heart disease.[75] Because of this low rate of progression, evidence to show that BE screening and surveillance are effective in reducing EAC-related mortality is challenging to generate. Although surveillance may be associated with earlier-stage EAC and may provide a small survival benefit, potential confounding biases (length and lead time) could account for this observation.[28,76] A large prospective randomized study to assess the effectiveness of surveillance in BE to reduce EAC-related mortality is ongoing.[77]

An area of controversy in BE is related to its diagnosis and whether the presence of an irregular Z line dictates obtaining a biopsy and instituting lifelong surveillance if IM is seen. In a study of 102 patients with an irregular Z line followed for a median of 70 months, only 2 patients developed LGD as the most advanced pathologic condition, although 8.8% of patients were subsequently diagnosed with short-segment

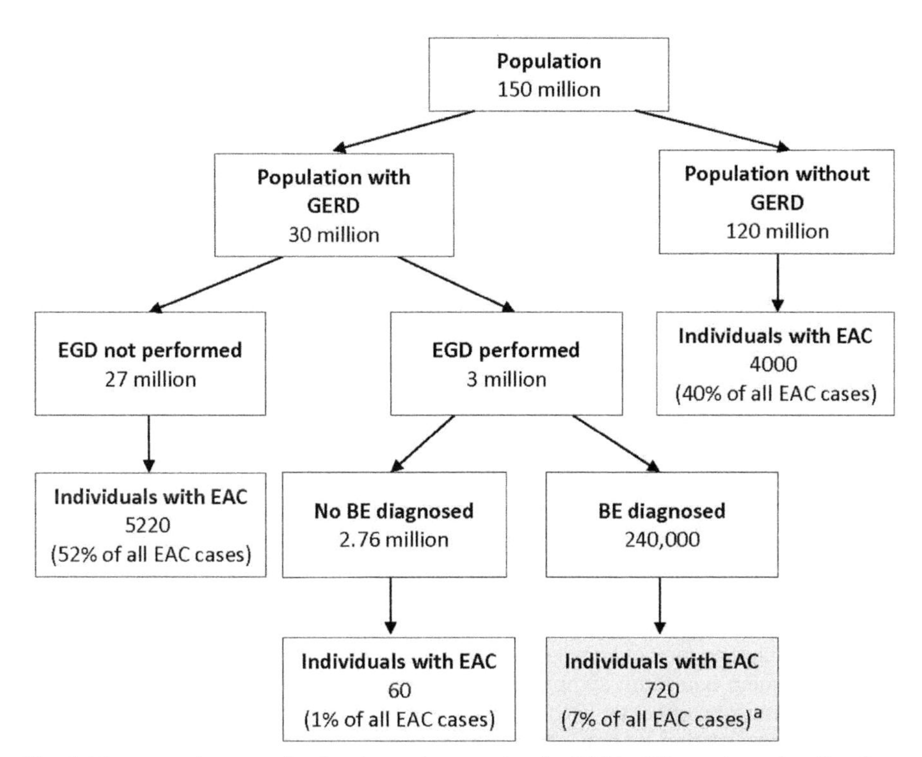

Fig. 1. The current approach of endoscopic screening for BE identifies only a minority of patients with EAC. [a] Only 7% of all EAC cases are diagnosed via current screening approaches. (*Adapted from* Vaughan TL., Fitzgerald RC. Precision prevention of oesophageal adenocarcinoma. *Nat Rev Gastroenterol Hepatol* 2015:243–8; with permission.)

BE.[78] In another study of 86 patients with IM of the gastroesophageal junction followed for a median of 8 years, progression to LGD occurred in 6 (7%), and similarly, no patient progressed to HGD or cancer.[79] Although there is some trepidation on the part of societies to definitively define a Barrett's segment by an absolute length, the summary of this data is that, although arbitrary, BE should continue to be defined as a salmon-colored area of mucosa proximal to the gastroesophageal junction $\geq$1 cm with IM, although it is possible cases of HGD or cancer may develop from smaller segments. Such cases may include cancers of the gastroesophageal junction. Unfortunately, there is no recognized prelesion at this point that merits identification and surveillance.

One of the emerging trends in guidelines is reconsideration of the importance of chronic heartburn as a criterion. Although most current guidelines recommend that BE screening should be performed in patients with chronic GERD symptoms, only 1 society guideline presently (AGA) does not place undue emphasis on heartburn in its criteria. The minimization of heartburn as a key criterion comes from studies that show neither adequate sensitivity nor specificity of this symptom in identifying patients with BE or EAC. In fact, 40% to 50% of patients with BE or EAC do not report chronic GERD symptoms, such as heartburn or regurgitation, and therefore, do not benefit from enrollment in a screening followed by surveillance program (see **Fig. 1**).[30] In a prospective study applying several guidelines for Barrett's screening to a large patient population, GERD symptoms alone identified patients with BE with an AUC of only 0.579 and performed less well than other guideline criteria.[80]

Although long-standing GERD is certainly associated with an increased risk of BE, patients with BE often have fewer symptoms of GERD because of impaired esophageal sensitivity.[81,82] As discussed earlier, there are numerous other risk factors for BE besides chronic GERD.

One of the greatest challenges in EAC is shifting the vast number of patients with prevalent to incident EAC. In other words, most patients with EAC present de novo, without prior identification of BE and enrollment in surveillance program. Several studies have demonstrated that at best 15% of EACs are found during surveillance.[83–85] This dilemma rests in part on the above discussion documenting the poor performance of heartburn as an indicator of BE. Furthermore, there is also some evidence to suggest that there may be 2 phenotypes of EAC, one arising in a background of grossly visible BE and/or histologically identifiable IM and another form without.[86] The latter form may be associated with poorer outcomes. The true precursor to this latter form of EAC is not yet known, and hence, this may also reduce the pool of EAC that can be prevented by screening for BE for lack of identification of a clear endoscopic Barrett's segment.[86] Although this concept is emerging, it potentially confounds the approach of identifying patients with endoscopic evidence of BE.

Another aspect of improving BE and EAC screening is adherence to established guidelines for identifying patients at risk for BE and EAC who require endoscopy. Only about 10% of US patients with chronic reflux symptoms undergo endoscopic screening.[87,88] The cause of this low screening rate is multifactorial with potential explanations including lack of knowledge about BE by primary care physicians, the patient not bringing heartburn symptoms to the attention of the caregiver because of their mild nature or effective empiric treatment with medical therapy, or hesitancy with physician ordering or patients proceeding with endoscopy.[88,89] Nevertheless, this leads to most BE cases in the community remaining undiagnosed, which leaves most BE cases (the likely source of most EACs) outside of surveillance programs (see **Fig. 1**).[79]

The absence of a widely applicable minimally or noninvasive tool for BE screening is also a major challenge to implementing BE screening. Sedated endoscopy (EGD) is not ideal because it requires the procedure to be performed in an endoscopy suite and carries with it small but significant risks from sedation and the procedure itself.[90] Endoscopic screening is also associated with both direct (staff, monitoring, recovery) and indirect costs (lost productivity because of patient and family members needing time off work) with 1 study showing median 30-day costs from endoscopic screening to be $2000.[90] Although unsedated transnasal endoscopy (uTNE) is safe, well tolerated, accurate, less expensive, and cost-effective, its utilization remains limited likely because of a host of patient- and provider-related limitations.[91–94] To overcome this limitation, nonendoscopic and imaging-based techniques are being developed, including capsule sponge/balloon cytology sampling devices combined with biomarkers (such as TFF3 and methylated DNA markers), esophageal capsule endoscopy, and tethered capsule endomicroscopy.[94–98] Although these technologies are promising and continue to be investigated, standard endoscopy remains the mainstay for screening of BE at this time.

Another future direction for improving endoscopic screening in BE might be using physician extenders to perform endoscopy or uTNE. The evidence that using physician extenders to perform endoscopy will lead to cost savings is variable. In a multicenter UK modeling study, physicians were more cost-effective measured in quality-adjusted life-years (QALYs) than nurses in performing endoscopy.[99] Nevertheless, the ability to expand the work force capable of doing endoscopy has merit. In 2016, it was estimated that there are more than 450 nurses performing endoscopy in Europe.[100] One concern is whether the quality of physician extenders performing endoscopy will be adequate. However, multiple studies have demonstrated similar accuracy to physicians.[101,102] Studies have also shown success in training physician extenders to perform uTNE.

Screening with sedated EGD and uTNE has been shown to be cost-effective for patients with chronic GERD and other risk factors.[103–105] Screening is associated with gains in QALYs in patients with chronic reflux at costs comparable to other preventive measures.[106,107] Screening patients with chronic GERD with EGD costs $22,200 per QALY gained, which falls within willingness to pay threshold.[108] Regardless, the cost-effectiveness of BE screening is dynamic and likely to change with development of new screening modalities, improvements in risk stratification of patients, and decreases in procedural costs. Some investigators have proposed the routine use of EGD for BE screening at the time of screening colonoscopy at age 50. Although this strategy may result in a relatively high yield of BE, the cost-effectiveness of such a strategy in the general population remains unproven, but estimates place this strategy at close to 5 times the cost of using guideline criteria.[109]

SUMMARY

EAC incidence is steadily increasing over the past few decades and continues to have a poor 5-year survival of less than 20%. BE is the only known precursor to EAC. The risk of EAC in patients with BE is significantly higher compared with the general population. Endoscopic screening and surveillance are performed to identify patients earlier in the metaplasia-dysplasia-carcinoma sequence from BE to EAC followed by endoscopic therapy to prevent and/or treat EAC. Given that BE does not have any specific presenting signs or symptoms, it can only be detected via screening. Therefore, current guidelines suggest that BE screening should be considered in individuals who have multiple risk factors, including chronic GERD, age greater than 50 years, male sex, white race, central obesity, smoking use, and family history of BE or EAC. Importantly, it should be recognized that screening only patients with chronic GERD is likely not sufficient to identify all those at risk for BE and EAC. A major limitation remains the absence of a minimally invasive screening tool, which would enable the detection of a larger pool of BE patients at risk for developing EAC. New nonendoscopic biomarker-based and imaging-based techniques for BE screening may be on the horizon. Additional progress on dysplasia detection is also critical to make adequate progress in EAC prevention.

CLINICS CARE POINTS

1. Screening for Barrett's esophagus should be considered in those with multiple risk factors, including age greater than 50 years, male sex, chronic gastroesophageal reflux disease (>5 years and/or frequent symptoms), white race, central obesity, smoking, and first-degree relative with Barrett's esophagus or esophageal adenocarcinoma. Screening of the general population is not recommended at this time.
2. If initial evaluation for Barrett's esophagus is negative, repeat screening is not recommended at this time.
3. Screening needs to be coupled with improved techniques and technology for dysplasia detection to make real progress in improving EAC outcomes.

REFERENCES

1. American Cancer Society. Key statistics for esophageal cancer. Available at: https://www.cancer.org/cancer/esophagus-cancer/about/key-statistics.html. Accessed February 10, 2020.
2. Edgren G, Adami HO, Vainio EW, et al. A global assessment of the oesophageal adenocarcinoma epidemic. Gut 2013;62(10):1406–14.
3. Cook MB, Chow WH, Devesa SS. Oesophageal cancer incidence in the United States by race, sex, and histologic type, 1977-2005. Br J Cancer 2009;101(5): 855–9.
4. Nassri A, Zhu H, Muftah M, et al. Epidemiology and survival of esophageal cancer patients in an American Cohort. Cureus 2018;10(4):e2507.
5. Xie SH, Lagergren J. The male predominance in esophageal adenocarcinoma. Clin Gastroenterol Hepatol 2016;14(3):338–47.
6. Lagergren J, Lagergren P. Recent developments in esophageal adenocarcinoma. CA Cancer J Clin 2013;63(4):232–48.
7. Coleman HG, Xie SH, Lagergren J. The epidemiology of esophageal adenocarcinoma. Gastroenterology 2018;154(2):390–405.
8. Turati F, Tramacere I, La Vecchia C, et al. A meta-analysis of body mass index and esophageal and gastric cardia adenocarcinoma. Ann Oncol 2013;24: 609–17.
9. Tramacere I, La Vecchia C, Negri E. Tobacco smoking and esophageal and gastric cardia adenocarcinoma: a meta-analysis. Epidemiology 2011;22(3): 344–9.
10. Njei B, McCarty TR, Birk JW. Trends in esophageal cancer survival in United States adults from 1973 to 2009: a SEER database analysis. J Gastroenterol Hepatol 2016;31(6):1141–6.
11. Gavin AT, Francisci S, Foschi R, et al. Oesophageal cancer survival in Europe: a EUROCARE-4 study. Cancer Epidemiol 2012;36(6):505–12.
12. Spechler SJ, Souza RF. Barrett's esophagus. N Engl J Med 2014;371(9):836–45.
13. Runge TM, Abrams JA, Shaheen NJ. Epidemiology of Barrett's esophagus and esophageal adenocarcinoma. Gastroenterol Clin North Am 2015;44:203–31.
14. Cameron AJ, Ott BJ, Payne WS. The incidence of adenocarcinoma in columnar-lined (Barrett's) esophagus. N Engl J Med 1985;313(14):857–9.
15. Shaheen NJ, Richter JE. Barrett's oesophagus. Lancet 2009;373(9666):850–61.
16. Westhoff B, Brotze S, Weston A, et al. The frequency of Barrett's esophagus in high-risk patients with chronic GERD. Gastrointest Endosc 2005;61(2):226–31.
17. Ronkainen J, Aro P, Storskrubb T, et al. Prevalence of Barrett's esophagus in the general population: an endoscopic study. Gastroenterology 2005;129(6): 1825–31.
18. Spechler SJ. Barrett esophagus and risk of esophageal cancer: a clinical review. JAMA 2013;310:627–36.
19. Shaheen NJ, Falk GW, Iyer PG, et al. ACG clinical guideline: diagnosis and management of Barrett's esophagus. Am J Gastroenterol 2016;111(1):30–50.
20. Shaheen NJ, Sharma P, Overholt BF, et al. Radiofrequency ablation in Barrett's esophagus with dysplasia. N Engl J Med 2009;360(22):2277–88.
21. Wolf WA, Pasricha S, Cotton C, et al. Incidence of esophageal adenocarcinoma and causes of mortality after radiofrequency ablation of Barrett's esophagus. Gastroenterology 2015;149(7):1752–61.

22. Phoa KN, Pouw RE, Van Vilsteren FGI, et al. Remission of Barrett's esophagus with early neoplasia 5 years after radiofrequency ablation with endoscopic resection: a Netherlands cohort study. Gastroenterology 2013;145(1):96–104.
23. Pech O, Behrens A, May A, et al. Long-term results and risk factor analysis for recurrence after curative endoscopic therapy in 349 patients with high-grade intraepithelial neoplasia and mucosal adenocarcinoma in Barrett's oesophagus. Gut 2008;57(9):1200–6.
24. Jankowski JAZ, de Caestecker J, Love SB, et al. Esomeprazole and aspirin in Barrett's oesophagus (AspECT): a randomised factorial trial. Lancet 2018; 392(10145):400–8.
25. Husain NS, El-Serag HB. Chemoprevention of Barrett's oesophagus: a step closer with PPIs and aspirin. Nat Rev Clin Oncol 2018;15(12):728–30.
26. Prasad GA, Wu TT, Wigle DA, et al. Endoscopic and surgical treatment of mucosal (T1a) esophageal adenocarcinoma in Barrett's esophagus. Gastroenterology 2009;137(3):815–23.
27. Zehetner J, Demeester SR, Hagen JA, et al. Endoscopic resection and ablation versus esophagectomy for high-grade dysplasia and intramucosal adenocarcinoma. J Thorac Cardiovasc Surg 2011;141(1):39–47.
28. Codipilly DC, Chandar AK, Singh S, et al. The effect of endoscopic surveillance in patients with Barrett's esophagus: a systematic review and meta-analysis. Gastroenterology 2018;154(8):2068–86.
29. Taylor JB, Rubenstein JH. Meta-analyses of the effect of symptoms of gastroesophageal reflux on the risk of Barrett's esophagus. Am J Gastroenterol 2010;105:1730–7.
30. Lagergren J, Bergström R, Lindgren A, et al. Symptomatic gastroesophageal reflux as a risk factor for esophageal adenocarcinoma. N Engl J Med 1999; 340(11):825–31.
31. Shaheen N, Ransohoff DF. Gastroesophageal reflux, Barrett esophagus, and esophageal cancer: scientific review. JAMA 2002;287:1972–81.
32. Lieberman DA, Oehlke M, Helfand M. Risk factors for Barrett's esophagus in community-based practice. GORGE consortium. Gastroenterology Outcomes Research Group in Endoscopy. Am J Gastroenterol 1997;92(8):1293–7.
33. Qumseya BJ, Bukannan A, Gendy S, et al. Systematic review and meta-analysis of prevalence and risk factors for Barrett's esophagus. Gastrointest Endosc 2019;90(5):707–17.
34. Crews NR, Johnson ML, Schleck CD, et al. Prevalence and predictors of gastroesophageal reflux complications in community subjects. Dig Dis Sci 2016; 61(11):3221–8.
35. Rex DK, Cummings OW, Shaw M, et al. Screening for Barrett's esophagus in colonoscopy patients with and without heartburn. Gastroenterology 2003;125(6): 1670–7.
36. Gerson LB, Banerjee S. Screening for Barrett's esophagus in asymptomatic women. Gastrointest Endosc 2009;70(5):867–73.
37. Ward EM, Wolfsen HC, Achem SR, et al. Barrett's esophagus is common in older men and women undergoing screening colonoscopy regardless of reflux symptoms. Am J Gastroenterol 2006;101(1):12–7.
38. Qumseya B, Sultan S, Bain P, et al. ASGE guideline on screening and surveillance of Barrett's esophagus. Gastrointest Endosc 2019;90(3):335–59.
39. Rubenstein JH, Scheiman JM, Sadeghi S, et al. Esophageal adenocarcinoma incidence in individuals with gastroesophageal reflux: synthesis and estimates from population studies. Am J Gastroenterol 2011;106(2):254–60.

40. Chak A, Faulx A, Kinnard M, et al. Identification of Barrett's esophagus in relatives by endoscopic screening. Am J Gastroenterol 2004;99(11):2107–14.
41. Chak A, Lee T, Kinnard MF, et al. Familial aggregation of Barrett's oesophagus, oesophageal adenocarcinoma, and oesophagogastric junctional adenocarcinoma in Caucasian adults. Gut 2002;51(3):323–8.
42. Romero Y. Familial association in Barrett esophagus. Gastroenterol Hepatol (N Y) 2007;3(5):346–8.
43. Juhasz A, Mittal SK, Lee TH, et al. Prevalence of Barrett esophagus in first-degree relatives of patients with esophageal adenocarcinoma. J Clin Gastroenterol 2011;45(10):867–71.
44. Verbeek RE, Spittuler LF, Peute A, et al. Familial clustering of Barrett's esophagus and esophageal adenocarcinoma in a European cohort. Clin Gastroenterol Hepatol 2014;12(10):1656–63.
45. Romero Y, Cameron AJ, Schaid DJ, et al. Barrett's esophagus: prevalence in symptomatic relatives. Am J Gastroenterol 2002;97(5):1127–32.
46. Thrift AP, Shaheen NJ, Gammon MD, et al. Obesity and risk of esophageal adenocarcinoma and Barrett's esophagus: a Mendelian randomization study. J Natl Cancer Inst 2014;106(11):dju252.
47. Kamat P, Wen S, Morris J, et al. Exploring the association between elevated body mass index and Barrett's esophagus: a systematic review and meta-analysis. Ann Thorac Surg 2009;87(2):655–62.
48. D'Silva M, Bhasker AG, Kantharia NS, et al. High-percentage pathological findings in obese patients suggest that esophago-gastro-duodenoscopy should be made mandatory prior to bariatric surgery. Obes Surg 2018;28(9):2753–9.
49. Csendes A, Burgos AM, Smok G, et al. Endoscopic and histologic findings of the foregut in 426 patients with morbid obesity. Obes Surg 2007;17(1):28–34.
50. Corley DA, Kubo A, Levin TR, et al. Abdominal obesity and body mass index as risk factors for Barrett's esophagus. Gastroenterology 2007;133(1):34–41.
51. Gerson LB, Edson R, Lavori PW, et al. Use of a simple symptom questionnaire to predict Barrett's esophagus in patients with symptoms of gastroesophageal reflux. Am J Gastroenterol 2001;96(7):2005–12.
52. Ford AC, Forman D, Reynolds PD, et al. Ethnicity, gender, and socioeconomic status as risk factors for esophagitis and Barrett's esophagus. Am J Epidemiol 2005;162(5):454–60.
53. Falk GW, Thota PN, Richter JE, et al. Barrett's esophagus in women: demographic features and progression to high-grade dysplasia and cancer. Clin Gastroenterol Hepatol 2005;3(11):1089–94.
54. Abrams JA, Fields S, Lightdale CJ, et al. Racial and ethnic disparities in the prevalence of Barrett's esophagus among patients who undergo upper endoscopy. Clin Gastroenterol Hepatol 2008;6(1):30–4.
55. Sharma P, Weston AP, Morales T, et al. Relative risk of dysplasia for patients with intestinal metaplasia in the distal oesophagus and in the gastric cardia. Gut 2000;46(1):9–13.
56. Blot WJ, Devesa SS, Kneller RW, et al. Rising incidence of adenocarcinoma of the esophagus and gastric cardia. JAMA 1991;265(10):1287–9.
57. Cook MB, Kamangar F, Whiteman DC, et al. Cigarette smoking and adenocarcinomas of the esophagus and esophagogastric junction: a pooled analysis from the International BEACON Consortium. J Natl Cancer Inst 2010;102(17):1344–53.
58. Cameron AJ. Barrett's esophagus: prevalence and size of hiatal hernia. A*m J Gastroenterol* 1999;94(8):2054–9.

59. Edelstein ZR, Bronner MP, Rosen SN, et al. Risk factors for Barrett's esophagus among patients with gastroesophageal reflux disease: a community clinic-based case-control study. Am J Gastroenterol 2009;104(4):834–42.
60. Singh S, Sharma AN, Murad MH, et al. Central adiposity is associated with increased risk of esophageal inflammation, metaplasia, and adenocarcinoma: a systematic review and meta-analysis. Clin Gastroenterol Hepatol 2013; 11(11):1399–412.
61. Cook MB, Wild CP, Forman D. A systematic review and meta-analysis of the sex ratio for Barrett's esophagus, erosive reflux disease, and nonerosive reflux disease. Am J Epidemiol 2005;162(11):1050–61.
62. Alkaddour A, Palacio C, Vega KJ. Risk of histologic Barrett's esophagus between African Americans and non-Hispanic whites: a meta-analysis. United European Gastroenterol J 2018;6(1):22–8.
63. Andrici J, Cox MR, Eslick GD. Cigarette smoking and the risk of Barrett's esophagus: a systematic review and meta-analysis. J Gastroenterol Hepatol 2013; 28(8):1258–73.
64. Andrici J, Tio M, Cox MR, et al. Hiatal hernia and the risk of Barrett's esophagus. J Gastroenterol Hepatol 2013;28(3):415–31.
65. Rubenstein JH, Morgenstern H, Appelman H, et al. Prediction of Barrett's esophagus among men. Am J Gastroenterol 2013;108(3):353–62.
66. Thrift AP, Vaughan TL, Anderson LA, et al. External validation of the Michigan Barrett's Esophagus Prediction Tool. Clin Gastroenterol Hepatol 2017;15(7): 1124–6.
67. Thrift AP, Garcia JM, El-Serag HB. A multibiomarker risk score helps predict risk for Barrett's esophagus. Clin Gastroenterol Hepatol 2014;12(8):1267–71.
68. American Gastroenterological Association, Spechler SJ, Sharma P, et al. American gastroenterological association medical position statement on the management of Barrett's esophagus. Gastroenterology 2011;140(3):1084–91.
69. Shaheen NJ, Weinberg DS, Denberg TD, et al. Upper endoscopy for gastroesophageal reflux disease: best practice advice from the clinical guidelines committee of the American College of Physicians. Ann Intern Med 2012; 157(11):808–17.
70. Fitzgerald RC, Di Pietro M, Ragunath K, et al. British Society of Gastroenterology guidelines on the diagnosis and management of Barrett's oesophagus. Gut 2014;63(1):7–42.
71. Săftoiu A, Hassan C, Areia M, et al. Role of gastrointestinal endoscopy in the screening of digestive tract cancers in Europe: European Society of Gastrointestinal Endoscopy (ESGE) Position Statement. Endoscopy 2020;52(4):293–304.
72. National Cancer Institute. Surveillance, Epidemiology and ERP. Cancer stat facts: esophageal cancer. Available at: https://seer.cancer.gov/statfacts/html/esoph.html. Accessed February 10, 2020.
73. Vaughan TL, Fitzgerald RC. Precision prevention of oesophageal adenocarcinoma. Nat Rev Gastroenterol Hepatol 2015;12:243–8.
74. Hvid-Jensen F, Pedersen L, Drewes AM, et al. Incidence of adenocarcinoma among patients with Barrett's esophagus. N Engl J Med 2011;365(15):1375–83.
75. Solaymani-Dodaran M, Card TR, West J. Cause-specific mortality of people with Barrett's esophagus compared with the general population: a population-based cohort study. Gastroenterology 2013;144(7):1375–83.
76. Tramontano AC, Sheehan DF, Yeh JM, et al. The impact of a prior diagnosis of Barrett's esophagus on esophageal adenocarcinoma survival. Am J Gastroenterol 2017;112(8):1256–64.

77. Old O, Moayyedi P, Love S, et al. Barrett's Oesophagus Surveillance versus endoscopy at need Study (BOSS): protocol and analysis plan for a multicentre randomized controlled trial. J Med Screen 2015;22(3):158–64.
78. Itskoviz D, Levi Z, Boltin D, et al. Risk of neoplastic progression among patients with an irregular Z line on long-term follow-up. Dig Dis Sci 2018;63(6):1513–7.
79. Jung KW, Talley NJ, Romero Y, et al. Epidemiology and natural history of intestinal metaplasia of the gastroesophageal junction and Barrett's esophagus: a population-based study. Am J Gastroenterol 2011;106(8):1447–55.
80. Rubenstein JH, McConnell D, Waljee AK, et al. Validation and comparison of tools for selecting individuals to screen for Barrett's esophagus and early neoplasia. Gastroenterology 2020;158(8):2082–92.
81. Brandt MG, Darling GE, Miller L. Symptoms, acid exposure and motility in patients with Barrett's esophagus. Can J Surg 2004;47(1):47–51.
82. Byrne PJ, Mulligan ED, O'Riordan J, et al. Impaired visceral sensitivity to acid reflux in patients with Barrett's esophagus. The role of esophageal motility. Dis Esophagus 2003;16(3):199–203.
83. Dulai GS, Gornbein J, Kahn KL, et al. Preoperative prevalence of Barrett's esophagus in esophageal adenocarcinoma: a systematic review. Gastroenterology 2002;122(1):26–33.
84. Verbeek RE, Leenders M, Ten Kate FJW, et al. Surveillance of Barrett's esophagus and mortality from esophageal adenocarcinoma: a population-based cohort study. Am J Gastroenterol 2014;109(8):1215–22.
85. Cooper GS, Kou TD, Chak A. Receipt of previous diagnoses and endoscopy and outcome from esophageal adenocarcinoma: a population-based study with temporal trends. Am J Gastroenterol 2009;104(6):1356–62.
86. Sawas T, Killcoyne S, Iyer PG, et al. Identification of prognostic phenotypes of esophageal adenocarcinoma in 2 independent cohorts. Gastroenterology 2018;155(6):1720–8.
87. Peery AF, Dellon ES, Lund J, et al. Burden of gastrointestinal disease in the United States: 2012 update. Gastroenterology 2012;143(5):1179–87.e3.
88. Menezes A, Tierney A, Yang YX, et al. Adherence to the 2011 American Gastroenterological Association medical position statement for the diagnosis and management of Barrett's esophagus. Dis Esophagus 2015;28(6):538–46.
89. Pohl H, Robertson D, Welch HG. Repeated upper endoscopy in the Medicare population: a retrospective analysis. Ann Intern Med 2014;160(3):154–60.
90. Sami SS, Ragunath K, Iyer PG. Screening for Barrett's esophagus and esophageal adenocarcinoma: rationale, recent progress, challenges, and future directions. Clin Gastroenterol Hepatol 2015;13(4):623–34.
91. Sami SS, Dunagan KT, Johnson ML, et al. A randomized comparative effectiveness trial of novel endoscopic techniques and approaches for Barrett's esophagus screening in the community. Am J Gastroenterol 2015;110(1):148–58.
92. Sami SS, Iyer PG, Pophali P, et al. Acceptability, accuracy, and safety of disposable transnasal capsule endoscopy for Barrett's esophagus screening. Clin Gastroenterol Hepatol 2019;17(4):638–46.
93. Blevins CH, Iyer PG. Putting it through the nose: the ins and outs of transnasal endoscopy. Am J Gastroenterol 2016;111:1371–3.
94. Honing J, Kievit W, Bookelaar J, et al. Endosheath ultrathin transnasal endoscopy is a cost-effective method for screening for Barrett's esophagus in patients with GERD symptoms. Gastrointest Endosc 2019;89(4):712–22.

95. Iyer PG, Taylor WR, Johnson ML, et al. Highly discriminant methylated DNA markers for the non-endoscopic detection of Barrett's esophagus. Am J Gastroenterol 2018;113(8):1156–66.
96. Kadri PSR, Lao-Sirieix I, O'Donovan M, et al. Acceptability and accuracy of a non-endoscopic screening test for Barrett's oesophagus in primary care: cohort study. BMJ 2010;341(7773):595.
97. Moinova HR, LaFramboise T, Lutterbaugh JD, et al. Identifying DNA methylation biomarkers for non-endoscopic detection of Barrett's esophagus. Sci Transl Med 2018;10(424).
98. Gora MJ, Sauk JS, Carruth RW, et al. Tethered capsule endomicroscopy enables less invasive imaging of gastrointestinal tract microstructure. Nat Med 2013;19(2):238–40.
99. Richardson G, Bloor K, Williams J, et al. Cost effectiveness of nurse delivered endoscopy: findings from randomised multi-institution nurse endoscopy trial (MIINuET). BMJ 2009;338(7693):b270.
100. Pfeifer UG, Schilling D. Non-physician endoscopy: how far can we go? Visc Med 2016;32:13–20.
101. Meaden C, Joshi M, Hollis S, et al. A randomized controlled trial comparing the accuracy of general diagnostic upper gastrointestinal endoscopy performed by nurse or medical endoscopists. Endoscopy 2006;38(6):553–60.
102. Stephens M, Hourigan LF, Appleyard M, et al. Non-physician endoscopists: a systematic review. World J Gastroenterol 2015;21(16):5056–71.
103. Inadomi JM, Saxena N. Screening and surveillance for Barrett's esophagus: is it cost-effective? Dig Dis Sci 2018;63:2094–104.
104. Rubenstein JH, Inadomi JM, Brill JV, et al. Cost utility of screening for Barrett's esophagus with esophageal capsule endoscopy versus conventional upper endoscopy. Clin Gastroenterol Hepatol 2007;5(3):312–8.
105. Inadomi JM, Sampliner R, Lagergren J, et al. Screening and surveillance for Barrett esophagus in high-risk groups: a cost-utility analysis. Ann Intern Med 2003; 138(3):176–86.
106. Nietert PJ, Silverstein MD, Mokhashi MS, et al. Cost-effectiveness of screening a population with chronic gastroesophageal reflux. Gastrointest Endosc 2003; 57(3):311–8.
107. Gerson LB, Groeneveld PW, Triadafilopoulos G. Cost-effectiveness model of endoscopic screening and surveillance in patients with gastroesophageal reflux disease. Clin Gastroenterol Hepatol 2004;2(10):868–79.
108. Benaglia T, Sharples LD, Fitzgerald RC, et al. Health benefits and cost effectiveness of endoscopic and nonendoscopic cytosponge screening for Barrett's esophagus. Gastroenterology 2013;144(1):62–73.
109. Gupta N, Bansal A, Wani SB, et al. Endoscopy for upper GI cancer screening in the general population: a cost-utility analysis. Gastrointest Endosc 2011;74(3): 610–24.

Progress in Screening for Barrett's Esophagus

Beyond Standard Upper Endoscopy

Wei Keith Tan, MBChB[a,b,c,1], Anamay N. Sharma, MD[d,1], Amitabh Chak, MD[d], Rebecca C. Fitzgerald, MD, FRCP, FMedSci[a,e,*]

KEYWORDS

- Barrett's esophagus • Esophageal adenocarcinoma • Screening

KEY POINTS

- Screening for Barrett's esophagus to detect dysplasia and early stage cancer could lead to improved survival from esophageal adenocarcinoma, although there is still a lack of consensus on which key risk factors should be used to identify the target population for screening.
- There have been recent developments in non-endoscopic cell sampling devices, which when coupled with biomarkers are less-invasive than endoscopy with promise for use as a screening tool or diagnostic triage to endoscopy.
- Non-invasive liquid biopsies from blood or breath would be ideal and are also being investigated as potential tools for screening for Barrett's esophagus.

Video content accompanies this article at http://www.giendo.theclinics.com.

INTRODUCTION

Barrett's esophagus (BE) is currently the only known precursor to esophageal adenocarcinoma (EAC). BE is common with an estimated prevalence of 1% to 2% based on 2 large population-based studies conducted in Sweden and Italy.[1,2] The prevalence

[a] MRC Cancer Unit, University of Cambridge, Cambridge Biomedical Campus, Box 197, Cambridge CB2 0XZ, United Kingdom; [b] Department of Gastroenterology, Addenbrookes Hospital, Cambridge University NHS Foundation Trust, Hills Road, Cambridge CB2 0QQ, United Kingdom; [c] Department of Gastroenterology, Hinchingbrooke Hospital, North West Anglia Foundation Trust, Huntingdon, PE29 6NT, United Kingdom; [d] University Hospitals, Cleveland Medical Center, Case Western Reserve University School of Medicine, 10900 Euclid Avenue, Cleveland, OH 44106, USA; [e] Addenbrookes Hospital, Cambridge University NHS Foundation Trust, Hills Road, Cambridge, CB2 0QQ, United Kingdom
[1] Joint first author.
* Corresponding author. MRC Cancer Unit, University of Cambridge, Cambridge Biomedical Campus, Box 197, Cambridge, CB2 0XZ, United Kingdom
E-mail address: rcf29@mrc-cu.cam.ac.uk

Gastrointest Endoscopy Clin N Am 31 (2021) 43–58
https://doi.org/10.1016/j.giec.2020.08.004 **giendo.theclinics.com**
1052-5157/21/

among those with symptoms of chronic gastroesophageal reflux disease (GERD), however, is as high as 8% to 13%.[3] Because 1 in 4 people in Westernized nations suffer from symptoms of chronic GERD, the estimated prevalence of BE in the United States would be approximately 3 million, most of whom remain undiagnosed.[4]

Progression of BE to EAC often follows a prolonged course where it progresses through intermediate stages of dysplasia encompassing non-dysplastic BE (NDBE), to BE with low-grade dysplasia (LGD), high-grade dysplasia (HGD), intramucosal carcinoma, and finally, invasive EAC. However, not all of these stages may be diagnosed during surveillance, probably due to sampling bias. Each of these disease stages harbors increasing risk of malignant potential. Current estimates have shown that the risk of progression from NDBE to EAC remains low, with estimates ranging between 0.1% and 0.6% per patient-year.[5–9] However, once LGD has developed, the risk of cancer progression increases significantly although current estimates remain highly diverging, with ranges between 0.6% and 13.4% per patient-year.[6,8,10–13] This progression risk has resulted in widely accepted guidelines to treat dysplastic (LGD and HGD) BE endoscopically to prevent its progression to EAC.

Although recent trends have shown that the incidence of EAC has started to plateau, the prognosis of EAC remains poor, with an average 5-year survival of less than 20%.[14] This poor prognosis is attributed to the late presentation of patients harboring EAC, such that distant metastases are often apparent at the time of presentation. The most recent Surveillance, Epidemiology, and End Results (SEER) Program statistics have shown that approximately 40% of patients who have EAC also had distal metastasis at presentation.[14] Unfortunately, this trend of late-stage presentation of EAC has not improved in recent years, and this is likely to be the main contributing factor to the overall poor survival of EAC.

RATIONALE FOR SCREENING

Screening is the process of proactively inviting individuals to test for an underlying medical condition. The criteria for screening were determined by Wilson and Junger in 1968 and have been recently reviewed and updated.[15,16] The prevalence of the disease within the target population is an important consideration for screening, as well as whether diagnosis through a screening test permits earlier intervention to prevent the sequelae of developing a more serious condition. Also, for a screening program to be successful, it needs to be accurate, cost-effective, and ideally, minimally invasive to maximize uptake and minimize side effects.

The argument for screening is predicated on the notion that early detection and treatment will inherently decrease the risk of mortality from the disease. This effect has been seen in breast cancer, including the premalignant ductal carcinoma in-situ, where breast cancer mortality rates have declined by 40% from 1989 to 2016 following the introduction of mammographic screening.[17] For colorectal cancer, similar trends in a reduction in both incidence and mortality were observed, with a reduction of 32% and 34%, respectively, over the past 2 decades following the introduction of colonoscopic screening for adenomatous polyps.[18] These benefits need to be weighed against the rates of overdiagnosis and overtreatment, because it is often difficult to distinguish between indolent cases and those at high risk for progression.

In the context of EAC, population-based studies have demonstrated earlier-stage EAC diagnosis and improved survival from having a prior endoscopy before a diagnosis of EAC.[19–21] A retrospective cohort study of 777 patients with EAC showed that receipt of an upper endoscopy at least 1 year (designated as the screening endoscopy) before the diagnosis of EAC was associated with an earlier stage tumor (local or in-situ cancer) in 27% of cases compared with those without an endoscopy the preceding year.[19] Further, endoscopy was also associated with a reduced risk of death (relative hazard 0.73, 95% confidence interval [CI] 0.57–0.93).[19] Similarly, a large population-based study from the United States of more than 2700 patients between 1991 and 2002 showed that a diagnosis of BE was associated with a better odds of having early stage EAC (odds ratio 3.68, 95% CI 0.25–0.80) and a 55% survival benefit (hazard ratio 0.45, 95% CI 0.25–0.80).[20] Although lead-time and length-time bias have to be taken into consideration, the improved survival from an earlier stage cancer diagnosis is in line with current estimates that report that the 5-year relative survival for localized, regional, and distant disease is 46.7%, 25.1%, and 4.8%, respectively.[14]

Following a diagnosis of BE, current societal guidelines endorse periodic 3- to 5-yearly surveillance to detect cancer progression. Once dysplastic disease is identified, then endoscopic therapies encompassing resection of visible lesions using endoscopic mucosal resection or endoscopic submucosal dissection, often combined with ablation therapy such as radiofrequency or argon plasma, can be used to remove the lesion and associated BE.[22] However, only an estimated 10% of patients in the United States with recurrent GERD receive an endoscopy and hence most of the BE is undiagnosed. In the United States, approximately 17,000 cases of esophageal cancer will be diagnosed each year,[14] of which 10,000 (60%) would be EAC.[23] However, estimates have shown that only around 10% of EAC would be diagnosed through screening and surveillance of BE.[7,24] The remaining 90% of incident cases of EAC occurs among those with a history of chronic GERD and who have not undertaken a screening endoscopy, as well as among those without a history of GERD.[23] The obvious deficit of this current paradigm is that the emphasis is on the small proportion of clinically diagnosed BE in the population, ignoring the most of the subjects with prevalent BE in the community who remain undiagnosed or who are at risk of BE.

IDENTIFYING THE AT-RISK POPULATION

Symptoms-based screening using GERD is the easiest method to use because, as shown by a US modeling study, it focuses on around 20% of the adult population and accounts for 50% cases.[23] However, depending on the threshold used to define chronic GERD symptoms, a substantial proportion may be missed. In a multi-institutional study from the USA, around 61% of those with EAC and 38% of those with adenocarcinoma of cardia had a history of heartburn for more than 5 years. Only 36% of those with EAC and 24% with adenocarcinoma of cardia had weekly symptoms.[25] Similar findings were seen in a Swedish study where 60% of patients with EAC and 29% of patients with adenocarcinoma of cardia had chronic GERD.[26] Additional risk factors are therefore required to enrich the population.

Societal recommendations suggest selective screening by endoscopy for high-risk individuals although the risk factors required for screening differs between the guidelines (**Table 1**). The British Society of Gastroenterology and the American College of Gastroenterology (ACG) guidelines require at least 3 and 2 risk factors, respectively, including older age,[27] male sex,[28] Caucasian ethnicity,[29] and family history[30] in conjunction with symptoms of chronic GERD, to meet the threshold of screening.[31,32] These recommendations, however, were not as specific in the European and American Society of Gastrointestinal Endoscopy guidelines.[33,34] Only the ACG guidelines explicitly define the magnitude of each risk factor required to trigger

Table 1
Societal guidelines for the recommendations for Barrett's esophagus screening

	Risk Factors for Screening						
Guideline	GERD	Obesity	Smoking	Gender	Age	Ethnicity	Family History of BE or EAC
BSG[a] (2014)[31]	Yes	Yes	No	Male	>50	Caucasian	Yes[b]
ACG[c] (2016)[32]	Yes	Yes	Yes	Male	>50	Caucasian	Yes
ESGE[d] (2017)[46]	Yes	Yes	No	Male	>50	Caucasian	Yes
ASGE[e] (2019)[34]	Yes	Yes	No	Male	>50	Not included	Yes

[a] BSG, British Society of Gastroenterology; Criteria for screening: chronic GERD and ≥3 risk factors (age >50 years, Caucasian, male, obesity).
[b] Lower threshold for screening if positive first-degree family history.
[c] ACG, American College of Gastroenterology; Criteria for screening: chronic GERD (>5 years or at least weekly) and ≥2 risk factors (age >50 years, Caucasian, obesity, current or past history of smoking, and positive family history).
[d] ESGE, European Society of Gastrointestinal Endoscopy; criteria for screening: chronic GERD (>5 years) and multiple risk factors (≥50 years, Caucasian, male, obesity, and positive family history).
[e] ASGE, American Society of Gastrointestinal Endoscopy; Criteria for screening: positive family history alone (considered a 'high-risk' risk factor), or the presence of GERD and one or more risk factors (obesity, male, or age >50 years).

a screening endoscopy. These include the duration (>5 years) or frequency of GERD (weekly or more) and central obesity (waist circumference >102 cm or waist-to-hip ratio >0.9).

ENDOSCOPIC SCREENING USING PREDICTION MODELS

With the widespread availability of epidemiologic and demographic data, a potentially cost-effective method to identify patients who should receive endoscopic screening is through the use of prediction algorithms. Economic modeling studies have shown that selective screening of populations that harbor a combination of risk factors (men, older than 50 years with chronic GERD symptoms) followed by surveillance and subsequent treatment of those with dysplastic disease is cost-effective, with an incremental cost-effectiveness ratio of $12,000 per quality-adjusted life-year gained compared with no screening.[35–37]

Recently there have been efforts to amalgamate different risk factors associated with BE and EAC to develop more precise risk prediction algorithms. These include the Michigan Barrett's Esophagus pREdiction Tool (M-BERET),[38] the Gerson tool,[39] the Locke tool,[40] the Thrift tool,[41] the Nord-Trøndelag Health Study (HUNT)[42] tool, the Kunzman tool,[43] and others.[44] However, many of these prediction tools have not been previously validated externally, and few studies have directly compared these tools.

A recent study from Michigan prospectively validated and compared the accuracy of all predictions tools with regard to (1) the presence of BE at first endoscopy and (2) presence of early neoplasia.[45] They demonstrated that all these tools were better than GERD frequency and duration alone, in predicting the presence of BE.[45] However, the operating characteristics of these scores were at best, modest, with an area under the receiving operating curve (AuROC) ranging from 0.660 to 0.695 and none of the 5 tools was superior to one another.[45] When these tools were used to discriminate between early BE-related neoplasia (LGD, HGD, or T1a tumor) from no BE, which is arguably a more applicable clinical outcome, the M-BERET, HUNT, and Kunzman tool performed equally well, with an AuROC of 0.773, 0.796, and 0.763, respectively, suggesting that these scoring systems could potentially assist clinicians to streamline the need for an upper endoscopy to identify subjects at greatest risk of neoplasia.[45] As well as enriching the population to test, there is also a need to develop less-invasive and more cost-effective tools for BE screening that can be applied in the primary care setting.

TRANSNASAL ENDOSCOPY

Transnasal endoscopy (TNE) uses ultrathin nasoendoscope for imaging and sampling the esophagus and can be done under local anesthetic. In a randomized crossover study of cases and controls comparing TNE versus standard endoscopy, TNE diagnosed BE with sensitivity and specificity of 98% and 100%, respectively and was associated with less anxiety.[47] A multicenter, prospective, cross-sectional study demonstrated that TNE was well tolerated by patients, had shorter procedural time, and was safe.[48] More recently, a randomized controlled trial (RCT) evaluated community-based screening using 3 different endoscopic techniques with sedated EGD (sEGD), unsedated TNE via a mobile research van (muTNE), and unsedated TNE in the hospital outpatient setting (huTNE); muTNE and huTNE had comparable efficacy, participation rate, and safety profiles compared with sEGD.[49] TNE was associated with much shorter procedural and recovery time, and 80% of patients were willing to repeat the procedure if needed.[49]

A new endosheath technology has been developed, which uses a disposable sheath and eliminates the need for extensive cleaning between procedures, making it feasible to be applied in the office-based setting. In a pilot RCT comparing transnasal endosheath endoscopy (TEE) with standard endoscopy, the sensitivity and specificity of TEE for an endoscopic diagnosis of BE was 100%, whereas the sensitivity and specificity for a histologic diagnosis of BE was 66.7% and 100%, respectively.[50] The acceptability for TEE was higher than standard endoscopy, although the optical quality for standard endoscopy was significantly better.[50] An economic analysis has shown that TEE was more cost-effective than standard endoscopy when used to screen for BE, with an incremental cost-utility ratio of $29,400 versus $47,500, respectively.[51] Although the efficacy and safety profile of TEE is comparable with sedated EGD while being more cost-effective, this technology has not gained widespread acceptance, as it still requires an expert operator. The procedure is similar to endoscopy from the patients' perspective, and efforts to bring this modality into clinical practice have waned. To reduce the invasiveness of endoscopy, yet still obtain tissue sampling, there has been considerable interest in non-endoscopic sampling devices coupled with biomarkers.

CYTOSPONGE AND IMMUNOHISTOCHEMISTRY FOR TREFOIL FACTOR 3

Developed by the Fitzgerald laboratory since 2001, the Cytosponge is a novel, cell sampling device comprising a compressed mesh, encapsulated within a gelatinous capsule and attached to a thread (**Fig. 1**). The capsule is swallowed and on reaching the stomach, the gelatin dissolves allowing a spherical mesh to expand to roughly the diameter of the esophagus. The mesh is then withdrawn by slowly retracting the thread and as it is withdrawn, it samples up to one-million cells from the surface of the gastric cardia, esophagus, and oropharynx.[52] The cells are transported in an ethanol-based preservative, processed to a homogeneous clot, and then embedded

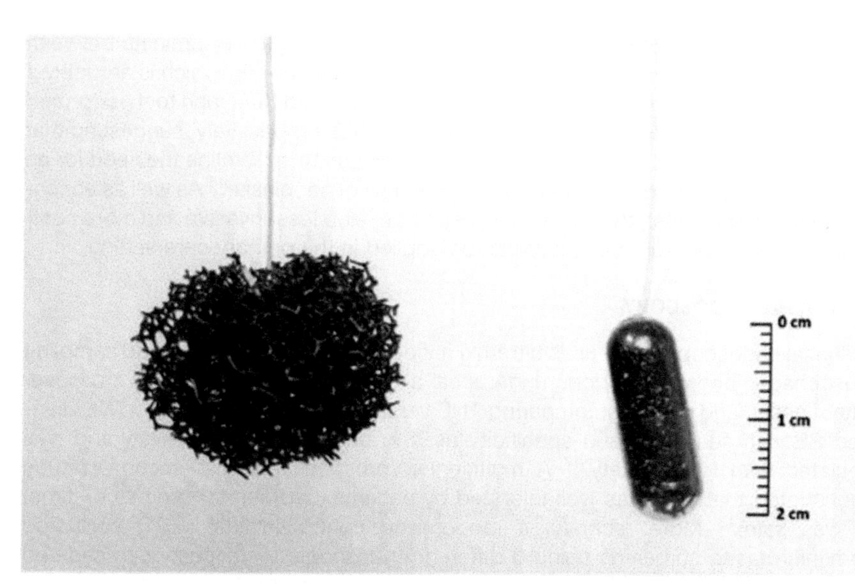

Fig. 1. Cytosponge expanded (left) and encapsulated (right) tethered to a thread.

into a standard paraffin block. Sections are stained with hematoxylin and eosin and immunohistochemistry for trefoilfactor 3 (TFF3), a specific biomarker for intestinal metaplasia (IM) identified by the same group.[53]

The Cytosponge-TFF3 technology has been rigorously tested in multiple different clinical studies comprising the Barrett's Esophagus Screening Trials (BEST) 1, 2, and 3. In a recent patient-level systematic review, the Cytosponge was shown to be safe, easy to swallow, and with a good acceptability profile.[54,55] The BEST1 study was a primary care–based prospective cohort study among patients with a previous prescription for acid suppressant medications for more than 6 months and showed that the Cytosponge was safe and well tolerated.[56] The follow-up BEST2 case-control study of 1110 patients showed that the Cytosponge had an overall sensitivity of 79.9% to detect BE, increasing to 87.2% for patients with circumferential BE greater than or equal to 3 cm.[57] This analysis was a per-protocol analysis including samples that had not reached the stomach, which is a quality control measure, and exclusion of these cases gives a sensitivity to 94%, and hence in the future when the gastric epithelium is not sampled, patients should be offered another Cytopsonge test. The specificity for diagnosing BE was 92.4%.[57] The BEST3 study was a randomized trial conducted within the primary care setting in England. This trial recruited greater than 13,000 patients and randomized 1:1 to either Cytosponge-TFF3 or usual care. The results showed that an offer of Cytosponge diagnosed 10 times more BE cases compared with usual care ($P<.0001$), and in a secondary endpoint analysis, cancer was detected at an earlier stage.[58] Microsimulation models have suggested that a Cytosponge-based screening strategy is cost-effective compared to endoscopy,[59,60] and further modeling studies using the BEST3 data are awaited.

More recently, the Cytosponge coupled with a multidimensional biomarker panel had the potential to discriminate between dysplastic and NDBE. The biomarker panel was composed of clinical parameters (age, length of BE, and BMI), atypia as well as the assessment of the tumor suppressor p53 immunohistochemistry, and a marker for aneuploidy called Aurora kinase A. These were incorporated into a regression model to stratify patients into 3 different risk categories—low-risk, moderate-risk, and high-risk and confirmed in an independent validation cohort. The low- and high-risk categories were highly predictive; however, a large proportion fell into the moderate-risk category limiting its usefulness.[61] Further work is underway to refine the stratification biomarkers with plans to perform a randomized trial in the surveillance setting.

ESOCHECK™ (LucidDx) BALLOON CAPSULE AND METHYLATED DNA MARKERS

Epigenetic changes such as aberrant cytosine methylation of CpG-rich islands have been associated with many cancers. Methylation of CpG islands in the first exon vimentin gene (methylated VIM [mVIM]) was shown to be a good biomarker for BE with a sensitivity of 91%.[62] More recently, genome wide epigenetic analysis using reduced representation bisulfite sequencing on biopsy samples from EAC, BE, EAC cell lines, and normal squamous epithelium was able to identify methylated markers that could complement mVIM.[63] High-frequency methylation within the CCNA1 locus on chromosome 13 was identified, and when tested as a methylation biomarker on 173 patients with and without BE, CCNA1 methylation (mCCNA1) was shown to be increased in BE-associated neoplasia compared with normal tissues, where it was detected in 81%, 68%, and 90% of patients with NDBE, BE, and EAC, respectively. Similar results were seen for methylation of the VIM locus where mVIM was detected in 100%, 63%, and 76.5% of NDBE, BE, and EAC cases, respectively. These 2 methylated marker panels (EsoGuard™ assay, LucidDx) were then combined and tested on cytologic brushings obtained from subjects with normal endoscopy (n = 54), erosive esophagitis (n = 8), NDBE (n = 31), dysplastic BE (n = 18), EAC (n = 48), and adenocarcinoma of the gastroesophageal junction (GEJ) (GEJCa, n = 14). Both markers had sensitivities and specificities greater than or equal to 90% for discriminating BE, EAC, and GEJCa from normal esophageal mucosa both in the discovery and validation sets with an AuROC greater than 0.95, making it promising as a tool for non-endoscopic screening. The advantage of methylated markers is that the assay can be automated and is quantitative.

Following the successful validation of these biomarkers on cytologic brushings, a novel balloon sampling device—the EsoCheck™ was then developed.[63] The balloon is swallowed in a pill-sized capsule, which attaches to a thin silicone catheter. Once in the stomach, the balloon is inflated using 5 to 6 cc of air and then gently withdrawn until the lower esophageal sphincter is encountered. The balloon is then dragged 3 to 6 cm through the distal esophagus to collect epithelium. The balloon is then deflated and inverts back into the capsule to protect the sample from contamination. Accompanied this article is a short video explaining use of EsoCheck™ (Video 1). In a pilot study of 156 patients, 82% successfully swallowed the capsule, and adequate samples were obtained in 74%. These adequate samples were then tested using the 2-marker EsoGuard™ assay (mVIM and mCCNA1) and achieved a sensitivity and specificity of 90.3% and 91.7%, respectively, for discriminating NDBE from unaffected controls (GERD, erosive esophagitis, and normal esophageal mucosa). The biomarker panel also detected 9 of 11 dysplasia and 7 of 8 cancers. Further, 93% of participants were willing to undergo the test again and 95% would recommend it to others (**Table 2**).

Balloon-assisted sampling of the distal esophagus combined with DNA methylation markers seems to be a promising, cost-effective, and minimally invasive alternative for

Table 2
Comparison between non-endoscopic devices and use of methylated biomarkers for diagnosing Barrett's esophagus

Device	Methylated Biomarkers	Number of Patients (Validation Cohort) BE (n)	Controls (n)	Sensitivity (%)	Specificity (%)
Cytosponge[64]	TFPI2	149	129	82.2	95.7
EsophaCap (Mayo)[65]	VAV3 and ZNF682	19	20	100	100
EsophaCap (Hopkins)[67]	P16, NELL1, AKAP12, TACI and Age	14	14	78.6	92.8
EsoCheck™[63]	EsoGuard™ Assay (CCNA1 and VIM)	50	36	90.3	91.7

BE screening with good acceptability and tolerability. Improvements in device design have been made and the results of multicenter trials are awaited.

METHYLATION BIOMARKERS APPLIED TO OTHER NONENDOSCOPIC CELL SAMPLING DEVICES

A panel of 4 hypermethylated genes, TFPI2, TWIST1, ZNF345, and ZNF569, has been shown to discriminate biopsies of NDBE from squamous esophagus and gastric cardia.[64] When tested on Cytosponge specimens comprising a validation cohort of 149 cases and 129 controls, these 4 genes were hypermethylated in patients with NDBE compared with reflux controls with TFPI2 having the best accuracy of diagnosing NDBE with a sensitivity and specificity of 82.2% and 95.7%, respectively.

Since the Cytosponge, other sponge-on-a-string (SOS) devices have surfaced for diagnosing BE. The EsophaCap (CapNostics, New Jersey, USA) is similar in concept to the Cytosponge, but with a smaller diameter of 2.5 cm and a finer sponge material. In a recent study by researchers from the Mayo Clinic, a 2-biomarker panel comprising VAV3 and ZNF682 were able to discriminate patients with known BE (n = 19) from controls (n = 20) based on adequate cytologic specimens obtained with the EsophaCap, achieving a sensitivity, specificity, and AuROC of 100%, 100%, and 1, respectively.[65] The biomarkers have now been further refined to include VAV3 and DOCK10 and are currently being tested in the ongoing SOS-2 trial (ClinicalTrials.gov: NCT02560623) among patients with and without BE. Preliminary results showed that the 2-biomarker combination yielded a sensitivity of 93%, specificity of 98%, and AuROC of 0.97 when tested on a cohort of BE (n = 90) and non-BE controls (n = 58). However, 11% of patients were unable to swallow the device.[66]

In a study from Johns Hopkins, which also used the EsophaCap device, researchers tested a methylation biomarker panel encompassing p16, NELL1, TAC1, and AKAP12 to diagnose BE.[67] Coupled with age, the researchers then fitted these MDMs onto a Lasso regression model for BE diagnosis, achieving sensitivity and specificity of 94.4% and 62.6%, respectively. This model was then validated on a separate cohort of 14 subjects with and 14 without BE, achieving an AuROC of 0.929, with a sensitivity of 78.6% and specificity of 92.8%.[67]

These methylation markers provide a quantitative approach to BE diagnosis, which is promising when coupled with an inexpensive and minimally invasive cell sampling device, thus making it feasible as a tool for large-scale screening. The assay thresholds, however, require standardization. It is also important to note that these studies were conducted on an enriched cohort of patients with BE (>50%), which differs from the desired screening population of BE where the prevalence of BE is much lower. Application of biomarkers on this enriched cohort introduces systematic bias, which may lead to overestimation of the operating characteristics of the biomarkers, and therefore, larger studies conducted on populations relevant to the BE screening population are required before these results can be translated into clinical practice. A large case-control study (ClinicalTrials.gov: NCT04214119) using the EsophaCap device with plans to enroll 2500 patients with and without BE is currently underway with results expected in 2026.

An alternative to a non-invasive cell sampling device is to use imaging that can be achieved using low-cost technology, potentially applicable in an office setting.

OPTICAL COHERENCE TOMOGRAPHY AND TETHERED CAPSULE ENDOMICROSCOPY

Optical coherence tomography (OCT) is an advanced imaging modality that uses infrared light and optical scattering, to produce high-resolution, cross-sectional images of the microscopic surface of the tissues.[68] This technology was shown to be able to accurately discriminate tissues with and without IM, achieving a sensitivity and specificity of 97% and 92%, respectively.[69]

More recently, tethered-capsule endomicroscopy (TCE), which incorporates the OCT technology has been developed.[70] This device uses an optomechanical pill, combined with optical frequency domain imaging and was able to obtain cross-sectional images of the esophageal mucosa to enable a diagnosis of BE-associated neoplasia. The capsule has a dimension of 11 $\times$ 24 mm and is tethered to a string.[71] Once swallowed, the device descends toward the stomach and multiple 30 $\times$ 7 μm resolution cross-sectional images are taken during transit, which is then used to reconstruct a 3-dimensional image.[71] The device is withdrawn by pulling the tether, and the device can then be disinfected for reuse.

In a feasibility study that tested the TCE on 38 patients with and without BE, 89% of patients were able to swallow the capsule.[71] The use of TCE was shown to correlate strongly in a blinded comparison with endoscopic measurement of the circumferential and maximum length of BE, achieving a correlation coefficient (r) of 0.7 to 0.83 and an interobserver agreement of greater than 0.84. Further studies are necessary to validate this technology in direct comparison to upper endoscopy in terms of efficacy and cost-effectiveness.

Ideally, a liquid biopsy from breath or blood would enable a minimally invasive and highly acceptable method for screening with the opportunity to readily perform repeat sampling to maximize sensitivity and for ongoing surveillance.

VOLATILE ORGANIC COMPOUNDS

Volatile organic compounds (VOCs) are byproducts of human and gut floral metabolism that can be detected in exhaled breath. Two current strategies for detecting VOCs include mass-spectrometric analysis, and the "electronic nose" or e-nose device.

A recent cross-sectional study, which used mass-spectrometry of VOCs and compared 81 patients with esophageal and gastric adenocarcinoma (GAC) and 129 controls (16 BE, 62 benign upper gastrointestinal [GI] disease, 51 normal GI tract), showed accurate discrimination of EAC and GAC from the normal upper GI tract, achieving AuROC of 0.97 (sensitivity 98% and specificity 91.7%) when comparing EAC versus normal upper GI tract, and 0.98 (sensitivity 100% and specificity 92.2%) when comparing GAC versus normal upper GI tract.[72] More recently, in a diagnostic validation study among 163 patients with EAC or GAC and 172 controls with benign upper GI endoscopy composed of patients with esophagitis, gastritis, benign gastric polyp, achalasia, and benign esophageal stricture, investigators showed that mass spectrometric VOCs analysis was able to diagnose EAC and GAC with greater than 80% sensitivity and specificity.[73]

A different technology using a portable “electronic nose” device resembling the mammalian olfaction was able to accurately diagnose BE among a cohort of 122 patients with a prior diagnosis of dysplastic BE who were at various stages of surveillance or treatment, achieving a sensitivity, specificity, and AuROC of 92%, 80%, and 79%, respectively.[74] In this study, there was a 95% rate of patient enrollment, suggesting high acceptability of the device. More recently, promising results from the Netherlands using this technology on a cohort of 129 patients with BE and 273 controls with GERD, esophagitis, and hiatal hernia, the e-nose was able to discriminate patients with BE from controls, achieving a sensitivity of 91%, specificity of 74%, and AuROC of 0.91, with the sensitivity of detecting BE increasing further to 96% for patients with BE maximum segment length greater than or equal to 3 cm.[75] Although both these VOCs analysis technologies hold promise, validation of these technologies among the target primary care population is required.

BLOOD-BASED BIOMARKERS

Circulating microRNAs (miRNA) are small, single-stranded, non-coding RNA fragments less than 25 nucleotides long, which regulates gene expression by binding to and inhibiting target messenger RNA and protein translation.[76] A recent systematic review of miRNAs for detecting BE identified 5 miRNAs, miRNA-192, -194, -203, -205, and -215 that hold promise for diagnosing BE.[77] Another study evaluating the differential expression of circulating miRNAs among patients with BE and controls showed that a combination of 4 miRNAs (miRNA-95-3p, -136-5p, -194-5p, and -451a) had an AuROC of 0.832 with a sensitivity of 78.4% and specificity of 85.7% to differentiate BE from controls.[78] Again these technologies were conducted among an enriched cohort of patients with BE, and validation of these results in the target screening population is required.

Circulating cell-free tumor DNA (ctDNA) is another novel approach, and a recent landmark study has shown that a PCR-based assay called CancerSeek, which detects circulating levels of proteins and mutations in ctDNA, was able to detect 5 cancer types (ovary, liver, stomach, pancreas, and esophagus) with sensitivities ranging from 69% to 98% and specificity of 99%.[79] The sensitivity of the test increases with the stage of cancer, achieving a sensitivity of 43%, 73%, and 78% for cancers presenting at stage 1, 2, and 3, respectively.[79] Disappointingly, however, the sensitivity for detecting stage 1 esophageal cancer was the lowest at 20%.[79] In a more recent study assessing methylation of circulating cell-free DNA to detect any cancer type across all stages that included 2482 participants with previously untreated cancer including esophageal cancer and 4207 participants without cancer, the sensitivity to detect cancer at stages 1,2, 3, and 4 were 18%, 43%, 81%, and 93%, respectively.[80] Although the concept of detecting ctDNA is promising, this technology requires further refinement to achieve the sensitivity required for detection of early cancer or premalignant disease.

SUMMARY

Significant progress has been made in identifying the at-risk population, as well as in the development of new technologies suitable for screening. Prediction algorithms relying on epidemiologic and demographic data are abundant, and work is now required to determine the target population to maximize the yield of screening in a manner that is cost-effective. Newer minimally invasive sampling devices coupled with biomarkers for diagnosis of BE are highly promising. In the future, the application of risk stratification biomarkers could further help to identify those at greatest risk to avoid unduly burdening endoscopy services. In the future, blood-based biomarkers and breath testing of organic compounds that are currently in development may pave the way for population-based screening if sufficient accuracy profiles can be achieved.

CLINICS CARE POINTS

- Mortality from EAC remains poor, with the overall 5-year survival being <20%.
- Population-based studies have shown that a diagnosis of BE was associated with having earlier stage EAC and an improved survival from EAC.
- Current societal recommendations suggest selective screening of high-risk patients by endoscopy depending on the presence of risk factors such as duration of GERD, obesity, smoking status, male gender, age>50 and positive family history.

DISCLOSURE

AC has founders shares and stock options in LucidDx, serves as a consultant to LucidDx, has sponsored research with LucidDx, and has a royalty interest in patents licensed by Case Western Reserve University to LucidDx. He is also a consultant for Interpace Diagnostics and receives research support from C2 Therapeutics/Pentax Inc. AC is supported by NIH grants U54 CA163060 and P50 CA150964. RCF is listed as an inventor on patents pertaining to Cytosponge and associated assays that have been licensed by the Medical Research Council to Civdien GI Solutions, now Medtronic. RCF has founders shares and serves as a consultant for Cyted Ltd. The laboratory of RCF is funded by a Core Programme Grant from the Medical Research Council (RG84369).

REFERENCES

1. Ronkainen J, Aro P, Storskrubb T, et al. Prevalence of Barrett's esophagus in the general population: an endoscopic study. Gastroenterology 2005;129(6): 1825–31.
2. Zagari RM, Fuccio L, Wallander MA, et al. Gastro-oesophageal reflux symptoms, oesophagitis and Barrett's oesophagus in the general population: the Loiano-Monghidoro study. Gut 2008;57(10):1354–9.
3. Westhoff B, Brotze S, Weston A, et al. The frequency of Barrett's esophagus in high-risk patients with chronic GERD. Gastrointest Endosc 2005;61(2):226–31.
4. El-Serag HB, Sweet S, Winchester CC, et al. Update on the epidemiology of gastro-oesophageal reflux disease: a systematic review. Gut 2014;63(6):871–80.
5. Desai TK, Krishnan K, Samala N, et al. The incidence of oesophageal adenocarcinoma in non-dysplastic Barrett's oesophagus: a meta-analysis. Gut 2012;61(7): 970–6.

6. Bhat S, Coleman HG, Yousef F, et al. Risk of malignant progression in Barrett's esophagus patients: results from a large population-based study. J Natl Cancer Inst 2011;103(13):1049–57.
7. Hvid-Jensen F, Pedersen L, Drewes AM, et al. Incidence of adenocarcinoma among patients with Barrett's esophagus. N Engl J Med 2011;365(15):1375–83.
8. de Jonge PJ, van Blankenstein M, Looman CW, et al. Risk of malignant progression in patients with Barrett's oesophagus: a Dutch nationwide cohort study. Gut 2010;59(8):1030–6.
9. Krishnamoorthi R, Ramos GP, Crews N, et al. Persistence of Nondysplastic Barrett's Esophagus Is Not Protective Against Progression to Adenocarcinoma. Clin Gastroenterol Hepatol 2017;15(6):950–2.
10. Curvers WL, ten Kate FJ, Krishnadath KK, et al. Low-grade dysplasia in Barrett's esophagus: overdiagnosed and underestimated. Am J Gastroenterol 2010; 105(7):1523–30.
11. Duits LC, Phoa KN, Curvers WL, et al. Barrett's oesophagus patients with low-grade dysplasia can be accurately risk-stratified after histological review by an expert pathology panel. Gut 2015;64(5):700–6.
12. Duits LC, van der Wel MJ, Cotton CC, et al. Patients with Barrett's esophagus and confirmed persistent low-grade dysplasia are at increased risk for progression to neoplasia. Gastroenterology 2017;152(5):993–1001.e1.
13. Lim CH, Treanor D, Dixon MF, et al. Low-grade dysplasia in Barrett's esophagus has a high risk of progression. Endoscopy 2007;39(7):581–7.
14. Howlader N, Noone A, Krapcho M, et al. SEER cancer statistics review, 1975-2016. Bethesda (MD): National Cancer Institute; 2019.
15. Wilson JMG, Jungner G. Principles and practices of screening for disease. Geneva, Switzerland: World Health Organization; 1968. Report No.: Public Health Papers No. 34. Available from: http://whqlibdoc.who.int/php/WHO_PHP_34.pdf.
16. Dobrow MJ, Hagens V, Chafe R, et al. Consolidated principles for screening based on a systematic review and consensus process. Can Med Assoc J 2018;190(14):E422–9.
17. Noone A, Howlader N, Krapcho M, et al. SEER cancer statistics review, 1975-2015. Bethesda (MD): National Cancer Institute; 2018.
18. Siegel RL, Fedewa SA, Anderson WF, et al. Colorectal cancer incidence patterns in the United States, 1974–2013. J Natl Cancer Inst 2017;109(8):djw322.
19. Cooper GS, Yuan Z, Chak A, et al. Association of prediagnosis endoscopy with stage and survival in adenocarcinoma of the esophagus and gastric cardia. Cancer 2002;95(1):32–8.
20. Cooper GS, Kou TD, Chak A. Receipt of previous diagnoses and endoscopy and outcome from esophageal adenocarcinoma: a population-based study with temporal trends. Am J Gastroenterol 2009;104(6):1356–62.
21. Kearney DJ, Crump C, Maynard C, et al. A case-control study of endoscopy and mortality from adenocarcinoma of the esophagus or gastric cardia in persons with GERD. Gastrointest Endosc 2003;57(7):823–9.
22. Shaheen NJ, Sharma P, Overholt BF, et al. Radiofrequency ablation in Barrett's esophagus with dysplasia. N Engl J Med 2009;360(22):2277–88.
23. Vaughan TL, Fitzgerald RC. Precision prevention of oesophageal adenocarcinoma. Nat Rev Gastroenterol Hepatol 2015;12(4):243–8.
24. Dulai GS, Guha S, Kahn KL, et al. Preoperative prevalence of Barrett's esophagus in esophageal adenocarcinoma: a systematic review. Gastroenterology 2002; 122(1):26–33.

25. Chak A, Faulx A, Eng C, et al. Gastroesophageal reflux symptoms in patients with adenocarcinoma of the esophagus or cardia. Cancer 2006;107(9):2160–6.
26. Lagergren J, Bergström R, Lindgren A, et al. Symptomatic gastroesophageal reflux as a risk factor for esophageal adenocarcinoma. N Engl J Med 1999;340(11): 825–31.
27. Rubenstein JH, Mattek N, Eisen G. Age- and sex-specific yield of Barrett's esophagus by endoscopy indication. Gastrointest Endosc 2010;71(1):21–7.
28. Rubenstein JH, Scheiman JM, Sadeghi S, et al. Esophageal adenocarcinoma incidence in individuals with gastroesophageal reflux: synthesis and estimates from population studies. Am J Gastroenterol 2011;106(2):254–60.
29. Corley DA, Kubo A, Levin TR, et al. Race, ethnicity, sex and temporal differences in Barrett's oesophagus diagnosis: a large community-based study, 1994-2006. Gut 2009;58(2):182–8.
30. Chak A, Lee T, Kinnard MF, et al. Familial aggregation of Barrett's oesophagus, oesophageal adenocarcinoma, and oesophagogastric junctional adenocarcinoma in Caucasian adults. Gut 2002;51(3):323–8.
31. Fitzgerald RC, di Pietro M, Ragunath K, et al. British Society of Gastroenterology guidelines on the diagnosis and management of Barrett's oesophagus. Gut 2014; 63(1):7–42.
32. Shaheen NJ, Falk GW, Iyer PG, et al. ACG clinical guideline: diagnosis and management of Barrett's esophagus. Am J Gastroenterol 2016;111(1):30.
33. Saftoiu A, Hassan C, Areia M, et al. Role of gastrointestinal endoscopy in the screening of digestive tract cancers in Europe: European Society of Gastrointestinal Endoscopy (ESGE) Position Statement. Endoscopy 2020;52(4):293–304.
34. Qumseya B, Sultan S, Bain P, et al. ASGE guideline on screening and surveillance of Barrett's esophagus. Gastrointest Endosc 2019;90(3):335–59.e2.
35. Gerson LB, Groeneveld PW, Triadafilopoulos G. Cost-effectiveness model of endoscopic screening and surveillance in patients with gastroesophageal reflux disease. Clin Gastroenterol Hepatol 2004;2(10):868–79.
36. Rubenstein JH, Inadomi JM, Brill JV, et al. Cost utility of screening for Barrett's esophagus with esophageal capsule endoscopy versus conventional upper endoscopy. Clin Gastroenterol Hepatol 2007;5(3):312–8.
37. Inadomi JM, Sampliner R, Lagergren J, et al. Screening and surveillance for Barrett esophagus in high-risk groups: a cost-utility analysis. Ann Intern Med 2003; 138(3):176–86.
38. Rubenstein JH, Morgenstern H, Appelman H, et al. Prediction of Barrett's esophagus among men. Am J Gastroenterol 2013;108(3):353.
39. Gerson LB, Edson R, Lavori PW, et al. Use of a simple symptom questionnaire to predict Barrett's esophagus in patients with symptoms of gastroesophageal reflux. Am J Gastroenterol 2001;96(7):2005–12.
40. Locke GR, Zinsmeister AR, Talley NJ. Can symptoms predict endoscopic findings in GERD? Gastrointest Endosc 2003;58(5):661–70.
41. Thrift AP, Kendall BJ, Pandeya N, et al. A clinical risk prediction model for Barrett esophagus. Cancer Prev Res 2012;5(9):1115–23.
42. Xie SH, Ness-Jensen E, Medefelt N, et al. Assessing the feasibility of targeted screening for esophageal adenocarcinoma based on individual risk assessment in a population-based cohort study in Norway (The HUNT Study). Am J Gastroenterol 2018;113(6):829–35.
43. Kunzmann AT, Thrift AP, Cardwell CR, et al. Model for Identifying Individuals at Risk for Esophageal Adenocarcinoma. Clin Gastroenterol Hepatol 2018;16(8): 1229–36.e4.

44. Liu X, Wong A, Kadri SR, et al. Gastro-esophageal reflux disease symptoms and demographic factors as a pre-screening tool for Barrett's esophagus. PLoS One 2014;9(4):e94163.
45. Rubenstein JH, McConnell D, Waljee AK, et al. Validation and Comparison of Tools for Selecting Individuals to Screen for Barrett's Esophagus and Early Neoplasia. Gastroenterology 2020;158(8):2082–92.
46. Weusten B, Bisschops R, Coron E, et al. Endoscopic management of Barrett's esophagus: European Society of Gastrointestinal Endoscopy (ESGE) position statement. Endoscopy 2017;49(02):191–8.
47. Shariff MK, Bird-Lieberman EL, O'Donovan M, et al. Randomized crossover study comparing efficacy of transnasal endoscopy with that of standard endoscopy to detect Barrett's esophagus. Gastrointest Endosc 2012;75(5):954–61.
48. Peery AF, Hoppo T, Garman KS, et al. Feasibility, safety, acceptability, and yield of office-based, screening transnasal esophagoscopy (with video). Gastrointest Endosc 2012;75(5):945–53.e2.
49. Sami SS, Dunagan KT, Johnson ML, et al. A randomized comparative effectiveness trial of novel endoscopic techniques and approaches for Barrett's esophagus screening in the community. Am J Gastroenterol 2015;110(1):148–58.
50. Shariff MK, Varghese S, O'Donovan M, et al. Pilot randomized crossover study comparing the efficacy of transnasal disposable endosheath with standard endoscopy to detect Barrett's esophagus. Endoscopy 2016;48(2):110–6.
51. Honing J, Kievit W, Bookelaar J, et al. Endosheath ultrathin transnasal endoscopy is a cost-effective method for screening for Barrett's esophagus in patients with GERD symptoms. Gastrointest Endosc 2019;89(4):712–22.e3.
52. Fitzgerald RC. Combining simple patient-oriented tests with state-of-the-art molecular diagnostics for early diagnosis of cancer. United Eur Gastroenterol J 2015;3(3):226–9.
53. Lao-Sirieix P, Boussioutas A, Kadri SR, et al. Non-endoscopic screening biomarkers for Barrett's oesophagus: from microarray analysis to the clinic. Gut 2009;58(11):1451–9.
54. Januszewicz W, Tan WK, Lehovsky K, et al. Safety and acceptability of a non-endoscopic esophageal sampling device–Cytosponge®: a systematic review of multi-center data. Clinical gastroenterology and hepatology: the official clinical practice journal of the American Gastroenterological Association 2019;17(4):647.
55. Iqbal U, Siddique O, Ovalle A, et al. Safety and efficacy of a minimally invasive cell sampling device ('Cytosponge') in the diagnosis of esophageal pathology: a systematic review. Eur J Gastroenterol Hepatol 2018;30(11):1261–9.
56. Kadri SR, Lao-Sirieix P, O'Donovan M, et al. Acceptability and accuracy of a non-endoscopic screening test for Barrett's oesophagus in primary care: cohort study. BMJ 2010;341:c4372.
57. Ross-Innes CS, Debiram-Beecham I, O'Donovan M, et al. Evaluation of a minimally invasive cell sampling device coupled with assessment of trefoil factor 3 expression for diagnosing Barrett's esophagus: a multi-center case–control study. PLoS Med 2015;12(1):e1001780.
58. Fitzgerald RC, di Pietro M, O'Donovan M, et al. Cytosponge-trefoil factor 3 versus usual care to identify Barrett's oesophagus in a primary care setting: a multicentre, pragmatic, randomised controlled trial. The Lancet 2020;396(10247):333–44.
59. Heberle CR, Omidvari AH, Ali A, et al. Cost Effectiveness of Screening Patients With Gastroesophageal Reflux Disease for Barrett's Esophagus With a Minimally

Invasive Cell Sampling Device. Clin Gastroenterol Hepatol 2017;15(9): 1397–404.e7.
60. Benaglia T, Sharples LD, Fitzgerald RC, et al. Health benefits and cost effectiveness of endoscopic and nonendoscopic cytosponge screening for Barrett's esophagus. Gastroenterology 2013;144(1):62–73.e6.
61. Ross-Innes CS, Chettouh H, Achilleos A, et al. Risk stratification of Barrett's oesophagus using a non-endoscopic sampling method coupled with a biomarker panel: a cohort study. Lancet Gastroenterol Hepatol 2017;2(1):23–31.
62. Moinova H, Leidner RS, Ravi L, et al. Aberrant vimentin methylation is characteristic of upper gastrointestinal pathologies. Cancer Epidemiol Biomarkers Prev 2012;21(4):594–600.
63. Moinova HR, LaFramboise T, Lutterbaugh JD, et al. Identifying DNA methylation biomarkers for non-endoscopic detection of Barrett's esophagus. Science translational medicine 2018;10(424).
64. Chettouh H, Mowforth O, Galeano-Dalmau N, et al. Methylation panel is a diagnostic biomarker for Barrett's oesophagus in endoscopic biopsies and non-endoscopic cytology specimens. Gut 2018;67(11):1942–9.
65. Iyer PG, Taylor WR, Johnson ML, et al. Highly discriminant methylated DNA markers for the non-endoscopic detection of Barrett's esophagus. Am J Gastroenterol 2018;113(8):1156–66.
66. Iyer PG, Lansing R, Johnson ML, et al. 878-Accurate Non-Endoscopic Detection of Barrett's Esophagus in a Multicenter Prospective Validation Cohort: The SOS 2 Trial. Gastroenterology 2018;154(6):S175–6.
67. Wang Z, Kambhampati S, Cheng Y, et al. Methylation biomarker panel performance in EsophaCap cytology samples for diagnosing Barrett's esophagus: a prospective validation study. Clin Cancer Res 2019;25(7):2127–35.
68. Ughi GJ, Gora MJ, Swager AF, et al. Automated segmentation and characterization of esophageal wall in vivo by tethered capsule optical coherence tomography endomicroscopy. Biomed Opt Express 2016;7(2):409–19.
69. Poneros JM, Brand S, Bouma BE, et al. Diagnosis of specialized intestinal metaplasia by optical coherence tomography. Gastroenterology 2001;120(1):7–12.
70. Gora MJ, Sauk JS, Carruth RW, et al. Tethered capsule endomicroscopy enables less invasive imaging of gastrointestinal tract microstructure. Nat Med 2013; 19(2):238–40.
71. Gora MJ, Quénéhervé L, Carruth RW, et al. Tethered capsule endomicroscopy for microscopic imaging of the esophagus, stomach, and duodenum without sedation in humans (with video). Gastrointest Endosc 2018;88(5):830–40.e3.
72. Kumar S, Huang J, Abbassi-Ghadi N, et al. Mass Spectrometric Analysis of Exhaled Breath for the Identification of Volatile Organic Compound Biomarkers in Esophageal and Gastric Adenocarcinoma. Ann Surg 2015;262(6):981–90.
73. Markar SR, Wiggins T, Antonowicz S, et al. Assessment of a Noninvasive Exhaled Breath Test for the Diagnosis of Oesophagogastric Cancer. JAMA Oncol 2018; 4(7):970–6.
74. Chan DK, Zakko L, Visrodia KH, et al. Breath Testing for Barrett's Esophagus Using Exhaled Volatile Organic Compound Profiling With an Electronic Nose Device. Gastroenterology 2017;152(1):24–6.
75. Peters Y, Schrauwen RW, Tan AC, et al. Detection of Barrett's oesophagus through exhaled breath using an electronic nose device. Gut 2020;69(7): 1169–72.
76. Wang H, Peng R, Wang J, et al. Circulating microRNAs as potential cancer biomarkers: the advantage and disadvantage. Clin Epigenet 2018;10(1):1–10.

77. Mallick R, Patnaik SK, Wani S, et al. A Systematic Review of Esophageal MicroRNA Markers for Diagnosis and Monitoring of Barrett's Esophagus. Dig Dis Sci 2016;61(4):1039–50.
78. Bus P, Kestens C, Ten Kate FJW, et al. Profiling of circulating microRNAs in patients with Barrett's esophagus and esophageal adenocarcinoma. J Gastroenterol 2016;51(6):560–70.
79. Cohen JD, Li L, Wang Y, et al. Detection and localization of surgically resectable cancers with a multi-analyte blood test. Science 2018;359(6378):926–30.
80. Liu M, Oxnard G, Klein E, et al. Sensitive and specific multi-cancer detection and localization using methylation signatures in cell-free DNA. Ann Oncol 2020;31: 745–59.

Best Practices in Surveillance for Barrett's Esophagus

Joseph R. Triggs, MD, PhD, Gary W. Falk, MD, MS*

KEYWORDS

- Barrett's esophagus • Surveillance • Intestinal metaplasia • Dysplasia
- Esophageal adenocarcinoma

KEY POINTS

- Barrett's esophagus is the precursor lesion to esophageal adenocarcinoma, and the goal of endoscopic surveillance is the early detection of dysplasia and cancer to improve patient outcomes.
- Meticulous visual inspection of the Barrett's segment with both high-definition white light and chromoendoscopy is recommended to increase the identification of high-risk lesions.
- Visible lesions should be biopsied or removed, preferably by endoscopic mucosal resection, followed by standardized Seattle protocol biopsies for the remaining Barrett's segment.

INTRODUCTION

Barrett's esophagus (BE) is a premalignant condition characterized by the replacement of the normal esophageal squamous epithelium with metaplastic intestinal-type columnar epithelium.[1] This change occurs due to the repetitive exposure of the distal esophagus to refluxate, which results in chronic injury and metaplastic changes.[2,3] Once these changes are identified, endoscopic surveillance aims to decrease the burden of invasive esophageal adenocarcinoma (EAC) by early detection of dysplasia and early-stage adenocarcinoma, which then are amenable to endoscopic eradication therapy (EET). Early detection of precancerous or neoplastic changes is attractive due to the high mortality rate of EAC, with an overall 5-year survival rate of less than 20% and less than 5% when patients have distant disease at the

J.R. Triggs: No disclosures; G.W. Falk: Research support from Lucid and Interpace NIH support: NCI U54 CA163004. Consulting for Lucid, Interpace and Cernostics.
Division of Gastroenterology, Hospital of the University of Pennsylvania, University of Pennsylvania, Perelman School of Medicine, Perelman Center for Advanced Medicine, 7th Floor South Pavilion, 3400 Civic Center Boulevard, Philadelphia, PA 19104, USA
* Corresponding author.
E-mail address: gary.falk@pennmedicine.upenn.edu

Gastrointest Endoscopy Clin N Am 31 (2021) 59–75
https://doi.org/10.1016/j.giec.2020.08.003
giendo.theclinics.com

time of diagnosis.[4] These numbers are even more concerning given the rising incidence of EAC over the past 3 decades.[5] This article reviews the rationale for surveillance of BE as well as the recommended surveillance techniques to optimize outcomes.

RATIONALE FOR SURVEILLANCE

The basic premise of endoscopic surveillance in BE is the fact that intestinal metaplasia is the precursor lesion for EAC. In order to accurately make recommendations regarding BE surveillance, the risk of progression from BE to EAC must first be understood. Initial data suggested a 30-fold to 40-fold increase in the relative risk of development of EAC in patients with BE.[6] Subsequent studies, however, have lowered these estimates.[7–13] A 2011 study from Denmark included patients diagnosed with BE between 1992 and 2009.[14] They identified 11,028 patients with BE during the study period and followed them for a median of 5.2 years. Excluding patients who developed EAC within the first year after diagnosis, they found 131 cases of EAC with an incidence of 1.2 cases per 1000 person-years and an annual risk of progression of 0.12%. A subsequent meta-analysis, which included 57 studies and 58,547 patient-years of follow-up, similarly found a reduction in the risk of progression from nondysplastic BE (NDBE) to EAC, with a pooled annual incidence of 0.33%.[15] Although the absolute risk of yearly progression in these studies is low, the relative risk is significantly elevated for patients with NDBE compared with those without BE, supporting the role for surveillance in this population.

In contrast to these findings in NDBE, the rate of progression to high-grade dysplasia (HGD) and/or EAC is considerably higher for patients with low-grade dysplasia (LGD), with estimates ranging from 1.7% to 13% per year.[13,16–20] In a 2014 systematic review and meta-analysis of 24 studies, 2694 patients were identified with a pooled annual incidence of progression to EAC of 0.54% (95% CI, 0.32%–0.76%) and 1.73% (95% CI, 0.99%–2.47%) for progression to HGD and/or EAC. Prior to the availability of EET, the role of surveillance was solely to diagnose cancer at an earlier stage due to improved survival seen with the detection of early-stage cancer.[21] Although this remains a key factor in the argument for surveillance today, current EET aims to treat precursors of invasive cancer, that is, LGD, HGD, and intramucosal cancer, with the goal of reducing the burden of later stage disease. This approach is safe, cost effective, and now considered standard of care for patients with LGD, HGD, or intramucosal cancer.[20]

To assess the role for surveillance in improving patient outcomes, early studies compared the diagnosis of EAC in patients with BE undergoing surveillance to those diagnosed with EAC based on symptoms. Although these studies showed a reduction in EAC-associated mortality in patients undergoing surveillance, they were relatively small retrospective cohort studies, and the indication for the initial surveillance endoscopy often was unavailable, making it unclear if patients were truly asymptomatic during these initial assessments.[22–27] A series of subsequent studies, however, has reinforced these early findings, suggesting that endoscopic surveillance does reduce EAC-related mortality.[28–30] These data include a Dutch multicenter prospective cohort study that followed 783 patients with at least 2 cm of BE and demonstrated 6.7% (53) went on to develop HGD or EAC during surveillance. When compared with the Dutch cancer registry for EAC in the general population, the diagnosis of EAC was made significantly earlier in patients in a surveillance program. Furthermore, those with neoplastic progression in the surveillance group had improved survival compared with those diagnosed with EAC outside of a surveillance program.[31] Similarly, a large cohort study of 29,536 patients diagnosed with BE at Veterans Affairs hospitals between 2004 and 2009 identified 424 patients who developed EAC during a mean follow-up of 5 years. Of these, 424 patients, 209 (49.3%) were diagnosed as part of a surveillance program. Patients in the surveillance program were more likely to be diagnosed at an early stage, survived longer and had a lower cancer-related mortality compared to those not undergoing surveillance: 34% compared with 54%, respectively ($P<0.001$).[32]

Complicating much of these data is the fact that these studies are susceptible to both lead-time bias and length-time bias, which may overestimate the true benefit of surveillance. In a 2015 study by Bhat and colleagues,[30] however, survival analyses were adjusted for lead-time bias using a sojourn time of 2.5 years (the difference between mean age of EAC diagnosis for those with and without prior BE diagnosis), and sensitivity analyses were performed to estimate the effects of length-time biases. Although these corrections reduced the estimated benefit of survival, it was not eliminated.[30] Despite these findings, there have been several studies that have demonstrated no benefit for surveillance. An often cited 2013 study by Corley and colleagues[27] identified 38 patients with BE who died of EAC (cases) and compared them to 101 living patients (controls) with BE matched for age, sex, and duration of follow-up. This study found no reduction in the risk of death in those individuals undergoing surveillance with an adjusted odds ratio of 0.99 (95% CI, 0.26–2.75). This study, like others with similar findings, however, was relatively small with incomplete assessment regarding surveillance protocols and patient inclusion criteria making it hard to draw definitive conclusions from them.[33,34] One larger study by Tramontano and colleagues[35] included almost 5000 patients with EAC in the Surveillance, Epidemiology, and End Results database and linked this to Medicare data to identify patients with a diagnosis of BE as a proxy for endoscopic screening and surveillance. They corrected for lead-time bias and demonstrated a hazard ratio for cancer-related mortality among patients with a prior diagnosis of BE controlling for cancer stage and treatment type to be 0.89 (95% CI, 0.78–1.01). Although the hazard ratio in this study spans one, suggesting there may not be a benefit to surveillance, the study controlled for 2 of the plausible mechanisms through which cancer mortality could be reduced—(1) stage of diagnosis and (2) subsequent treatment type—and therefore likely underestimates the benefit of surveillance.[35] In an effort to assess the efficacy of BE surveillance more thoroughly, a 2018 meta-analysis by Codipilly and colleagues[36] provided a pooled analysis of 12 cohort studies and showed lower EAC-related and all-cause mortality among patients with surveillance-detected EAC compared with symptom-detected EAC (relative risk, 0.73 [95% CI, 0.57–0.94]; hazard ratio 0.59 [95% CI, 0.45–0.76]). These benefits, however, either were attenuated or eliminated by adjustment for lead-time bias and length-time bias. Despite limitations of the available data and the lack of randomized controlled trials, practice guidelines around the world uniformly recommend endoscopic surveillance for BE. The results are awaited of an ongoing multicenter randomized trial in the United Kingdom, which includes 3400 patients with BE who are undergoing either endoscopic surveillance every 2 years or nonsurveillance. which hopefully should shed further light on this debate.[37]

Finally, several cost-effectiveness studies have demonstrated the utility of surveillance for NDBE and EET for LGD and HGD.[38–41] A 2012 study constructed a decision analytical Markov model for patients with NDBE, LGD, or HGD and compared 3 treatment strategies: (1) surgery when cancer was detected (no surveillance); (2) surveillance with EET when HGD was detected; and (3) initial EET followed by endoscopic surveillance.[38] This study demonstrated that for patients with NDBE, surveillance with EET at HGD was the most cost-effective strategy. Both surveillance with EET at HGD and EET initially, however, were more cost effective than surgery when cancer was detected without surveillance. This study also demonstrated that upfront EET for both LGD and HGD was the more cost-effective strategy. Furthermore, a comparative modeling approach found surveillance and treatment protocols for men with BE prevented 23% to 75% of cases of EAC and decreased mortality by 31% to 88%. These results were reduced for women given the lower incidence of disease. EET for LGD, if confirmed on repeat endoscopy, a 3-year surveillance interval for men with NDBE and a 5-year surveillance interval for women with NDBE were the optimal strategies identified in this study at a willingness-to-pay threshold of $100,000 per quality-adjusted life-year.[42]

SURVEILLANCE TECHNIQUE

Counseling Patients

Once a decision has been made to proceed with surveillance, the next step should focus on patient education and counseling to inform them of the risks and potential benefits of entering into a surveillance program. This is a critical step because surveillance endoscopy programs take a commitment from both patients and providers to optimize outcomes and reduce the morbidity and mortality associated with EAC. Unfortunately, patients often miscalculate their own risk of progression, which not only can have an impact their physical health but also on their mental health.[43,44] A 2009 systematic review found patients with BE had a significant reduction in their health-related quality of life and are at risk for depression, anxiety and stress. This study found that a diagnosis of BE was associated with an increase in health care use and spending.[45] This increase, however, may not necessarily be due to BE per se, because BE patients are at a 21% to 71% increased risk of all-cause mortality, and the largest causes of death among patients with BE are nonesophageal neoplasms and cardiac disease.[46,47]

Surveillance Intervals

As part of counseling, patient education also should include a discussion of the process of surveillance, which includes timing of repeat endoscopy. Current surveillance intervals largely are driven by expert opinion and each of the 3 major United States gastrointestinal (GI) societies (American Gastroenterological Association, American College of Gastroenterology [ACG], American Society for Gastrointestinal Endoscopy [ASGE]) have guidelines that include recommendations regarding surveillance intervals. All three US societies recommend an interval of 3 years to 5 years for patients with NDBE (**Table 1**).[4,48,49] Several international guidelines now recommend, however, a stratified approach for NDBE based on the length of the metaplastic segment.[50–52] Support for this type of stratified approach comes from several studies that have demonstrated an increased risk of BE progression based on segment length.[53,54] The European Society of Gastrointestinal Endoscopy guidelines recommend no surveillance for an irregular Z-line (<1 cm), 5 years for greater than or equal to 1 cm and less than 3 cm, 3 years for greater than or equal to 3 cm and less than 10 cm and referral to an expert center for greater than 10 cm. The British Society of Gastroenterology and Australian guidelines each recommend intervals of 2 years to 3 years for an NDBE segment greater than 3 cm and 3 years to 5 years for a segment less than 3 cm. Other risk-prediction models have included a variety of demographic, clinical, and endoscopic factors along with a wide range of biomarkers. None has been sufficiently validated to warrant their use in clinical practice and dysplasia remains the only clinically applicable predictor of risk for progression.

Table 1
Best practice surveillance intervals and treatment recommendations based on Barrett histologic grade[a]

Histologic Grade	Best Practice Recommendations
NDBE	Repeat upper endoscopy in 3–5 y for surveillance.
Indefinite dysplasia	Optimize acid suppression therapy and repeat endoscopy in 3–6 mo. If confirmed, yearly surveillance endoscopy.
LGD	Confirm histologic grade with expert GI pathologist. If confirmed and persistent on second endoscopy treat with EET. For those not undergoing EET, yearly surveillance.
HGD	Confirm histologic grade with expert GI pathologist. If confirmed, treat with EET, including EMR for visible lesions. Endoscopy every 3–6 mo for those not undergoing eradication therapy.

[a] Based on current ACG and ASGE guidelines.

For patients with indefinite dysplasia, current guidelines recommend repeat upper endoscopy within 3 months to 6 months after optimization of acid suppression medications to reduce inflammation and confirm the diagnosis. Data on the risk of progression to HGD/EAC for indefinite dysplasia are variable. A recent systematic review and meta-analysis, however, found a pooled incidence of 1.5 per 100 person-years (95% CI, 1.0–2.0) or 1.5% annual risk for progression to HGD/EAC.[11] This is similar to the risk of progression for LGD, which suggests that yearly surveillance may be appropriate. No guidelines currently recommend EET for patients with indefinite dysplasia. EET, however, is recommended as a treatment option for patients with expert GI pathologist–confirmed LGD or HGD.[20,49] Based on patient preference or increased risk due to comorbidities, patients with LGD or HGD may not undergo EET and instead could undergo surveillance every 6 months to 12 months or every 3 months, respectively.[48] If LGD is confirmed and endoscopic therapy is not performed, annual surveillance should be continued until 2 examinations in a row are negative for dysplasia. Despite the concern for missed lesions at the time of the index endoscopy, current guidelines suggest patients need not undergo repeat endoscopy for surveillance at 1 year if diagnosed with NDBE on their index examination.[4,49,55]

Pathology Confirmation

Current surveillance recommendations are based on the pathologic grade of dysplasia. Guidelines suggest that a standard five-tier system for dysplasia should be used: (1) negative for dysplasia, (2) indefinite dysplasia, (3) LGD, (4) HGD, and (5) carcinoma.[56] This system is problematic, however, given the high degree of interobserver variability among pathologists, especially for indefinite dysplasia and LGD.[57] Despite attempts to standardize the diagnosis and grading of dysplasia, several studies have suggested that community-based pathologists have difficulties in the interpretation of both NDBE and dysplasia.[58] Specifically, 2 studies from the Netherlands have highlighted these difficulties. In a study of 147 patients diagnosed with LGD in the community, 85% were downgraded to no dysplasia when the samples were reviewed by 2 GI pathologists with extensive experience with BE neoplasia.[59] Further work by the same group examined an additional 293 patients diagnosed with LGD in the community and 73% were downgraded to indefinite dysplasia or NDBE.[60] For these reasons, it is recommended that all cases of dysplasia be confirmed by a second pathologist with expertise in BE. It also is important that patients diagnosed with any level of dysplasia be on optimal acid suppression regimens at the time of tissue sampling, because this can reduce inflammation and leads to more accurate pathologic diagnoses.

Endoscopic Approach

Initial evaluation of the BE segment should begin with careful inspection of the anatomic landmarks to orient the endoscopist. This includes identification of the diaphragmatic hiatus, the gastroesophageal junction (top of the gastric folds), and the squamocolumnar junction. These locations (referenced as distance [centimeters] from incisors) should be documented. Further assessment and documentation of the BE segment should include the Prague C & M criteria (**Fig. 1**) for describing the extent of the BE segment and the Paris classification for visible lesions.[61,62] These classification systems have been validated and allow physicians to readily communicate with each other regarding the risk of progression and the potential risk for invasive cancer.[12,63] Careful inspection with high-definition white light of the entire Barrett's segment, including retroflexed view of the cardia is a key part of a careful examination. Compared with standard definition white light, high-definition white light has been shown to improve dysplasia detection with an odds ratio of 3.27 (95% CI, 1.27–8.40) and is recommended in current guidelines.[4,49,64]

After thorough cleaning, the esophagus should be examined partially insufflated to best aid in visualization and lesion detection. Under-insufflation can result in missed esophageal surface area and over-insufflation can result in the flattening of raised areas, which can result in missed lesions. During visual inspection, particular attention should be paid to the right hemisphere of the esophagus extending from the 12:00 position to the 6:00 position with the patient in left lateral position and the endoscope in a neutral position. Two studies have demonstrated an increased risk of advanced neoplasia in this location.[65,66] One study of 119 patients with HGD or intramucosal cancer demonstrated that 84.9% developed in the right hemisphere compared with 15.1% of in the left hemisphere.[66] Inspection time also is a critical component of a

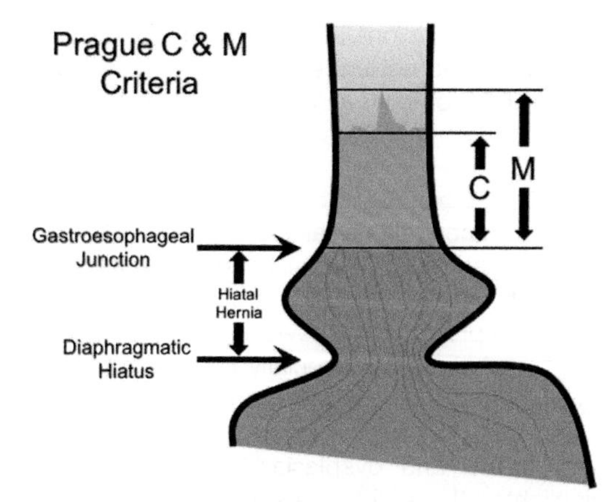

Fig. 1. Gastroesophageal landmarks with Prague C & M criteria. The distance from the gastroesophageal junction (top of the gastric folds) to the top of the circumferential metaplastic tissue ends is the C value in centimeters and the distance from the gastroesophageal junction to the maximal extent of the metaplastic tissue is the M value in centimeters. Islands are not included in the Prague C & M criteria and should be documented separately in the endoscopic report.

thorough examination and can have an impact on the quality of the examination and ability to detect dysplasia. In a study of 112 patients undergoing surveillance by 11 different endoscopists, longer inspection times were associated with a higher likelihood of diagnosing HGD or EAC (P = .001). The same study also found a direct correlation between inspection time per centimeter of the metaplastic segment and the detection of HGD or EAC with a trend toward those endoscopists whose inspection time was greater than 1 minute per centimeter having improved detection rates of HGD or EAC, 40.2% versus 6.7%, respectively (P = .06).[67]

Advanced Imaging

After careful inspection with high-definition white light, current guidelines from the ASGE recommend evaluation with chromoendoscopy, either dye based or electronic.[4,68] This is a slight departure from the 2015 ACG guidelines, which did not recommend the routine use of dye-based chromoendoscopy.[49] Neither guideline recommends the regular use of other advanced imaging techniques including confocal laser endomicroscopy, volumetric laser endomicroscopy, spectroscopy, or molecular imaging. Based on the 2016 ASGE meta-analysis, only acetic acid and virtual chromoendoscopy (in the form of narrow band imaging [NBI]) met the ASGE Preservation and Incorporation of Valuable Endoscopic Innovations thresholds for recommendation.[69] Acetic acid chromoendoscopy is performed by the topical application of dilute acetic acid to the esophageal mucosa and has excellent performance characteristics for the detection of dysplasia (sensitivity, 96.6% [95% CI, 95.2%–97.7%]; specificity, 84.6% [95% CI, 68.5%–93.2%]).[68,69] Furthermore, the use of acetic acid in combination with targeted biopsies has been shown to be cost-effective in a study of high-risk patients when compared with random biopsy sampling.[70] However, given the additional cost needed for spray catheters and solution, the difficulty in applying acetic acid evenly, and the time consuming nature of dye-based chromoendoscopy, electronic chromoendoscopy may be the preferred advanced imaging technique.[71,72]

Electronic chromoendoscopy uses various light filters or postprocessing techniques to increase the ability to detect advanced neoplasia without the need for special dyes. Although NBI (Olympus, Center Valley, Pennsylvania) is the most extensively studied, each of the 3 major endoscopic platforms has a version of electronic chromoendoscopy (Fujinon Intelligent Color Enhancement [Fujinon, Wayne, New Jersey] and i-scan [Pentax Medical, Montvale, New Jersey]). NBI has been shown to increase the detection of dysplasia as well as reduce the number of biopsies needed per patient.[73,74] To aid in the ability to identify dysplasia and cancer on NBI, the Barrett's International NBI Group has developed and validated an NBI classification system in patients with BE. The system, which includes the assessment under NBI imaging of the mucosal pattern and the vascular pattern as either regular or irregular, has a greater than 90% accuracy and high level of interobserver agreement (**Figs. 2** and **3**, **Table 2**).[75] Ideally, the use of chromoendoscopy would supplant the need for random biopsies during surveillance. Neither the ASGE nor ACG guidelines, however, support this practice, in part because a majority of the data supporting the use of electronic chromoendoscopy come from large academic centers with expertise in BE, thereby limiting the generalizability of these data.[4,49]

Tissue Acquisition

Mucosal abnormalities identified on high-definition white light examination and/or chromoendoscopy should be sampled separately for pathologic processing and assessment, preferably using endoscopic mucosal resection (EMR) techniques for larger areas.[20] These abnormalities include ulceration, erosion, plaque, nodule, or

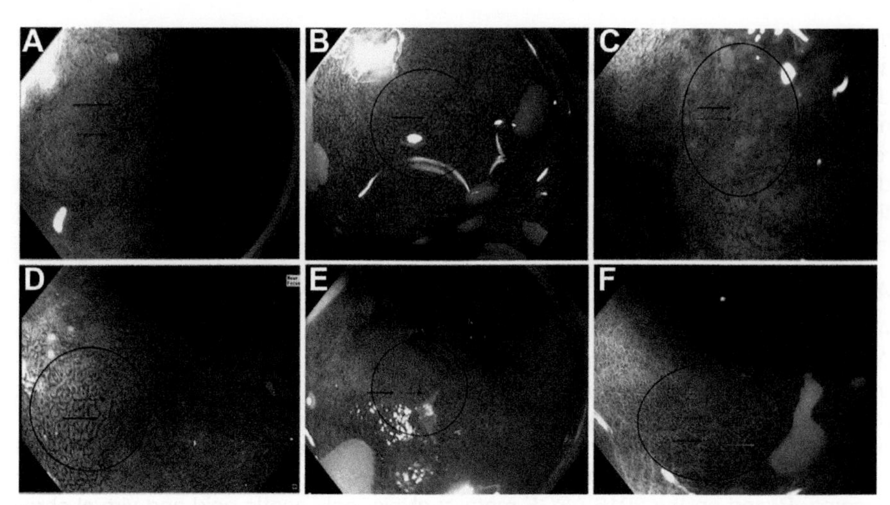

Fig. 2. (*A*) High-resolution images of NDBE using NBI. Circular mucosal patterns (*solid arrow*) are arranged in an orderly fashion and blood vessels clearly follow the mucosal architecture (*dashed arrows*). (*B*) High-resolution images of NDBE using NBI. Circular mucosal patterns are arranged in an orderly fashion and blood vessels clearly follow the normal architecture of mucosa (*solid arrow*). (*C*) High-resolution images of NDBE using NBI. Circular mucosal patterns (*solid arrow*) are arranged in an orderly fashion and blood vessels clearly follow the architecture of mucosal ridges (*dashed arrows*). (*D*) High-resolution images of NDBE using NBI. Note the ridge/villous mucosal patterns (*solid arrow*) that are arranged in an orderly fashion and blood vessels that are arranged in a regular fashion between the mucosal ridges (*dashed arrows*). (*E*) High-resolution images of NDBE using NBI. Circular mucosal patterns (*solid arrow*) are arranged in an orderly fashion and blood vessels follow the architecture of the mucosa (*dashed arrows*). (*F*) High-resolution images of NDBE using NBI. Circular (*solid black arrow*) and ridge/villous (*red arrow*) mucosal patterns are arranged in an orderly fashion and blood vessels follow the mucosal ridge architecture (*dashed arrows*). (*From* Sharma P, Bergman JJ, Goda K, et al. Development and Validation of a Classification System to Identify High-Grade Dysplasia and Esophageal Adenocarcinoma in Barrett's Esophagus Using Narrow-Band Imaging. Gastroenterology 2016;150:591-8; with permission.)

other luminal irregularity because there is an association between these lesions and underlying malignancy (**Fig. 4**).[76] There also is evidence that EMR leads to more consistent pathologic assessment of dysplasia and interobserver agreement compared with biopsy samples.[63,77] EMR in these cases is both diagnostic and therapeutic. In patient care settings where EMR is not offered, these findings should prompt consideration for referral to a tertiary care center. These changes are distinct from those of erosive esophagitis. The presence of ongoing inflammation during surveillance is a relative contraindication to tissue sampling due to the difficulty in distinguishing between dysplasia and reparative changes when these areas are sampled. Patients with ongoing inflammation should have their acid suppression regimen optimized and undergo reevaluation in 8 weeks to 12 weeks.

In addition to sampling visible lesions, guidelines recommend Seattle protocol biopsies, which include 4-quadrant biopsies every 2 cm throughout the entire length of the metaplastic segment or every 1 cm in patients with known or suspected dysplasia. Although this biopsy protocol is time consuming, data suggest that the number of biopsies strongly correlates with diagnostic yield and that this type of standardized biopsy sampling increases the detection of dysplasia and EAC.[78–80] A cohort

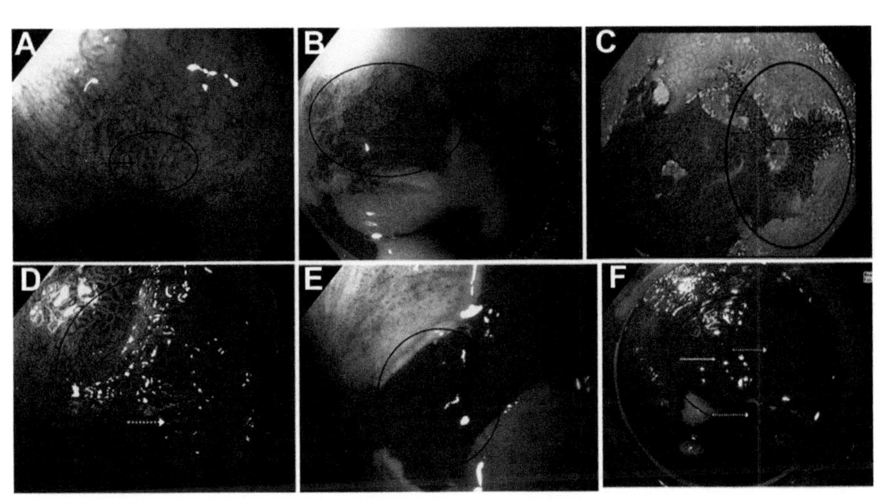

Fig. 3. (*A*) High-resolution images of dysplastic BE using NBI. Irregular mucosal and vascular patterns in BE patient using NBI. Note the irregular mucosal (*black arrow*) and vascular patterns (*red arrow*). (*B*) High-resolution images of dysplastic BE using NBI There are irregular mucosal (*black arrow*) and vascular patterns (*red arrow*). Vessels do not follow the normal architecture of the mucosa. (*C*) High-resolution images of dysplastic BE using NBI. There are irregular mucosal (*solid black arrow*) and vascular patterns (*dashed arrows*). In contrast, red arrow shows area on the mucosa with vessels arranged in a regular fashion following the normal architecture of the mucosa. (*D*) High-resolution images of NDBE using NBI. Note the presence of ridge/villous mucosal patterns (*solid arrow*) that are arranged in an orderly fashion and blood vessels that are arranged in a regular fashion between the mucosal ridges (*dashed arrows*). Focally or diffusely distributed vessels do not follow the normal architecture of the mucosa. (*E*) High-resolution images of dysplastic BE using NBI. There is an irregular mucosal and vascular pattern (*solid arrow*). The *dashed arrows* show regularly arranged mucosal and vascular pattern. (*F*) High-resolution images of dysplastic BE using NBI. There are irregular mucosal (*solid arrow*) and vascular patterns (*dashed arrows*). (*From* Sharma P, Bergman JJ, Goda K, et al. Development and Validation of a Classification System to Identify High-Grade Dysplasia and Esophageal Adenocarcinoma in Barrett's Esophagus Using Narrow-Band Imaging. Gastroenterology 2016;150:591-8; with permission.)

Table 2
Consensus-driven narrow band imaging classification of Barrett epithelium

Morphologic Characteristics	Classification
Mucosal pattern	
Circular, ridged/villous, or tubular patterns	Regular
Absent or irregular patterns	Irregular
Vascular pattern	
Blood vessels situated regularly along or between mucosal ridges and/or those showing normal, long, branching patterns	Regular
Focally or diffusely distributed vessels not following normal architecture of the mucosa	Irregular

From Sharma P, Bergman JJ, Goda K, et al. Development and Validation of a Classification System to Identify High-Grade Dysplasia and Esophageal Adenocarcinoma in Barrett's Esophagus Using Narrow-Band Imaging. Gastroenterology 2016;150:591-8; with permission.

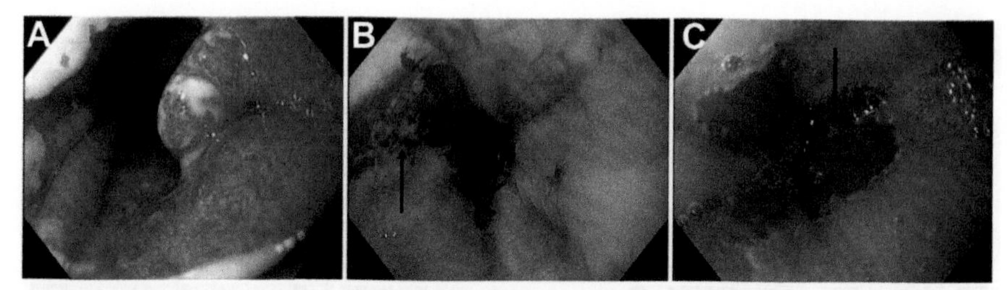

Fig. 4. (*A*) Barrett segment with Paris Is lesion removed by mucosal resection. The histopathologic diagnosis was high-grade dysplasia. (*B*) Barrett segment, with arrow indicating Paris IIa lesion. The histopathologic diagnosis was moderately differentiated adenocarcinoma, stage T1a (invasion to muscularis mucosa) without lymphovascular invasion. Mucosal resection of this lesion was considered curative. (*C*) Barrett segment with erosion marked by arrow. Diagnostic and therapeutic (curative) mucosal resection revealed well-differentiated adenocarcinoma stage T1a.

study of patients with long-segment BE compared 180 patients with 4-quadrant biopsies every 2 cm to 182 patients with nonsystematic biopsies over the course of 10 years. The 4-quadrant biopsy protocol significantly outperformed the nonsystematic cohort with LGD identified in 18.9% versus 1.6% (P<.001) of patients and HGD identified in 2.8% versus 0% (P = .03) of patients.[81] Unfortunately, despite the recommendation from multiple GI societies and good data in support of the Seattle protocol, adherence to this recommendation remains problematic.[82,83] Specifically, data from the GI quality improvement consortium registry assessed compliance to the Seattle protocol in more than 58,000 endoscopies for screening or surveillance and found that approximately 20% of endoscopies performed were nonadherent, with the odds ratio of nonadherence increasing by 31% per 1 cm of BE length.[84] Patients in whom adequate biopsies are obtained and BE is suspected endoscopically without confirmation of intestinal metaplasia histologically should be considered for repeat examination in 1 year to 2 years, because approximately 30% of these patients can be expected to have intestinal metaplasia on repeat examination.[85,86]

Wide-Area Transepithelial Sampling

Unlike standard brush biopsies, which have been shown to be of little utility in the detection of dysplasia, the 2019 ASGE guideline provided a conditional recommendation for the use of wide-area transepithelial sampling (WATS) with computer-assisted 3-dimensional analysis for patients with known or suspected BE in addition to Seattle protocol biopsy sampling.[4,87] This technology uses a stiff wire brush to sample a larger area of the esophagus compared with standard biopsy-based sampling. The analysis is performed first by a computer, which reconstructs an image of the sample and identifies concerning areas for review by a cytopathologist. A 2018 randomized controlled trial of WATS either before or after targeted and Seattle protocol biopsies included 16 BE referral centers and 160 patients undergoing surveillance endoscopy or referred for eradication therapy.[88] The primary outcome was the diagnosis of HGD/EAC, which with the addition of WATS was 14.4% (95% CI, 7.5%–21.2%) higher compared with biopsies alone. The study demonstrated no significant difference based on the order of sampling and an increase in procedural time of only 4.5 minutes. There are several limitations, however, which raise questions regarding its generalizability, including the inclusion of only BE expert centers and the high-risk patient population sampled that included 55% of patients with known dysplasia and more than 15% with HGD or carcinoma. The systematic review conducted as part of the updated ASGE guideline included 6 studies, both for screening and surveillance, and included 6271 patients with BE.[4,88] Targeted and Seattle protocol biopsies identified 125 cases of dysplasia and WATS identified an additional 137 cases with a relative increase in dysplasia detection of 48% (95% CI, 34%–60%).[4] Although this is an impressive increase in the number of cases in which dysplasia was detected, the clinical context and definition of dysplasia are not uniform. Studies to date also have assessed only the role of WATS as an adjunct to standard biopsy protocols. The cost effectiveness of this technology and its potential as a stand-alone assessment to replace the Seattle protocol remain in question. Furthermore, it is unclear if dysplasia based on cytology has the same clinical importance as dysplasia detected by histology. Therefore, future studies are needed with long-term outcomes data before this technology likely becomes adopted more widely.

PITFALLS IN SURVEILLANCE

Although all GI professional society guidelines currently recommend surveillance for BE, proper application and execution of this recommendation remain challenging. A recent systematic review and meta-analysis attempted to address this issue by reviewing adherence rates to the appropriate clinical guidelines, including performance of surveillance, surveillance interval, biopsy protocol, landmark identification, and histopathologic information reported. Pooled adherence rates varied widely from 18%to 89%, with adherence to surveillance intervals and the recommended biopsy protocol at approximately 50%.[89] These numbers are of particular concern because shorter surveillance intervals add significant cost to an already costly endeavor, and inadequate biopsy regimens can lead to missed lesions and, therefore, missed cancers.[55,82,90] Overall poor adherence to the appropriate guidelines results in poor utilization of resources and poorer health outcomes for patients. Therefore, it is critical that endoscopists use the appropriate technique for surveillance with slow, meticulous examination of the metaplastic segment in both high-definition white light and NBI at appropriate intervals with the recommended biopsy protocol.

FUTURE PROSPECTS

BE surveillance is both time consuming and costly. This cost at least in part is due to the low absolute risk of progression and large numbers of patients in surveillance programs that likely will never develop advanced lesions requiring treatment. Ideally, those at high-risk for progression could be identified and efforts focused on them while lengthening surveillance intervals for those at low risk or not surveying them at all. Future work will continue to expand on risk stratification tools to aid in the ability to identify the at-risk population using both clinical data and biomarkers.[11,91–95] Further development of enhanced imaging techniques, especially artificial intelligence, also may allow for optimized detection of dysplasia and early cancer while also reducing operator variability.[69,96,97]

SUMMARY

The goal of well-done endoscopic surveillance of BE is the detection of dysplasia and early EAC, thereby decreasing the morbidity and mortality associated with advanced-stage EAC. High-quality surveillance includes counseling patients and careful inspection of the entire metaplastic segment with both high-definition white light and NBI followed by appropriate tissue sampling for all mucosal abnormalities and systematic biopsies of the remaining tissue. Diagnoses of dysplasia should be confirmed by a second experienced GI pathologist, and patients should be appropriately triaged to the recommended surveillance intervals or EET as appropriate.

REFERENCES

1. Spechler SJ, Souza RF. Barrett's esophagus. N Engl J Med 2014;371:836–45.
2. Shaheen N, Ransohoff DF. Gastroesophageal reflux, barrett esophagus, and esophageal cancer: scientific review. JAMA 2002;287:1972–81.
3. Que J, Garman KS, Souza RF, et al. Pathogenesis and cells of origin of barrett's esophagus. Gastroenterology 2019;157:349–64.e1.
4. Qumseya B, Sultan S, Bain P, et al. ASGE guideline on screening and surveillance of Barrett's esophagus. Gastrointest Endosc 2019;90:335–59.e2.
5. Coleman HG, Xie SH, Lagergren J. The epidemiology of esophageal adenocarcinoma. Gastroenterology 2018;154:390–405.
6. Spechler SJ, Goyal RK. Barrett's esophagus. N Engl J Med 1986;315:362–71.
7. Wani S, Falk G, Hall M, et al. Patients with nondysplastic Barrett's esophagus have low risks for developing dysplasia or esophageal adenocarcinoma. Clin Gastroenterol Hepatol 2011;9:220–7.
8. Wani S, Puli SR, Shaheen NJ, et al. Esophageal adenocarcinoma in Barrett's esophagus after endoscopic ablative therapy: a meta-analysis and systematic review. Am J Gastroenterol 2009;104:502–13.
9. Sikkema M, de Jonge PJ, Steyerberg EW, et al. Risk of esophageal adenocarcinoma and mortality in patients with Barrett's esophagus: a systematic review and meta-analysis. Clin Gastroenterol Hepatol 2010;8:235–44.
10. Yousef F, Cardwell C, Cantwell MM, et al. The incidence of esophageal cancer and high-grade dysplasia in Barrett's esophagus: a systematic review and meta-analysis. Am J Epidemiol 2008;168:237–49.
11. Krishnamoorthi R, Mohan BP, Jayaraj M, et al. Risk of progression in Barrett's esophagus indefinite for dysplasia: a systematic review and meta-analysis. Gastrointest Endosc 2020;91:3–10.e3.
12. Chandrasekar VT, Hamade N, Desai M, et al. Significantly lower annual rates of neoplastic progression in short- compared to long-segment non-dysplastic Barrett's esophagus: a systematic review and meta-analysis. Endoscopy 2019;51: 665–72.
13. O'Byrne LM, Witherspoon J, Verhage RJJ, et al. Barrett's Registry Collaboration of academic centers in Ireland reveals high progression rate of low-grade dysplasia and low risk from nondysplastic Barrett's esophagus: report of the RIBBON network. Dis Esophagus 2020. https://doi.org/10.1093/dote/doaa009.
14. Hvid-Jensen F, Pedersen L, Drewes AM, et al. Incidence of adenocarcinoma among patients with Barrett's esophagus. N Engl J Med 2011;365:1375–83.
15. Desai TK, Krishnan K, Samala N, et al. The incidence of oesophageal adenocarcinoma in non-dysplastic Barrett's oesophagus: a meta-analysis. Gut 2012; 61:970.
16. Phoa K, van Vilsteren FI, Weusten BM, et al. Radiofrequency ablation vs endoscopic surveillance for patients with barrett esophagus and low-grade dysplasia: A randomized clinical trial. JAMA 2014;311:1209–17.
17. Wani S, Falk GW, Post J, et al. Risk factors for progression of low-grade dysplasia in patients with barrett's esophagus. Gastroenterology 2011;141:1179–86.e1.

18. Duits LC, van der Wel MJ, Cotton CC, et al. Patients with barrett's esophagus and confirmed persistent low-grade dysplasia are at increased risk for progression to neoplasia. Gastroenterology 2017;152:993–1001.e1.
19. Singh S, Manickam P, Amin AV, et al. Incidence of esophageal adenocarcinoma in Barrett's esophagus with low-grade dysplasia: a systematic review and meta-analysis. Gastrointest Endosc 2014;79:897–909.
20. Wani S, Qumseya B, Sultan S, et al. Endoscopic eradication therapy for patients with Barrett's esophagus-associated dysplasia and intramucosal cancer. Gastrointest Endosc 2018;87:907–31.e9.
21. Rustgi A, El-Serag HB. Esophageal carcinoma. N Engl J Med 2015;372:1472–3.
22. Incarbone R, Bonavina L, Saino G, et al. Outcome of esophageal adenocarcinoma detected during endoscopic biopsy surveillance for Barrett's esophagus. Surg Endosc 2002;16:263–6.
23. Ferguson MK, Durkin A. Long-term survival after esophagectomy for Barrett's adenocarcinoma in endoscopically surveyed and nonsurveyed patients. J Gastrointest Surg 2002;6:29–35 [discussion: 36].
24. van Sandick JW, van Lanschot JJ, Kuiken BW, et al. Impact of endoscopic biopsy surveillance of Barrett's oesophagus on pathological stage and clinical outcome of Barrett's carcinoma. Gut 1998;43:216–22.
25. Peters JH, Clark GW, Ireland AP, et al. Outcome of adenocarcinoma arising in Barrett's esophagus in endoscopically surveyed and nonsurveyed patients. J Thorac Cardiovasc Surg 1994;108:813–21 [discussion: 821–2].
26. Cooper GS, Yuan Z, Chak A, et al. Association of prediagnosis endoscopy with stage and survival in adenocarcinoma of the esophagus and gastric cardia. Cancer 2002;95:32–8.
27. Corley DA, Levin TR, Habel LA, et al. Surveillance and survival in Barrett's adenocarcinomas: a population-based study. Gastroenterology 2002;122:633–40.
28. Cooper GS, Kou TD, Chak A. Receipt of previous diagnoses and endoscopy and outcome from esophageal adenocarcinoma: a population-based study with temporal trends. Am J Gastroenterol 2009;104:1356–62.
29. Verbeek RE, Leenders M, Ten Kate FJ, et al. Surveillance of Barrett's esophagus and mortality from esophageal adenocarcinoma: a population-based cohort study. Am J Gastroenterol 2014;109:1215–22.
30. Bhat SK, McManus DT, Coleman HG, et al. Oesophageal adenocarcinoma and prior diagnosis of Barrett's oesophagus: a population-based study. Gut 2015; 64:20–5.
31. Kastelein F, van Olphen SH, Steyerberg EW, et al. Impact of surveillance for Barrett's oesophagus on tumour stage and survival of patients with neoplastic progression. Gut 2016;65:548–54.
32. El-Serag HB, Naik AD, Duan Z, et al. Surveillance endoscopy is associated with improved outcomes of oesophageal adenocarcinoma detected in patients with Barrett's oesophagus. Gut 2016;65:1252.
33. Corley DA, Mehtani K, Quesenberry C, et al. Impact of endoscopic surveillance on mortality from Barrett's esophagus-associated esophageal adenocarcinomas. Gastroenterology 2013;145:312–9.e1.
34. Rubenstein JH, Sonnenberg A, Davis J, et al. Effect of a prior endoscopy on outcomes of esophageal adenocarcinoma among United States veterans. Gastrointest Endosc 2008;68:849–55.
35. Tramontano AC, Sheehan DF, Yeh JM, et al. The impact of a prior diagnosis of barrett's esophagus on esophageal adenocarcinoma survival. Am J Gastroenterol 2017;112:1256–64.

36. Codipilly DC, Chandar AK, Singh S, et al. The effect of endoscopic surveillance in patients with barrett's esophagus: a systematic review and meta-analysis. Gastroenterology 2018;154:2068–86.e5.
37. Old O, Moayyedi P, Love S, et al. Barrett's Oesophagus Surveillance versus endoscopy at need Study (BOSS): protocol and analysis plan for a multicentre randomized controlled trial. J Med Screen 2015;22:158–64.
38. Hur C, Choi SE, Rubenstein JH, et al. The cost effectiveness of radiofrequency ablation for Barrett's esophagus. Gastroenterology 2012;143:567–75.
39. Gordon LG, Mayne GC, Hirst NG, et al. Cost-effectiveness of endoscopic surveillance of non-dysplastic Barrett's esophagus. Gastrointest Endosc 2014;79: 242–56.e6.
40. Phoa KN, Rosmolen WD, Weusten B, et al. The cost-effectiveness of radiofrequency ablation for Barrett's esophagus with low-grade dysplasia: results from a randomized controlled trial (SURF trial). Gastrointest Endosc 2017;86:120–9.e2.
41. Kastelein F, van Olphen S, Steyerberg EW, et al. Surveillance in patients with long-segment Barrett's oesophagus: a cost-effectiveness analysis. Gut 2015; 64:864–71.
42. Omidvari AH, Ali A, Hazelton WD, et al. Optimizing management of patients with barrett's esophagus and low-grade or no dysplasia based on comparative modeling. Clin Gastroenterol Hepatol 2020;18(9):1961–9.
43. Kruijshaar ME, Siersema PD, Janssens AC, et al. Patients with Barrett's esophagus perceive their risk of developing esophageal adenocarcinoma as low. Gastrointest Endosc 2007;65:26–30.
44. Shaheen NJ, Green B, Medapalli RK, et al. The perception of cancer risk in patients with prevalent Barrett's esophagus enrolled in an endoscopic surveillance program. Gastroenterology 2005;129:429–36.
45. Crockett SD, Lippmann QK, Dellon ES, et al. Health-related quality of life in patients with Barrett's esophagus: a systematic review. Clin Gastroenterol Hepatol 2009;7:613–23.
46. Solaymani-Dodaran M, Card TR, West J. Cause-specific mortality of people with Barrett's esophagus compared with the general population: a population-based cohort study. Gastroenterology 2013;144:1375–83, 1383.e1.
47. Erichsen R, Horvath-Puho E, Lund JL, et al. Mortality and cardiovascular diseases risk in patients with Barrett's oesophagus: a population-based nationwide cohort study. Aliment Pharmacol Ther 2017;45:973–82.
48. Spechler SJ, Sharma P, Souza RF, et al. American Gastroenterological Association medical position statement on the management of Barrett's esophagus. Gastroenterology 2011;140:1084–91.
49. Shaheen NJ, Falk GW, Iyer PG, et al. ACG Clinical Guideline: Diagnosis and Management of Barrett/'s Esophagus. Am J Gastroenterol 2016;111:30–50.
50. Whiteman DC, Appleyard M, Bahin FF, et al. Australian clinical practice guidelines for the diagnosis and management of Barrett's esophagus and early esophageal adenocarcinoma. J Gastroenterol Hepatol 2015;30:804–20.
51. Fitzgerald RC, di Pietro M, Ragunath K, et al. British Society of Gastroenterology guidelines on the diagnosis and management of Barrett's oesophagus. Gut 2014; 63:7–42.
52. Weusten B, Bisschops R, Coron E, et al. Endoscopic management of Barrett's esophagus: European Society of Gastrointestinal Endoscopy (ESGE) Position Statement. Endoscopy 2017;49:191–8.

53. Sikkema M, Looman CW, Steyerberg EW, et al. Predictors for neoplastic progression in patients with Barrett's Esophagus: a prospective cohort study. Am J Gastroenterol 2011;106:1231–8.
54. Anaparthy R, Gaddam S, Kanakadandi V, et al. Association between length of Barrett's esophagus and risk of high-grade dysplasia or adenocarcinoma in patients without dysplasia. Clin Gastroenterol Hepatol 2013;11:1430–6.
55. Visrodia K, Singh S, Krishnamoorthi R, et al. Magnitude of missed esophageal adenocarcinoma after barrett's esophagus diagnosis: a systematic review and meta-analysis. Gastroenterology 2016;150:599.e15.
56. Montgomery E, Bronner MP, Goldblum JR, et al. Reproducibility of the diagnosis of dysplasia in Barrett esophagus: a reaffirmation. Hum Pathol 2001;32:368–78.
57. Kerkhof M, van Dekken H, Steyerberg EW, et al. Grading of dysplasia in Barrett's oesophagus: substantial interobserver variation between general and gastrointestinal pathologists. Histopathology 2007;50:920–7.
58. Alikhan M, Rex D, Khan A, et al. Variable pathologic interpretation of columnar lined esophagus by general pathologists in community practice. Gastrointest Endosc 1999;50:23–6.
59. Curvers WL, ten Kate FJ, Krishnadath KK, et al. Low-grade dysplasia in Barrett's esophagus: overdiagnosed and underestimated. Am J Gastroenterol 2010;105: 1523–30.
60. Duits LC, Phoa KN, Curvers WL, et al. Barrett's oesophagus patients with low-grade dysplasia can be accurately risk-stratified after histological review by an expert pathology panel. Gut 2015;64:700–6.
61. Endoscopic Classification Review Group. Update on the paris classification of superficial neoplastic lesions in the digestive tract. Endoscopy 2005;37:570–8.
62. Sharma P, Bergman JJ, Goda K, et al. Development and validation of a classification system to identify high-grade dysplasia and esophageal adenocarcinoma in barrett's esophagus using narrow-band imaging. Gastroenterology 2016;150: 591–8.
63. Peters FP, Brakenhoff KP, Curvers WL, et al. Histologic evaluation of resection specimens obtained at 293 endoscopic resections in Barrett's esophagus. Gastrointest Endosc 2008;67:604–9.
64. Sami SS, Subramanian V, Butt WM, et al. High definition versus standard definition white light endoscopy for detecting dysplasia in patients with Barrett's esophagus. Dis Esophagus 2015;28:742–9.
65. Kariyawasam VC, Bourke MJ, Hourigan LF, et al. Circumferential location predicts the risk of high-grade dysplasia and early adenocarcinoma in short-segment Barrett's esophagus. Gastrointest Endosc 2012;75:938–44.
66. Enestvedt BK, Lugo R, Guarner-Argente C, et al. Location, location, location: does early cancer in Barrett's esophagus have a preference? Gastrointest Endosc 2013;78:462–7.
67. Gupta N, Gaddam S, Wani SB, et al. Longer inspection time is associated with increased detection of high-grade dysplasia and esophageal adenocarcinoma in Barrett's esophagus. Gastrointest Endosc 2012;76:531–8.
68. Sharma P, Savides TJ, Canto MI, et al. The American Society for Gastrointestinal Endoscopy PIVI (Preservation and Incorporation of Valuable Endoscopic Innovations) on imaging in Barrett's Esophagus. Gastrointest Endosc 2012;76:252–4.
69. Thosani N, Abu Dayyeh BK, Sharma P, et al. ASGE Technology Committee systematic review and meta-analysis assessing the ASGE Preservation and Incorporation of Valuable Endoscopic Innovations thresholds for adopting real-time

imaging-assisted endoscopic targeted biopsy during endoscopic surveillance of Barrett's esophagus. Gastrointest Endosc 2016;83:684–98.e7.

70. Bhandari P, Kandaswamy P, Cowlishaw D, et al. Acetic acid-enhanced chromoendoscopy is more cost-effective than protocol-guided biopsies in a high-risk Barrett's population. Dis Esophagus 2012;25:386–92.
71. Olliver JR, Wild CP, Sahay P, et al. Chromoendoscopy with methylene blue and associated DNA damage in Barrett's oesophagus. Lancet 2003;362:373–4.
72. Kondo H, Fukuda H, Ono H, et al. Sodium thiosulfate solution spray for relief of irritation caused by Lugol's stain in chromoendoscopy. Gastrointest Endosc 2001;53:199–202.
73. Wolfsen HC, Crook JE, Krishna M, et al. Prospective, controlled tandem endoscopy study of narrow band imaging for dysplasia detection in Barrett's Esophagus. Gastroenterology 2008;135:24–31.
74. Sharma P, Hawes RH, Bansal A, et al. Standard endoscopy with random biopsies versus narrow band imaging targeted biopsies in Barrett's oesophagus: a prospective, international, randomised controlled trial. Gut 2013;62:15–21.
75. Sharma P, Dent J, Armstrong D, et al. The development and validation of an endoscopic grading system for Barrett's esophagus: the Prague C & M criteria. Gastroenterology 2006;131:1392–9.
76. Reid BJ, Blount PL, Feng Z, et al. Optimizing endoscopic biopsy detection of early cancers in Barrett's high-grade dysplasia. Am J Gastroenterol 2000;95: 3089–96.
77. Mino-Kenudson M, Hull MJ, Brown I, et al. EMR for Barrett's esophagus-related superficial neoplasms offers better diagnostic reproducibility than mucosal biopsy. Gastrointest Endosc 2007;66:660–6 [quiz: 767].
78. Fitzgerald RC, Saeed IT, Khoo D, et al. Rigorous surveillance protocol increases detection of curable cancers associated with Barrett's esophagus. Dig Dis Sci 2001;46:1892–8.
79. Qumseya BJ, Wang H, Badie N, et al. Advanced imaging technologies increase detection of dysplasia and neoplasia in patients with Barrett's esophagus: a meta-analysis and systematic review. Clin Gastroenterol Hepatol 2013;11: 1562–70.e1-2.
80. Nachiappan A, Ragunath K, Card T, et al. Diagnosing dysplasia in Barrett's oesophagus still requires Seattle protocol biopsy in the era of modern video endoscopy: results from a tertiary centre Barrett's dysplasia database. Scand J Gastroenterol 2020;55:9–13.
81. Abela JE, Going JJ, Mackenzie JF, et al. Systematic four-quadrant biopsy detects Barrett's dysplasia in more patients than nonsystematic biopsy. Am J Gastroenterol 2008;103:850–5.
82. Abrams JA, Kapel RC, Lindberg GM, et al. Adherence to biopsy guidelines for Barrett's esophagus surveillance in the community setting in the United States. Clin Gastroenterol Hepatol 2009;7:736–42 [quiz: 710].
83. Curvers WL, Peters FP, Elzer B, et al. Quality of Barrett's surveillance in The Netherlands: a standardized review of endoscopy and pathology reports. Eur J Gastroenterol Hepatol 2008;20:601–7.
84. Wani S, Williams JL, Komanduri S, et al. Endoscopists systematically undersample patients with long-segment Barrett's esophagus: an analysis of biopsy sampling practices from a quality improvement registry. Gastrointest Endosc 2019; 90:732–41.e3.

85. Harrison R, Perry I, Haddadin W, et al. Detection of intestinal metaplasia in Barrett's esophagus: an observational comparator study suggests the need for a minimum of eight biopsies. Am J Gastroenterol 2007;102:1154–61.
86. Khandwalla HE, Graham DY, Kramer JR, et al. Barrett's esophagus suspected at endoscopy but no specialized intestinal metaplasia on biopsy, what's next? Am J Gastroenterol 2014;109:178–82.
87. Kumaravel A, Lopez R, Brainard J, et al. Brush cytology vs. endoscopic biopsy for the surveillance of Barrett's esophagus. Endoscopy 2010;42:800–5.
88. Vennalaganti PR, Kaul V, Wang KK, et al. Increased detection of Barrett's esophagus-associated neoplasia using wide-area trans-epithelial sampling: a multicenter, prospective, randomized trial. Gastrointest Endosc 2018;87:348–55.
89. Roumans CAM, van der Bogt RD, Steyerberg EW, et al. Adherence to recommendations of Barrett's esophagus surveillance guidelines: a systematic review and meta-analysis. Endoscopy 2020;52:17–28.
90. Wani S, Williams JL, Komanduri S, et al. Over-utilization of repeat upper endoscopy in patients with non-dysplastic barrett's esophagus: a quality registry study. Am J Gastroenterol 2019;114:1256–64.
91. Vaughan TL, Onstad L, Dai JY. Interactive decision support for esophageal adenocarcinoma screening and surveillance. BMC Gastroenterol 2019;19:109.
92. Konda VJA, Souza RF. Biomarkers of Barrett's Esophagus: From the Laboratory to Clinical Practice. Dig Dis Sci 2018;63:2070–80.
93. Davison JM, Goldblum J, Grewal US, et al. Independent blinded validation of a tissue systems pathology test to predict progression in patients with barrett's esophagus. Am J Gastroenterol 2020;115(6):843–52.
94. Critchley-Thorne RJ, Davison JM, Prichard JW, et al. A tissue systems pathology test detects abnormalities associated with prevalent high-grade dysplasia and esophageal cancer in barrett's esophagus. Cancer Epidemiol Biomarkers Prev 2017;26:240–8.
95. Dong J, Buas MF, Gharahkhani P, et al. Determining risk of barrett's esophagus and esophageal adenocarcinoma based on epidemiologic factors and genetic variants. Gastroenterology 2018;154:1273–81.e3.
96. de Souza LA Jr, Palm C, Mendel R, et al. A survey on Barrett's esophagus analysis using machine learning. Comput Biol Med 2018;96:203–13.
97. Falk GW. 2017 David Sun Lecture: screening and surveillance of barrett's esophagus: where are we now and what does the future hold? Am J Gastroenterol 2019;114:64–70.

Cost-Effectiveness of Screening, Surveillance, and Endoscopic Eradication Therapies for Managing the Burden of Esophageal Adenocarcinoma

Joel H. Rubenstein, MD, MSc[a,b,c], John M. Inadomi, MD[d,*]

KEYWORDS

• Systematic review • Health care costs • Costs and analysis • Cost-benefit analysis

KEY POINTS

- Screening for Barrett's esophagus and esophageal adenocarcinoma in men with symptoms of gastroesophageal reflux is a cost-effective strategy.
- Screening modalities that do not require sedation (eg, cytosponge, transnasal endoscopy) may be more cost-effective than screening with standard, sedated endoscopy.
- Endoscopic eradication therapy is the most cost-effective strategy for managing patients with Barrett's esophagus and high-grade dysplasia or early adenocarcinoma.
- Endoscopic eradication therapy for patients with nondysplastic Barrett's esophagus provides little benefit and is more expensive than the generally accepted willingness to pay in the United States.
- The optimal endoscopic surveillance interval for nondysplastic Barrett's esophagus is likely 3 years among men and 5 years among women.

INTRODUCTION

Many potential strategies for reducing the morbidity and mortality of esophageal adenocarcinoma have been used, more have been proposed, and even more could be imagined.[1] However, directly comparing all of the possible strategies prospectively, for instance in randomized trials, is impractical due to cost, duration of

[a] Center for Clinical Management Research, Ann Arbor Veterans Affairs Medical Center, 2215 Fuller Road, Ann Arbor, MI 48105, USA; [b] Division of Gastroenterology, Department of Internal Medicine, University of Michigan Medical School, Ann Arbor, MI, USA; [c] Rogel Cancer Center, University of Michigan, Ann Arbor, MI, USA; [d] Department of Internal Medicine, University of Utah School of Medicine, 30 North 1900 East, Suite 4C104, Salt Lake City, UT 84132, USA
* Corresponding author.
E-mail address: john.inadomi@hsc.utah.edu

Gastrointest Endoscopy Clin N Am 31 (2021) 77–90
https://doi.org/10.1016/j.giec.2020.08.005
giendo.theclinics.com

follow-up required, difficulties in measuring clinically important outcomes, and in some instances, potential ethical considerations. Medical decision analysis avoids these practical limitations by mathematically comparing outcomes of competing strategies of management based on probability theory, typically using computer simulation models. Cost-effectiveness analysis (CEA) includes costs in these comparisons (**Box 1** for definitions). Here, the authors aim to review the available CEAs comparing strategies to manage the burden of esophageal adenocarcinoma, with focus on screening and surveillance of Barrett's esophagus.

METHODS

A previously published systematic review on this topic included publications between 8/2001 and 8/2016 and had identified 24 relevant publications.[3] The authors updated the systematic review by searching in PubMed from 1/2016 to 2/2020 with the following Medical Subject Headings: [Barrett esophagus or esophageal neoplasms] and [Health Care Costs or "Costs and Analysis" or Cost-Benefit Analysis or CEA.mp]. Eligible studies were published in English and presented results of a CEA comparing strategies of screening, surveillance, endoscopic therapy, or chemoprevention with outcomes expressed as quality-adjusted life-years (QALYs). The search identified 71 articles, 7 of which were relevant and unique to the publications identified in the earlier systematic review.[4–10] Because endoscopic eradication therapy (EET) has

Box 1
Definitions of terms used in cost-effectiveness analyses

- Cost: resources forgone to provide medical care. Often differ from charges, which also depend on bargaining power, profit structures, and accounting inaccuracies.
- Utility: quantification of patient preferences for specific health states, ranging from 0 (death) to 1 (perfect health).
- Quality Adjusted Life Years (QALYs): the product of years of life multiplied by utility.
- Incremental Cost-Effectiveness Ratio (ICER): difference in cost divided by the difference in outcomes (often expressed in units of $/QALY).
- Willingness-to-Pay (WTP) threshold: the cost society is willing to pay for an outcome. In the United States, the WTP is typically accepted as $100,000/QALY.[2]
- Dominant strategy: a strategy that is both more effective and less costly than its comparator strategy.
- Domination by extension: in the situation where the ICER between strategy B versus A is greater than the ICER between strategy C versus B, strategy B is dominated by extension by strategy C.
- Optimal strategy: the most effective strategy with an ICER no greater than the WTP compared with the next most effective strategy.
- Base case analysis: analysis with all the inputs (transitions, costs, utilities) set at their point estimate.
- Sensitivity analysis: examines the degree of uncertainty regarding assumptions by varying inputs in the model, which can be performed by varying one variable at a time (1-way sensitivity analysis) or multiple variables (multivariable sensitivity analysis) at a time.
- Monte Carlo simulation: a multivariable sensitivity analysis where the model is run thousands of times with each input sampled again from its probability distribution in each run of the model.

such profound impact on the modeled outcomes of managing the burden from esophageal adenocarcinoma, the authors consider CEAs assessing EET first and then address CEAs assessing screening, surveillance, and chemoprevention.

Comparative modeling exercises conduct CEAs in multiple independent models using the same population, strategies, time horizon, outcomes, and some shared baseline assumptions. This offers unique advantages to assess the robustness of the results from individual models and identify structural differences in models that may lead to different outcomes. The National Cancer Institute Cancer Intervention and Surveillance Modeling Network (CISNET) Esophageal Working Group encompasses 3 models that are each calibrated to the US Surveillance, Epidemiology, and End Results (SEER) cancer registry.[11] The CISNET Esophageal Working Group has published several such comparative modeling exercises, which the authors highlight.

ENDOSCOPIC ERADICATION THERAPIES FOR BARRETT'S ESOPHAGUS OR EARLY ADENOCARCINOMA

Before the advent of endoscopic resection and radiofrequency ablation, there were 4 CEAs that demonstrated photodynamic therapy to be the optimal management of Barrett's esophagus with high-grade dysplasia, compared with strategies of surveillance or esophagectomy.[3] The earlier systematic review identified 5 CEAs comparing EET in high-grade dysplasia, including endoscopic resection, radiofrequency ablation, and argon plasma coagulation to surveillance, or esophagectomy, and the updated review identified 3 additional CEAs.[3,5,6,9] The setting for these analyses were the United States, Great Britain, and Spain. Each of these studies identified EET as the optimal strategy, and some even reported that EET was a dominant strategy (more effective and less costly). Two CEAs have examined EET for early esophageal adenocarcinomas (T1a or T1b).[4,12] Both found that EET was optimal in T1a (intramucosal) adenocarcinomas, regardless of life expectancy or other factors. For T1b (submucosal) adenocarcinoma, EET was also optimal in many scenarios, including in settings of shorter life expectancy from age and comorbidities, greater operative mortality, or worse quality of life following esophagectomy compared with EET.

The cost-effectiveness of EET for Barrett's esophagus with low-grade dysplasia has been a topic of important interest in recent years. The prior systematic review identified 2 CEAs assessing EET for low-grade dysplasia, and the authors identified 3 subsequent publications (**Table 1**).[5,8,9,13,14] The studies by Hur and colleagues and Esteban and colleagues both found that EET for low-grade dysplasia was optimal at their specified willingness-to-pay (WTP) thresholds and was robust to all sensitivity analyses considered.[5,14] Inadomi and colleagues considered a strategy of discontinuing surveillance following EET for low-grade dysplasia that had resulted in complete eradication of intestinal metaplasia and found the strategy to dominate EET with continued surveillance[13]; however, subsequent data regarding the durability of EET reduce the likelihood that such a strategy would be adopted in the current environment.[15] As part of the CISNET comparative modeling group, Kroep and colleagues directly compared 2 independent models that shared similar inputs but differed in their structure. One of the models found EET for low-grade dysplasia optimal, but the other found it too expensive.[9] Finally, Omidvari and colleagues compared results from all 3 CISNET esophageal cancer models (including updates of the same 2 from Kroep, plus a third model) for 78 different strategies of management of 60-year-old patients with Barrett's esophagus with either no dysplasia or low-grade dysplasia.[8] The investigators simultaneously varied 3 factors in the

Table 1
Cost-effectiveness of endoscopic eradication therapy for Barrett's esophagus with low-grade dysplasia

Author, Year	Population	Strategies	QALYs	Cost	ICER	Optimal Strategy
Inadomi et al,[13] 2009	50 y/o with BE LGD	None	14.71	$687		
		RFA without surveillance if CEIM	15.78	$12,540	$11,147/QALY	RFA without surveillance if CEIM
		APC then surveillance	15.73	$13,881	(Dominated)	
		RFA then surveillance	15.78	$14,409	(Dominated)	
		Surveillance, esophagectomy for Ca	15.38	$16,210	(Dominated)	
		PDT then surveillance	15.75	$28,017	(Dominated)	
Hur et al,[14] 2012	50 y/o with BE LGD that is confirmed and persistent on repeat endoscopy	Surveillance, RFA for HGD	16.88	$26,517		
		RFA then surveillance	16.99	$28,486	$18,231/QALY	RFA then surveillance
		Surveillance, esophagectomy for Ca	16.71	$33,963	(Dominated)	
Kroep et al,[9] 2017 EACMo	60 y/o man with BE	None	14.78	$3931		
		Surveillance, EET for HGD	14.98	$8113	$21,132/QALY	Surveillance, EET for HGD
		Surveillance, esophagectomy for Ca	14.86	$10,483	(Dominated)	
		Surveillance, EET for LGD	14.99	$11,014	$299,642/QALY	
		EET for NDBE	15.00	$14,159	$399,020/QALY	
Kroep et al,[9] 2017 MISCAN-EAC	60 y/o man with BE	None	14.83	$3383		
		Surveillance, EET for HGD	15.01	$6475	$16,475/QALY	
		Surveillance, EET for LGD	15.05	$7116	$18,950/QALY	Surveillance, EET for LGD
		Surveillance, esophagectomy for Ca	14.90	$9022	(Dominated)	
		EET for NDBE	15.07	$11,209	$198,000/QALY	
Esteban et al,[5] 2018	65 y/o with BE LGD	Surveillance	9.15	€13,259		
		RFA ± EMR then surveillance	9.71	€20,464	€12,865/QALY	RFA ± EMR then surveillance
Omidvari et al,[8] 2019 MISCAN-EAC	60 y/o with BE ND or LGD	78 strategies varying surveillance interval, confirmation of LGD, and EET for LGD	78 strategies	78 strategies	78 strategies	EET for LGD if confirmed by expert pathologist on repeat EGD after high-dose acid suppression

Abbreviations: APC, argon plasma coagulation; BE, Barrett's esophagus; Ca, cancer; CEIM, complete eradication of intestinal metaplasia; EACMo, CISNET Esophageal Adenocarcinoma Model (originally developed at Massachusetts General Hospital and subsequently at Columbia University); EET, endoscopic eradication therapy; EGD, esophagogastroduodenoscopy; EMR, endoscopic mucosal resection; HGD, high-grade dysplasia; ICER, incremental cost-effectiveness ratio; LGD, low-grade dysplasia; MISCAN-EAC, CISNET Micosimulation Screening Analysis – Esophageal Adenocarcinoma Model from Erasmus University and University of Washington; MSCE-EAC, CISNET multisage clonal expansion for esophageal adenocarcinoma from fred Hutchinson Cancer Research Center; ND, non-

strategies tested in these analyses: endoscopic surveillance intervals, whether low-grade dysplasia was managed by endoscopic surveillance or be EET, and whether low-grade dysplasia should undergo repeat endoscopy after high-dose proton pump inhibitor therapy with pathology confirmed by an expert pathologist before initiating EET. The models included a strategy in which an initial diagnosis of low-grade dysplasia prompted an 8-week trial of high-dose proton pump inhibitor, after which endoscopy with biopsies was repeated to examine the effect of false-positive tests for low-grade dysplasia. This is because of the common clinical finding that the inflammatory and regeneration features of gastroesophageal reflux disease can mimic the histopathological appearance of dysplasia.[16] Each of the 3 independent models found that EET for low-grade dysplasia was optimal, but only if the confirmatory endoscopy was performed, demonstrating the adverse impact of overtreatment of false-positive diagnoses of low-grade dysplasia. The findings were robust to sensitivity analyses, including sex.

The question of whether to perform EET for nondysplastic Barrett's esophagus has been addressed by 3 publications encompassing 5 models (**Table 2**).[9,13,14] Four studies found that EET for nondysplastic Barrett's esophagus resulted in increases in average QALYs (range: 0.01, 0.16) compared with EET only for dysplasia, but one found that EET for nondysplastic Barrett's esophagus led to a reduction of 0.17 QALYs on average (dominated), and 3 found the strategy to be cost-prohibitive with incremental cost-effectiveness ratios (ICERs) of $124,796 to $399,020 per QALY. The only study that found EET for nondysplastic Barrett's esophagus to be optimal was in the setting of discontinuing surveillance after complete eradication of intestinal metaplasia and not considering surveillance intervals other than every 5 years.[13] In contrast to the other studies on this topic, that particular study reported the greatest benefit from EET of nondysplastic Barrett's esophagus but was the only one that had not calibrated the cancer incidence to the incidence observed in the US SEER cancer registry, possibly resulting in overestimation of the benefit.

SCREENING FOR BARRETT'S ESOPHAGUS AND ESOPHAGEAL ADENOCARCINOMA

Most of the earlier CEAs of screening for Barrett's esophagus and esophageal adenocarcinoma used data that predated the widespread use of EET. Because EET of dysplasia and early adenocarcinoma dramatically alters the cost-effectiveness of management of Barrett's esophagus, the authors only considered subsequent cost-effectiveness analyses that included strategies of EET downstream from screening in this review (**Table 3**). The prior systematic review identified 3 publications examining the cost-effectiveness of screening that included downstream EET; the authors identified 2 subsequent publications reporting results from 3 additional models.[3,7,10] Five of the models assessed screening in a population of middle-aged men with symptoms of gastroesophageal reflux. All of those models found that endoscopic screening was cost-effective. The other model assessed endoscopic screening in the entire general population at the time of screening colonoscopy and included identification and treatment of early esophageal squamous cell carcinoma and gastric adenocarcinoma; that study also found screening simultaneously for both cancers was the optimal strategy.[17] Four of the models also assessed alternative screening modalities (cytosponge in 3 and unsedated transnasal endoscopy in 1), reporting that those less-invasive modalities had very similar effectiveness as conventional sedated endoscopic screening, but at lower cost, resulting in the alternative screening modalities to be the optimal strategy. For cytosponge, the results were sensitive to the prevalence of Barrett's esophagus (screening is not cost-effective if the prevalence is very low) and the

Table 2
Cost-effectiveness of endoscopic eradication therapy for nondysplastic Barrett's esophagus

Author, Year	Population	Strategies	QALY	Cost	ICER	Optimal Strategy
Inadomi et al,[13] 2009	50 y/o with NDBE	None	15.19	$471		
		RFA without surveillance if CEIM	15.83	$10,876	$16,286/QALY	RFA without surveillance if CEIM
		Surveillance, RFA for dysplasia	15.67	$10,933	(Dominated)	
		APC then surveillance	15.77	$12,512	(Dominated)	
		MPEC then surveillance	15.81	$12,691	(Dominated)	
		RFA then surveillance	15.83	$13,268	(Dominated)	
Hur et al,[14] 2012	50 y/o with NDBE	Surveillance, RFA for HGD	16.93	$16,435		Surveillance, RFA for HGD
		Surveillance, esophagectomy for Ca	16.87	$19,315	(Dominated)	
		RFA then surveillance	17.00	$24,422	$124,796	
Kroep et al,[9] 2017 EACMo	60 y/o man with BE	None	14.78	$3931		
		Surveillance, EET for HGD	14.98	$8113	$21,132/QALY	Surveillance, EET for HGD
		Surveillance, esophagectomy for Ca	14.86	$10,483	(Dominated)	
		Surveillance, EET for LGD	14.99	$11,014	$299,642/QALY	
		EET for NDBE	15.00	$14,159	$399,020/QALY	
Kroep et al,[9] 2017 MISCAN-EAC	60 y/o man with BE	None	14.83	$3383		
		Surveillance, EET for HGD	15.01	$6475	$16,475/QALY	
		Surveillance, EET for LGD	15.05	$7116	$18,950/QALY	Surveillance, EET for LGD
		Surveillance, esophagectomy for Ca	14.90	$9022	(Dominated)	
		EET for NDBE	15.07	$11,209	$198,000/QALY	
Kroep et al,[9] 2017 MSCE-EAC	60 y/o man with BE	None	14.32	$6246		
		Surveillance, EET for HGD	14.56	$10,479	$17,288/QALY	Surveillance, EET for HGD
		EET for NDBE	14.39	$13,586	(Dominated)	
		Surveillance, esophagectomy for Ca	14.59	$14,495	$182,093/QALY	

Abbreviations: APC, argon plasma coagulation; BE, Barrett's esophagus; Ca, cancer; CEIM, complete eradication of intestinal metaplasia; EACMo, CISNET Esophageal Adenocarcinoma Model (originally developed at Massachusetts General Hospital and subsequently at Columbia University); EET, endoscopic eradication therapy; HGD, high-grade dysplasia; ICER, incremental cost-effectiveness ratio; LGD, low-grade dysplasia; MISCAN-EAC, CISNET Micosimulation Screening Analysis—Esophageal Adenocarcinoma Model from Erasmus University and University of Washington; MPEC, multipolar electrocoagulation; MSCE-EAC, CISNET multisage clonal expansion for esophageal adenocarcinoma from Fred Hutchinson Cancer Research Center; ND, nondysplastic; QALY, quality-adjusted life-year; RFA, radiofrequency ablation.

Table 3
Cost-effectiveness of screening for Barrett's esophagus and esophageal adenocarcinoma

Author, Year	Population	Strategies	QALY	Cost	ICER	Optimal Strategy
Gerson et al,[25] 2004	50 y/o man with heartburn	No screening, EET for Ca	18.16 LYs[a]	$655	Reference	
		No screening, esophagectomy for Ca	18.13	$668	Dominated	
		EGD Scr & Surv of dysplasia, EET for Ca	18.21	$1614	Dominated Ext	
		EGD Scr & Surv of dysplasia, esophagectomy for Ca	18.16	$1617	Dominated	
		EGD Scr & Surv of LGD, EET for HGD	18.21	$1623	Dominated	
		EGD Scr & Surv of LGD, esophagectomy for HGD	18.17	$1626	Dominated	
		EGD Scr & Surv of NDBE, esophagectomy for Ca	18.19	$1852	Dominated	
		EGD Scr & Surv of NDBE, esophagectomy for HGD	18.21	$1883	Dominated	
		EGD Scr & Surv of NDBE, EET for Ca	18.25	$1890	Dominated Ext	
		EGD Scr & Surv of NDBE, EET for HGD	18.27	$1920	$11,500/LY	Scr & Surv of NDBE, EET for HGD
Gupta et al,[17] 2011	50 y/o undergoing screening colonoscopy	No screening	18.08	$480	Reference	
		EGD Screening, EET for HGD	18.08	$933	Dominated Ext	
		EGD Scr & Surv of NDBE, EET for HGD	18.08	$961	$95,590/QALY	Scr & Surv of NDBE, EET for HGD
Benaglia et al,[18] 2013	50 y/o man with GERD	No screening	17.96	$132	Reference	
		Cytosponge Scr, EGD Surv, EET for HGD	17.98	$373	$15,724/QALY	Cytosponge Scr, EGD Surv, EET for HGD
		EGD Scr, EGD Surv, EET for HGD	17.98	$431	Dominated	
Heberle et al,[10] 2017 EACMo	60 y/o man with GERD	No screening	15.08	$762	Reference	
		Cytosponge Scr, EGD Surv, EET for HGD	15.10	$1485	$33,057/QALY	Cytosponge Scr, EGD Surv, EET for HGD
		EGD Scr, EGD Surv, EET for HGD	15.10	$2090	$330,361/QALY	

(*continued on next page*)

Table 3
(*continued*)

Author, Year	Population	Strategies	QALY	Cost	ICER	Optimal Strategy
Heberle et al,[10] 2017 MISCAN-EAC	60 y/o man with GERD	No screening	15.08	$704	Reference	
		Cytosponge Scr, EGD Surv, EET for HGD	15.11	$1598	$26,358/QALY	Cytosponge Scr, EGD Surv, EET for HGD
		EGD Scr, EGD Surv, EET for HGD	15.12	$2186	$330,361/QALY	
Honing et al,[7] 2018	50 y/o white man with GERD	No screening	18.43	$1436	Reference	
		mTNE Scr, EGD Surv, EET for LGD	18.47	$2425	$29,446/QALY	mTNE Scr, EGD Surv, EET for LGD
		uTNE Scr, EGD Surv, EET for LGD	18.47	$2494	Dominated	
		EGD Scr, EGD Surv, EET for LGD	18.47	$2957	Dominated	

Abbreviations: Ca, cancer; EACMo, CISNET Esophageal Adenocarcinoma Model (originally developed at Massachusetts General Hospital and subsequently at Columbia University); EET, endoscopic eradication therapy; EGD, esophagogastroduodenoscopy; Ext, by extension; GERD, gastroesophageal reflux disease; HGD, high-grade dysplasia; ICER, incremental cost-effectiveness ratio; LGD, low-grade dysplasia; MISCAN-EAC, CISNET Micosimulation Screening Analysis—Esophageal Adenocarcinoma Model from Erasmus University and University of Washington; mTNE, mobile van transnasal endoscopy; QALY, quality-adjusted life-year; Scr, screening; Surv, surveillance; uTNE, unsedated transnasal endoscopy.

[a] Gerson and colleagues reported absolute life-years, not QALYs.

accuracy of cytosponge (conventional endoscopy is optimal if cytosponge is less accurate than reported in efficacy studies).[10,18] Also, in a sensitivity analysis, Heberle and colleagues found that endoscopic screening was dominated by cytosponge screening among women with symptoms of gastroesophageal reflux.[10] Further studies are needed to validate the accuracy of cystosponge and similar less invasive screening technologies in detecting Barrett's esophagus. In addition, studies are needed that assess the cost-effectiveness of screening stratified by age, sex, race, and other risk factors.

CHEMOPREVENTION

The Aspirin and Esomeprazole Chemoprevention in Barrett's metaplasia Trial (AspECT) demonstrated that high-dose (80 mg daily) compared with low-dose (20 mg daily) esomeprazole led to a significant reduction in a defined composite outcome composed of overall mortality or progression to high-grade dysplasia or cancer in patients with Barrett's esophagus.[19] Aspirin was not observed to reduce the composite outcome; however, a subanalysis of participants who did not take concomitant nonsteroidal antiinflammatory drugs was able to demonstrate improved outcomes among aspirin users. Unfortunately, the authors could not identify any CEAs of chemoprevention that included EET for dysplastic Barrett's esophagus. Importantly, Hur and colleagues found that chemoprevention with aspirin (assumed to decrease cancer incidence by 50%, which is more effective than found in AspECT) dominated no therapy and that endoscopic surveillance (without EET) costs more than $1 million per QALY gained compared with aspirin. Further CEAs that include EET for dysplasia are needed that incorporate estimates of efficacy from AspECT.[20]

SURVEILLANCE OF NONDYSPLASTIC BARRETT'S ESOPHAGUS

The prior systematic review identified only one CEA comparing intervals of endoscopic surveillance and no surveillance in the setting of EET for dysplasia (**Table 4**).[21] Kastelein and colleagues compared strategies of no surveillance, or surveillance at 1, 2, 3, 4, or 5 years, all in the setting of offering EET for high-grade dysplasia. Using a Dutch health care perspective and WTP of €35,000/QALY, they concluded that the optimal strategy was surveillance every 5 years.[21] Most recently, Omidvari and colleagues compared results from 3 CISNET models for 78 different strategies of management of 60-year-old patients with Barrett's esophagus with either no dysplasia or low-grade dysplasia, stratified by sex, and using a US population with a WTP of $100,000/QALY.[8] These strategies simultaneously varied surveillance intervals for nondysplastic Barrett's esophagus (1, 2, 3, 4, 5, 10 years or no surveillance) and management of low-grade dysplasia (the latter described earlier and in **Table 1**). For men, 2 of the models found the optimal surveillance interval in nondysplastic Barrett's esophagus to be 3 years and one found it to be 2 years; averaging the costs and QALYs across models led to 3-year intervals being optimal, and this remained so in 100% of probabilistic sensitivity analyses. For women, 2 of the models found the optimal interval to be 4 years and the other model found it to be 5 years; however, the average result was 5 years (due to difference in the magnitude of the predicted results across models).

There is much interest in developing tissue-based biomarkers to guide surveillance or initiation of EET. The authors identified 2 CEAs addressing the use of such biomarkers. First, Gordon and colleagues compared strategies for management of nondysplastic Barrett's esophagus of no surveillance, surveillance every 2 years, and strategies guided by results of a panel of tissue-based biomarkers including

Table 4
Cost-effectiveness of surveillance strategies of nondysplastic Barrett's esophagus

Author, Year	Population	Strategies	QALY	Cost	ICER	Optimal Strategy
Gordon et al,[22] 2014	50 y/o with NDBE	No Surveillance	12.04	$5226	Reference	
		Biomarker[a] + RFA/−no surv	10.47	$7652	Dominated	
		Biomarker[a] + surv q 6 mo/−no surv	12.19	$11,087	$38,307	Biomarker[a] + surv q 6 mo/ −no surv
		Biomarker[a] + surv q 6 mo/−surv 5 y then q2 y	12.19	$12,587	Dominated	
		Surveillance q2 y	12.19	$14,659	$1,946,085/QALY	
Kastelein et al,[21] 2015	55 y/o man with NDBE	None	12.62	€5695	Reference	
		Surveillance q5 y, RFA HGD	12.87	€7019	€5283/QALY	NDBE surveillance q5 y, HGD RFA[a]
		Surveillance q4 y, RFA HGD	12.89	€7821	€62,619/QALY	
		Surveillance q3 y, RFA HGD	12.90	€9005	€105,755/QALY	
		Surveillance q2 y, RFA HGD	12.90	€10,984	€324,420/QALY	
		Surveillance q1 y, RFA HGD	12.89	€15,074	Dominated	
Omidvari et al,[8] 2019 MISCAN-EAC	60 y/o man with BE ND or LGD	78 strategies varying surveillance interval, confirmation of LGD, and EET for LGD	78 strategies	78 strategies	78 strategies	NDBE surveillance q2 y, LGD confirmed then EET
Omidvari et al,[8] 2019 EACMo	60 y/o man with BE ND or LGD	78 strategies varying surveillance interval, confirmation of LGD, and EET for LGD	78 strategies	78 strategies	78 strategies	NDBE surveillance q3 y, LGD confirmed then EET
Omidvari et al,[8] 2019 MSCE-EAC	60 y/o man with BE ND or LGD	78 strategies varying surveillance interval, confirmation of LGD, and EET for LGD	78 strategies	78 strategies	78 strategies	NDBE surveillance q3 y, LGD confirmed then EET
Omidvari et al,[8] 2019 MISCAN-EAC	60 y/o woman with BE ND or LGD	78 strategies varying surveillance interval, confirmation of LGD, and EET for LGD	78 strategies	78 strategies	78 strategies	NDBE surveillance q4 y, LGD confirmed then EET
Omidvari et al,[8] 2019 EACMo	60 y/o woman with BE ND or LGD	78 strategies varying surveillance interval, confirmation of LGD, and EET for LGD	78 strategies	78 strategies	78 strategies	NDBE surveillance q5 y, LGD confirmed then EET

Omidvari et al,[8] 2019 MSCE-EAC	60 y/o woman with BE ND or LGD	78 strategies varying surveillance interval, confirmation of LGD, and EET for LGD	78 strategies	78 strategies	78 strategies	NDBE surveillance q4 y, LGD confirmed then EET
Hao et al,[23] 2019	62 y/o with BE ND, indefinite dysplasia, or LGD	Surv q3 y ND, Surv q1 y LGD, EET HGD	4.08	$7254		
		TissueCypher: low-risk surv q 5 y, intermediate-risk surv q 3 y + EET HGD, high-risk EET	4.08	$7470	$52,483	TissueCypher low-risk surv q 5 y, intermediate-risk surv q 3 y + EET HGD, high-risk EET

Abbreviations: BE, Barrett's esophagus; EACMo, CISNET Esophageal Adenocarcinoma Model (originally developed at Massachusetts General Hospital and subsequently at Columbia University); EET, endoscopic eradication therapy; HGD, high-grade dysplasia; ICER, incremental cost-effectiveness ratio; LGD, low-grade dysplasia; MISCAN-EAC, CISNET Micosimulation Screening Analysis—Esophageal Adenocarcinoma Model from Erasmus University and University of Washington; MSCE-EAC, CISNET multisage clonal expansion for esophageal adenocarcinoma from Fred Hutchinson Cancer Research Center; ND, non-dysplastic; QALY, quality-adjusted life-year; RFA, radiofrequency ablation; Surv, surveillance.

[a] Using Dutch health care perspective and WTP of €35,000/QALY.

methylation-specific polymerase chain reaction and flow cytometry for alterations in p53, p16, aneuploidy, and tetraploidy.[22] They found the optimal strategy was one in which patients with an abnormal biomarker panel underwent repeat surveillance at 6 months, and those with normal biomarkers discontinued surveillance. However, the strategy was optimal in only 61% of scenarios in the probabilistic sensitivity analysis, and the accuracy of the biomarker panel still requires validation.

Second, a commercially available risk prediction multibiomarker assay (TissueCypher Cernostics, Inc. Pittsburgh, PA) was compared with usual care using standard endoscopic surveillance and biopsies in a hypothetical cohort of patients with Barrett's esophagus and no dysplasia and indeterminate or low-grade dysplasia in a hybrid decision tree/Markov decision model to compare costs and QALYs between strategies over a 5-year time frame.[23] The performance of the multibiomarker assay was based on a nested case-control validation study reporting the positive and negative predictive values for the prediction of progression of patients with Barrett's esophagus and no-, indeterminate-, or low-grade dysplasia to high-grade dysplasia or cancer over a 5-year period.[24] Cancer mortality was predicted to decrease by 37.6% with an incremental cost-effectiveness ratio of $52,483 per QALY gained compared with standard endoscopic surveillance. Sensitivity analysis demonstrated robustness of the conclusions as long as the sensitivity of the assay to predict progression to high-grade dysplasia or cancer was 51% or greater, and probabilistic sensitivity analysis illustrated the cost-effectiveness of the assay strategy in 57.3% of simulations using a WTP threshold of $100,000 per QALY gained. The limitations of the study included a short time horizon for the analysis (5 years) and test characteristics of the assay that were based on a single validation nested case-control study that required estimation of the positive and negative predictive values of the assay to be adjusted for disease prevalence.

DISCUSSION

Decision analyses are useful for comparing multiple potential clinical management trials when conducting trials would be impractical. For instance, the study by Omidvari and colleagues compared 78 different potential strategies with follow-up of approximately 15 years on average—a feat not conceivable for a randomized trial—and providing results much sooner than an observational study comparing strategies.[8] CEA adds a dimension of the economic consequences of implementing strategies to reduce cancer mortality, which is an increasingly important factor, as the competition for health care resources increases. Comparative modeling is useful for identifying strategies that should be accepted as standard of care versus those that need more investigation. For instance, all of the CEAs described in this review found that EET for high-grade dysplasia is optimal, indicating the robustness of that finding. Through sensitivity analyses, CEAs also identify the key remaining questions that must be answered in order to provide strong recommendations for clinical care and direct investigators to pursue research in areas where further empirical data are required to determine optimal strategies. For instance, the sensitivity analyses for CEAs regarding Cytosponge and other tissue biomarker assays illustrate the need to validate test characteristics across multiple independent populations to ensure their results are generalizable to the entirety of the US and global populations. Future CEAs are particularly needed to address screening strategies stratified by risk of esophageal adenocarcinoma, the role of chemoprevention in the setting of EET, and the role of surveillance following EET.

SUMMARY

The authors conducted a review of cost-effectiveness analyses in management of Barrett's esophagus, identifying which clinical management strategies should be incorporated into standard clinical care and also identifying which strategies need additional empirical data.

CLINICS CARE POINTS

- Older men with chronic symptoms of gastroesophageal reflux should be offered endoscopic screening.
- Men with nondysplastic Barrett's esophagus should undergo surveillance every 3 years and women likely every 5 years.
- Patients found to have high-grade dysplasia or T1a adenocarcinoma should undergo EET.
- Patients with T1b adenocarcinoma can be considered for EET.
- Patients with low-grade dysplasia likely should undergo EET if it is confirmed on second endoscopy after 8 weeks of high-dose acid suppression therapy.

DISCLOSURE

Research effort provided for J.H. Rubenstein and J.M. Inadomi by the National Institutes for Health (U01CA152926, U01CA199336, U54CA163059). J.H. Rubenstein has served as a consultant to the American Gastroenterological Association Institute for work related to TissueCypher. J.M. Inadomi is on the scientific advisory board of Cernostics, which developed and produces TissueCypher.

REFERENCES

1. Codipilly DC, Chandar AK, Singh S, et al. The Effect of Endoscopic Surveillance in Patients With Barrett's Esophagus: A Systematic Review and Meta-analysis. Gastroenterology 2018;154:2068–86.e5.
2. Ubel PA, Hirth RA, Chernew ME, et al. What is the price of life and why doesn't it increase at the rate of inflation? Arch Intern Med 2003;163:1637–41.
3. Saxena N, Inadomi JM. Effectiveness and Cost-Effectiveness of Endoscopic Screening and Surveillance. Gastrointest Endosc Clin N Am 2017;27:397–421.
4. Chu JN, Choi J, Tramontano A, et al. Surgical vs Endoscopic Management of T1 Esophageal Adenocarcinoma: A Modeling Decision Analysis. Clin Gastroenterol Hepatol 2018;16:392–400.e7.
5. Esteban JM, Gonzalez-Carro P, Gornals JB, et al. Economic evaluation of endoscopic radiofrequency ablation for the treatment of dysplastic Barrett's esophagus in Spain. Rev Esp Enferm Dig 2018;110:145–54.
6. Filby A, Taylor M, Lipman G, et al. Cost-effectiveness analysis of endoscopic eradication therapy for treatment of high-grade dysplasia in Barrett's esophagus. J Comp Eff Res 2017;6:425–36.
7. Honing J, Kievit W, Bookelaar J, et al. Endosheath ultrathin transnasal endoscopy is a cost-effective method for screening for Barrett's esophagus in patients with GERD symptoms. Gastrointest Endosc 2019;89:712–22.e3.
8. Omidvari AH, Ali A, Hazelton WD, et al. Optimizing Management of Patients with Barrett's Esophagus and Low-grade or No Dysplasia Based On Comparative Modeling: Optimizing Barrett's esophagus management. Clin Gastroenterol Hepatol 2020;18(9):1961–9.

9. Kroep S, Heberle CR, Curtius K, et al. Radiofrequency Ablation of Barrett's Esophagus Reduces Esophageal Adenocarcinoma Incidence and Mortality in a Comparative Modeling Analysis. Clin Gastroenterol Hepatol 2017;15:1471–4.
10. Heberle CR, Omidvari AH, Ali A, et al. Cost Effectiveness of Screening Patients With Gastroesophageal Reflux Disease for Barrett's Esophagus With a Minimally Invasive Cell Sampling Device. Clin Gastroenterol Hepatol 2017;15: 1397–1404 e7.
11. CISNET Esophageal Cancer Model Profiles. Available at: https://cisnet.cancer.gov/esophagus/profiles.html. Accessed May 1, 2018.
12. Pohl H, Sonnenberg A, Strobel S, et al. Endoscopic versus surgical therapy for early cancer in Barrett's esophagus: a decision analysis. Gastrointest Endosc 2009;70:623–31.
13. Inadomi JM, Somsouk M, Madanick RD, et al. A cost-utility analysis of ablative therapy for Barrett's esophagus. Gastroenterology 2009;136:2101–14.
14. Hur C, Choi SE, Rubenstein JH, et al. The cost effectiveness of radiofrequency ablation for Barrett's esophagus. Gastroenterology 2012;143:567–75.
15. Shaheen NJ, Overholt BF, Sampliner RE, et al. Durability of radiofrequency ablation in Barrett's esophagus with dysplasia. Gastroenterology 2011;141:460–8.
16. Wani S, Rubenstein JH, Vieth M, et al. Diagnosis and Management of Low-Grade Dysplasia in Barrett's Esophagus: Expert Review From the Clinical Practice Updates Committee of the American Gastroenterological Association. Gastroenterology 2016;151:822–35.
17. Gupta N, Bansal A, Wani SB, et al. Endoscopy for upper GI cancer screening in the general population: a cost-utility analysis. Gastrointest Endosc 2011;74: 610–24.e2.
18. Benaglia T, Sharples LD, Fitzgerald RC, et al. Health benefits and cost effectiveness of endoscopic and nonendoscopic cytosponge screening for Barrett's esophagus. Gastroenterology 2013;144:62–73.
19. Jankowski JAZ, de Caestecker J, Love SB, et al. Esomeprazole and aspirin in Barrett's oesophagus (AspECT): a randomised factorial trial. Lancet 2018;392: 400–8.
20. Hur C, Nishioka NS, Gazelle GS. Cost-effectiveness of aspirin chemoprevention for Barrett's esophagus. J Natl Cancer Inst 2004;96:316–25.
21. Kastelein F, van Olphen S, Steyerberg EW, et al. Surveillance in patients with long-segment Barrett's oesophagus: a cost-effectiveness analysis. Gut 2014; 64(6):864–71.
22. Gordon LG, Mayne GC, Hirst NG, et al. Cost-effectiveness of endoscopic surveillance of non-dysplastic Barrett's esophagus. Gastrointest Endosc 2014;79: 242–56.e6.
23. Hao J, Critchley-Thorne R, Diehl DL, et al. A Cost-Effectiveness Analysis Of An Adenocarcinoma Risk Prediction Multi-Biomarker Assay For Patients With Barrett's Esophagus. Clinicoecon Outcomes Res 2019;11:623–35.
24. Critchley-Thorne RJ, Duits LC, Prichard JW, et al. A Tissue Systems Pathology Assay for High-Risk Barrett's Esophagus. Cancer epidemiology, biomarkers & prevention : a publication of the American Association for Cancer Research. cosponsored by the. Am Soc Prev Oncol 2016;25:958–68.
25. Gerson LB, Groeneveld PW, Triadafilopoulos G. Cost-effectiveness model of endoscopic screening and surveillance in patients with gastroesophageal reflux disease. Clin Gastroenterol Hepatol 2004;2:868–79.

Advanced Imaging and Sampling in Barrett's Esophagus

Artificial Intelligence to the Rescue?

Maarten R. Struyvenberg, MD[a], Albert J. de Groof, MD[a], Jacques J. Bergman, MD, PhD[a], Fons van der Sommen, PhD[b], Peter H.N. de With, PhD[b], Vani J.A. Konda, MD[c], Wouter L. Curvers, MD, PhD[d,*]

KEYWORDS

- Barrett's esophagus • Early neoplasia • Endoscopy • Artificial intelligence

KEY POINTS

- Endoscopic detection of early Barrett's esophagus (BE) neoplasia can be improved via usage of high-definition endoscopes, structured BE surveillance protocols, and web-based teaching tools.
- Currently, advanced imaging techniques do not significantly increase the diagnostic yield of BE neoplasia compared with high-resolution endoscopy using high-definition white light endoscopy with random quadratic biopsies.
- Artificial intelligence systems have the potential to overcome the endoscopist-dependent limitations by serving as a second-reader using real-time image interpretation.
- In the future, wide field sampling techniques aided by artificial intelligence may risk stratify patients for more patient-tailored surveillance strategies.

INTRODUCTION

Barrett's esophagus (BE) is a known risk factor for the development of esophageal adenocarcinoma. Therefore, patients with BE undergo regular endoscopic surveillance, in order to detect neoplasia at an early stage. However, these early neoplastic

[a] Department of Gastroenterology and Hepatology, Amsterdam UMC, University of Amsterdam, Meibergdreef 9, 1105 AZ Amsterdam, the Netherlands; [b] Department of Electrical Engineering, VCA group, Eindhoven University of Technology, Groene Loper 19, 5612 AP Eindhoven, the Netherlands; [c] Department of Gastroenterology and Hepatology, Baylor University Medical Center, 3500 Gaston Ave, Dallas, TX 75246, USA; [d] Department of Gastroenterology and Hepatology, Catharina Hospital Eindhoven, Michelangelolaan 2, 5623 EJ Eindhoven, the Netherlands

* Corresponding author. Department of Gastroenterology and Hepatology, Catharina Hospital Eindhoven, Michelangelolaan 2, Eindhoven 5623 EJ, the Netherlands.

E-mail address: wouter.curvers@catharinaziekenhuis.nl

Gastrointest Endoscopy Clin N Am 31 (2021) 91–103
https://doi.org/10.1016/j.giec.2020.08.006
1052-5157/21/

lesions are often subtle, focally distributed, and poorly visible endoscopically. In addition, BE surveillance, consisting of inspection with white light endoscopy (WLE) and quadratic random biopsies, suffers from sampling error of random biopsies, and early lesions are often missed, as endoscopists rarely encounter early neoplastic lesions.[1]

To increase BE neoplasia detection, many new endoscopic imaging and sampling techniques have been developed over the past decades. These techniques include magnification endoscopy, chromoendoscopy, optical chromoscopy, optical coherence tomography, molecular imaging, and sampling techniques such as wide-area transepithelial sampling with computer-assisted 3-dimensional analysis (WATS-3D). However, none of these techniques have truly exceeded the Preservation and Incorporation of Valuable endoscopic Innovations (PIVI) criteria for BE neoplasia detection (per patient sensitivity $\geq$90%, negative predictive value $\geq$98% and specificity $\geq$80%) in large prospective trials.[2] Furthermore, BE surveillance still suffers from challenges of standard diagnosis, both in terms of endoscopy and histology, and challenges of imaging-based detection regarding technical limitations and observer variation.

Over the past years, artificial intelligence (AI) has gained popularity in endoscopy, as it has the ability to automatically recognize informative patterns in imagery. AI is not limited by a long learning curve or variation in intra- and interobserver agreement. In addition, AI does not suffer from fatigue in contrast to endoscopists who may be affected by the time of the endoscopy, their mental state, time pressure, or cumbersome procedures. Recent studies have used AI for colon polyp classification and detection of BE neoplasia, showing promising diagnostic performance.[3,4] Moreover, AI may also be used to increase reproducibility in histologic diagnosis (ie, low-grade dysplasia) without the use of multiple expert BE pathologists, for improved analysis of sampling techniques such as WATS-3D and for risk-stratification of early neoplasia progression using computer models. Therefore, in the future, AI may change gastrointestinal practice.

In this review, the authors discuss the recent advances and challenges of advanced imaging and sampling techniques for the detection of BE neoplasia and subsequently provide the construct for how AI may be implemented to overcome some of the deficiencies associated with BE surveillance.

ARTIFICIAL INTELLIGENCE

AI is a wide branch of computer sciences that emphasizes on the development of intelligent machines that mimic human behavior. Over the last decade, AI has been applied in self-driving cars, facial recognition, natural language processing, and medicine. AI aims to develop a generic form of autonomous learning and has shown promising results in medical fields such as pathology, radiology, and dermatology.[5–7] To assist in the interpretation of medical imagery, computer-aided detection (CAD) systems are trained to autonomously learn to distinguish features and are not hampered by human perceptual biases. Especially via deep learning techniques with artificial neural networks, these CAD systems offer many potential advantages for the endoscopic practice.[8]

When interpreting medical imagery, an important distinction is made between CAD and computer-aided diagnosis (CADx). CAD algorithms are produced to *detect* pathology (ie, detection of esophageal cancer), in contrast to CADx algorithms that are developed to *classify* pathology (ie, characterization as nondysplastic or neoplastic). Another applications in the field of BE surveillance in the future may be the development of risk stratification algorithms for neoplastic progression based on clinical patient characteristics in combination with endoscopic and histopathological information. In addition to CAD and CADx, AI can also be used for improving or monitoring endoscopic quality, for example, by indicating the amount of surface area that was inadequately visualized or missed during a colonoscopy or EGD.[9,10] This quality assurance may turn out to be of vital importance, as AI technologies can only detect what is shown to them and cannot make up for suboptimal preparation or poor imaging by the endoscopist.

Although the introduction of artificial neural networks in endoscopy sounds very promising, its application is associated with pitfalls such as overfitting and selection bias. To address these scientific problems, researchers should be encouraged to provide a complete description of the data acquisition process and reduce the risk of overfitting by using multiple large and heterogeneous datasets, preferably collected in different studies. Furthermore, patient privacy and data ownership form a challenge in AI, as there is currently no standardized understanding of legislation. Finally, in clinical practice, AI tools may also lead to an increase in the amount of false-positive predictions, resulting in, for example, the resection of many clinically irrelevant and benign polyps. As a consequence, this may increase the length of endoscopic procedures, medical costs, and patient burden.

In the future, these fast and autonomic CAD systems may revolutionize endoscopic practice. Yet, studies reporting on the implementation of clinically relevant improved outcomes of AI in daily endoscopic practice are rare. Therefore, in vivo clinical testing of new AI tools in a large controlled setting should be performed before clinical implementation.

ENDOSCOPIC IMAGING: WHITE LIGHT ENDOSCOPY AND OPTICAL CHROMOSCOPY

Background

The standard of care in endoscopic BE surveillance is high-resolution endoscopy using high-definition white light endoscopy (HD-WLE) with random biopsy analysis for detection of dysplasia. The endoscopic detection of early BE neoplasia is challenging however, because early lesions are mostly subtle and flat. Therefore, preprocessing optical chromoscopy techniques, including narrow band imaging (NBI; Olympus Corp, Tokyo, Japan), blue light imaging (BLI; Fujifilm Co., Kanagawa, Japan), and optical enhancement (PENTAX Medical, Tokyo, Japan) have been developed, which allow for enhanced interpretation of mucosal and vascular patterns in patients with BE.

Recent Advances, Potential Applications, and Challenges of Artificial Intelligence

Detection

In community hospitals, the prevalence of BE neoplasia is low (<5.0%), and therefore endoscopists are often not familiar with the endoscopic appearance of early neoplastic lesions in BE.[1,11] The lack of endoscopic recognition of early BE neoplasia is therefore often the rate-limiting factor. This endoscopic recognition of early neoplasia by endoscopists may be improved by the use of high-definition white light endoscopy and systematic surveillance protocols. Furthermore, web-based teaching tools (ie, the BORN module) have demonstrated improved detection and delineation of early BE neoplasia in nonexpert endoscopists and may further improve BE surveillance in the future when universally adapted.[12]

In addition, 2 recent meta-analyses evaluating optical chromoscopy for surveillance of nondysplastic BE reported that NBI-targeted biopsies can be incorporated into routine clinical practice, at least when performed by endoscopists with expertise in advanced imaging techniques, as the PIVI thresholds were met.[13,14] However, these studies were performed by experts endoscopists in tertiary care hospitals where the prevalence of neoplasia was high and results were evaluated per image as opposed to per patient. Given these limitations, guidelines currently do not recommend replacing HD-WLE examination with random quadratic biopsies for optical chromoscopy evaluation with targeted biopsies only.

To address these pitfalls and improve detection of BE neoplasia using HD-WLE and optical chromoscopy techniques, AI forms a very promising tool. CAD systems have already shown high diagnostic accuracy for the detection of BE neoplasia using these techniques.[15,16] A recent study using HD-WLE overview images showed an accuracy, sensitivity, and specificity of 86%, 90%, and 83% for the detection of BE neoplasia using a deep-learning CAD system.[4] More importantly, the CAD system outperformed 53 endoscopists who evaluated the same images. Subsequently, the performance of this CAD system was evaluated in a pilot study during live endoscopic procedures and demonstrated high accuracy for the detection of BE neoplasia with only a small number of false-positive predictions.[17] **Fig. 1** provides different image examples of how the CAD algorithm was applied during the live clinical procedures.

Characterization

Optical chromoscopy techniques may be used for more enhanced inspection of the mucosal and vascular pattern characteristics, as shown in **Fig. 2**. However, recent studies evaluating diagnostic criteria for BE characterization have shown disappointing outcomes.[18,19] The Barrett's International NBI Group developed a consensus-driven simplified NBI classification system for identification of BE neoplasia, resulting in a sensitivity of 80%, specificity of 88%, and a substantial

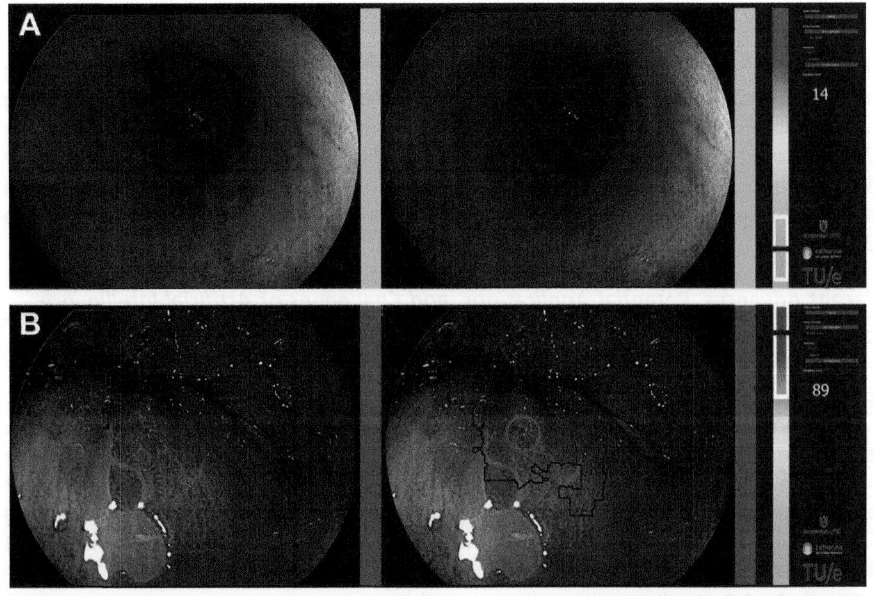

Fig. 1. Visualization of the graphical user interface of the computer-aided detection (CAD) algorithm. (*A*). Nondysplastic Barrett's segment, with a correct CAD algorithm prediction indicated using green bars (*B*). Neoplastic Barrett's segment with a correct CAD algorithm prediction indicated using red bars. The computers' delineation is shown in black and the preferred biopsy location using a red circle.

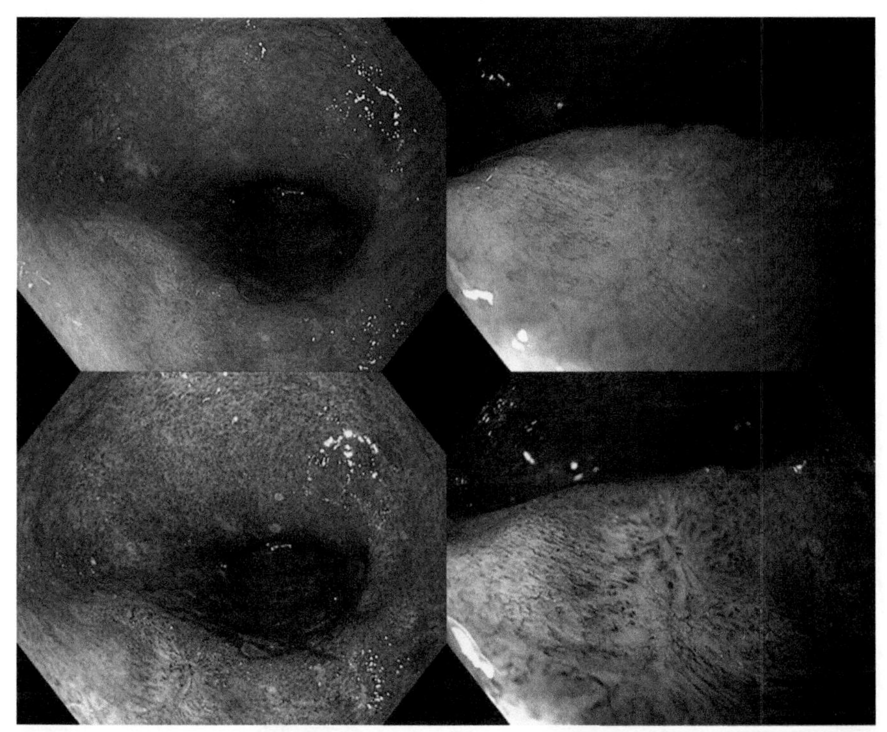

Fig. 2. Corresponding white light endoscopy (WLE) and optical chromoscopy overview and magnification images of an early neoplastic lesion in Barrett's esophagus.

interobserver agreement (kappa = 0.68).[20] However, only expert endoscopists evaluated these high-quality images, and images containing low-grade dysplasia and erosive esophagitis were excluded. Evaluation of these diverse NBI classifications systems is therefore suboptimal and the question remains if endoscopists are able to address the limitations of variation in intra- and interobserver agreement or AI should fill this gap.

In the near future, it is expected that most of the early neoplastic lesions in BE will be detected by HD-WLE in combination with CAD systems. However, in order to reduce the number of false-positive predictions associated with AI, the authors envision automated characterization of BE using optical chromoendoscopy in combination with CAD, to be of importance. Recently, improved characterization of BE was shown when NBI was supplemented by an AI tool[16] on still images, yet future studies should confirm these preliminary results.

Treatment decisions

Optical chromoscopy allows for enhanced visualization of the subtle differences in mucosal relief, including subtle elevations and depressions relative to the normal-appearing flat surrounding mucosa, compared with HD-WLE (**Fig. 3**). A recent study reported that BLI provided an improved visualization of surface relief and Paris classification compared with HD-WLE and that optical chromoscopy ensured more reliable delineation of BE neoplasia.[21]

AI might also be a promising ad-on for improving the evaluation of surface relief and allowing an enhanced delineation of the demarcation line before endoscopic resection.

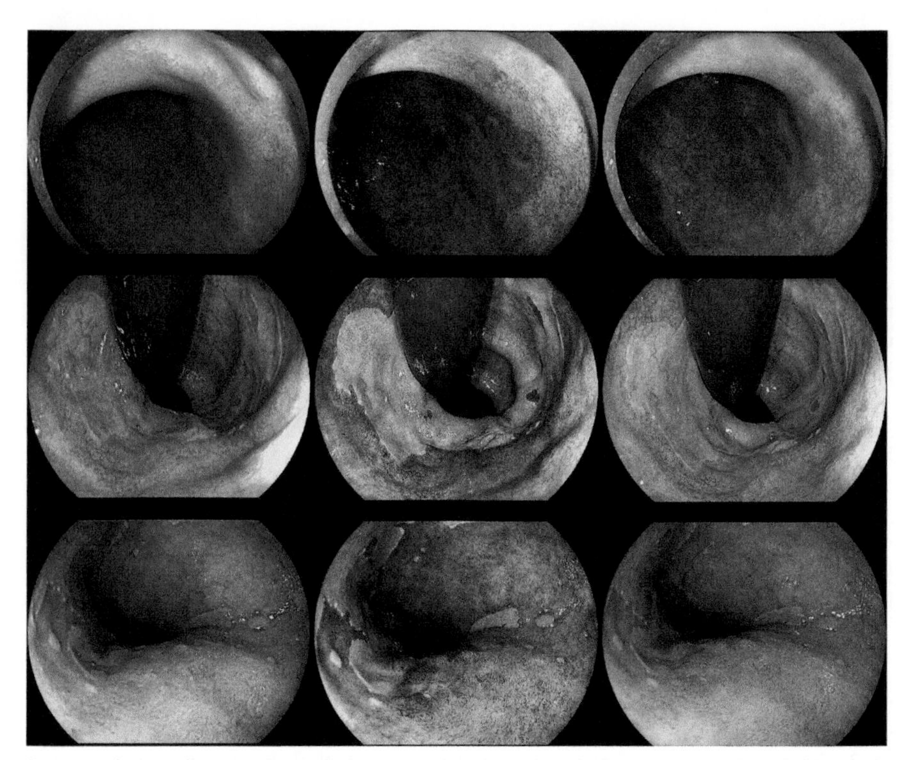

Fig. 3. Early neoplastic Barrett's lesions visualized in white light endoscopy (WLE), blue light imaging (BLI), and linked color imaging (LCI).

Future Role for Artificial Intelligence

AI systems have the potential to overcome the endoscopist-dependent limitations related to poor intra- and interobserver agreement. However, AI cannot make up for poor preparation or poor imaging, so quality improvement is another important potential area for AI. This quality improvement may increase the detection rates of both endoscopists and AI tools. In the near future of BE surveillance, the authors envision that most of the early neoplastic lesions will be detected by HD-WLE in combination with CAD systems. However, large prospective studies should investigate the real-time diagnostic performance of these CAD systems in clinical practice.

VOLUMETRIC LASER ENDOMICROSCOPY

Background

Volumetric laser endomicroscopy (VLE) is an advanced imaging technique that is based on optical coherence tomography. This balloon-based technique creates high-resolution cross-sectional images of the esophagus based on differences in optical scattering properties of different tissue structures,[22] as shown in **Fig. 4**. Using an imaging probe centered by a pliable balloon, a circumferential scan through 6 cm is made visualizing the esophageal mucosa and subsurface layers up to 3 mm deep with a near-microscopic resolution of 7 μm. In 96 seconds, a 3-dimensional esophageal scan is created, and subsequently suspicious areas in a BE segment can be targeted using the VLE laser marking tool, enabling biopsy correlation.[23] Therefore, this

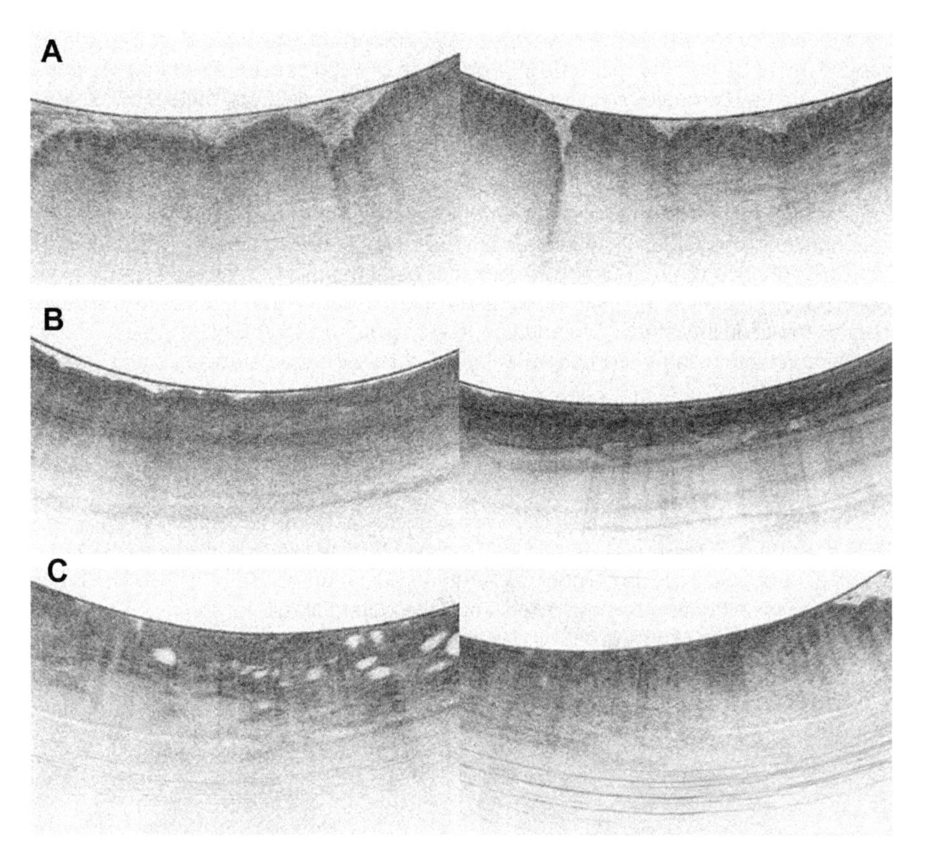

Fig. 4. Volumetric laser endomicroscopy (VLE) images (*A*). Gastric mucosa with the presence of a clear gastric pit-and-crypt pattern (*B*). Nondysplastic Barrett's esophagus with the presence of regular mucosal layering (*C*). Early Barrett's neoplasia showing the abnormal VLE features, multiple irregular glands, lack of mucosal layering, and high surface signal intensity.

technique has the potential to improve the detection of early BE neoplasia and eliminate the problem of sampling errors associated with random biopsies.

Recent Advances, Potential Applications, and Challenges of Artificial Intelligence

Detection and characterization

Until recently, most VLE studies have focused on the development of ex vivo VLE reviewing criteria for the detection of BE neoplasia, including the VLE-DA,[22] OCT-SI,[24] and the VLE-prediction score.[25] Abnormal VLE features were identified, which produced the highest likelihood for presence of BE neoplasia. Subsequent validation studies of these diagnostic VLE criteria demonstrated a high interobserver agreement and high diagnostic accuracy among VLE experts.[26,27] However, no histopathology correlation was provided by VLE laser marking, only preselected still images were assessed, and VLE images of low-grade dysplasia were not included. Another challenge for endoscopists include difficulty of differentiating normal submucosal structures from abnormal epithelial features. The true potential for VLE is detection of "endoscopically invisible" low- and high-grade dysplasia in a surveillance setting;

this has, however, not yet been reported. One important limitation of VLE in clinical practice might be that the real-time interpretation of 1200 consecutive circumferential VLE frames may be challenging for endoscopists in the endoscopy suite. To aid endoscopists, the VLE-system has recently been upgraded by incorporating an Intelligent Real-time Image Segmentation (IRIS) tool for enhanced and more systematic interpretation of VLE features,[28,29] as shown in **Fig. 5**. This technique uses computer-aided image enhancement to improve the endoscopic recognition of dysplastic VLE features, including highlighting glandular features and surface intensity. IRIS software may also enhance the real-time delineation of early neoplastic lesions, especially via improved appreciation of the demarcation line to better appreciate the epithelial area, as shown in this study.[29] In addition, CAD algorithms in VLE have already shown promising results using VLE images,[30,31] yet in vivo validation studies should confirm these findings.

Treatment decisions

VLE might also be used to guide endoscopic treatment, including radiofrequency ablation (RFA) and cryotherapy, by measuring the Barrett's epithelial thickness (BET).[32] In theory, there is a certain BET threshold that predicts failure of RFA and that this threshold may be higher for cryotherapy than for RFA. However, future studies are investigating this hypothesis and the potential role for AI.

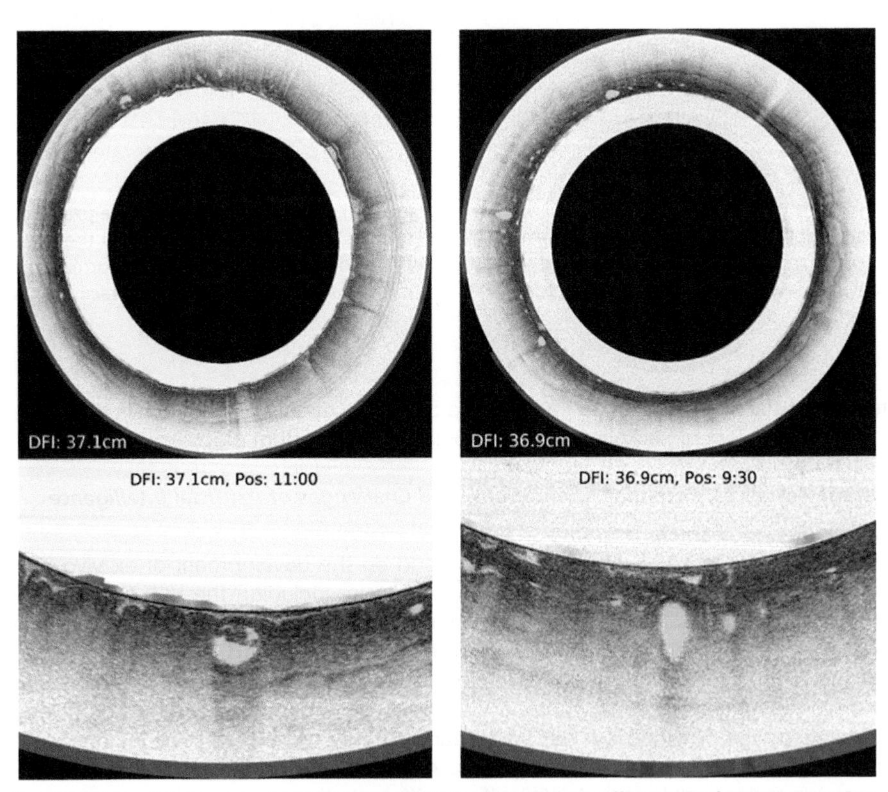

Fig. 5. Volumetric laser endomicroscopy (VLE) images with Intelligent Real-time Image Segmentation (IRIS). The abnormal VLE feature irregular glands are highlighted in blue, lack of mucosal layering in orange, and increased surface signal intensity in purple.

Future Role for Artificial Intelligence

The real-time diagnostic performance of VLE users for the detection of dysplastic BE is not adequately reported yet. Future studies should investigate the incremental yield of dysplasia detection in BE using VLE, VLE aided with AI, and compare this with a standardized random biopsy protocol. Furthermore, VLE in adjunct with AI may play an important role in more enhanced appreciation of the demarcation line and thus improved delineation of early neoplastic lesions. Next, VLE algorithms may also guide endoscopic treatment, yet this area needs further exploration. Another similar imaging technique with potential for implementation of AI is called tethered capsule endomicroscopy, a novel technique that rapidly acquires microscopic images of the entire esophagus in unsedated subjects.[33] In the future, such a screening tool may be applied in a primary care setting in patients who are at risk of BE (eg, age >55 years, longstanding acid reflux). This device should then preferably be used in combination with CAD algorithms for automated image interpretation, to refer patients for endoscopy if the result is suspicious for BE.

SAMPLING TECHNIQUES

Background

In absence of visible abnormalities in a Barrett's segment, random quadratic biopsies are obtained every 1 to 2 cm for risk stratification purposes. This Seattle biopsy protocol, however, only samples around 5% of the entire Barrett's segment, resulting in significant sampling error.[34] Therefore, wide field sampling of the BE segment has gained popularity. These techniques aim to risk stratify patients, reduce unnecessary endoscopies in patients with low risk of progression to BE neoplasia, and vice-versa select the high-risk group for more patient-tailored surveillance strategies. Another possibility for risk stratification is to improve conventional histologic assessment of biopsy specimens and usage of biomarker panels that may predict neoplastic progression before morphologic changes become visible for histologic assessment by pathologists. In this section, the authors primarily discuss the wide field sampling techniques.

Recent Advances, Potential Applications, and Challenges of Artificial Intelligence

Detection and treatment decisions

WATS-3D is a brush sampling technique that enables to sample an extensive area of the BE segment.[35] This brush technique is designed to allow for a transepithelial specimen of the esophageal mucosa in contrast to brush cytology. The addition of computer-assisted 3D tissue analysis, using AI algorithms, has made it possible to identify potentially abnormal cells based on cellular morphology and molecular diagnostics and subsequently display the cells on the glass slide.[36] WATS-3D in combination with random biopsies has shown increased detection rates of BE pathology ranging from indefinite/low-grade displasia to cancer in a multicenter community-based study.[37] In a multicenter randomized trial with a referral BE population, WATS-3D increased the detection of BE neoplasia approximately 4 times compared with the Seattle protocol.[36] Although WATS-3D may reduce sampling error during BE surveillance, the true clinical relevance remains unknown. In particular, it remains unclear how to interpret discrepancies between the standard biopsy diagnosis by a pathologist and the WATS-3D diagnosis.

A novel, less-invasive, and low-cost sampling technique called the Cytosponge provides a means of sampling the esophagus without the need for a sedated endoscopic procedure. A capsule on a string can be swallowed and subsequently expands into a sponge in the stomach. Sensitivity and specificity of the Cytosponge for diagnosing BE was around 90% in a primary care setting.[38,39] A recent study has reported that clinical characteristics in combination with a Cytosponge brush analyzed with a molecular biomarker panel was able to accurately identify patients with nondysplatic BE.[40] However, the analysis of a large variety of biomarkers is currently quite cumbersome and expensive. To account for these pitfalls, and to allow for a more reliable and faster analysis of multiple biomarkers, AI may be implemented to risk stratify patients and to predict neoplastic progression. In the future, patients who are at risk of BE (eg, age >55 years, long-standing acid reflux) may undergo screening with this tool. In Cytosponge-negative cases or low neoplastic progression risk, screening could be repeated after 3 to 5 years or even discontinued. In patients with a high neoplastic progression risk, an endoscopic procedure with possible endoscopic resection or ablation may be performed. This risk stratification would significantly reduce the amount of unnecessary endoscopies and shift the screening and surveillance of BE toward a primary care, nonendoscopic setting.

Future Role for Artificial Intelligence

In the future, AI may help to reduce intra- and interobserver variation in both endoscopists and pathologists. In particular, AI has proved to be effective in WATS-3D sampling, to allow for a more reliable assessment of transepithelial specimens. Larger areas of the BE segment may thus be analyzed in a shorter amount of time and with a higher degree of diagnostic certainty. Finally, a patient-tailored approach using clinical information in combination with endoscopic, histopathological, and biomarker information analyzed by AI algorithms may possibly change the endoscopic practice.

DISCUSSION

Because the current BE surveillance protocol is suboptimal and suffers from sampling error of random biopsies and a high miss-rate of early neoplastic lesions, many new endoscopic imaging and sampling techniques have been developed. None of these techniques, however, have exceeded the PIVI criteria for BE neoplasia detection in large prospective trials. In fact, these techniques have led to an increase in the amount of visible information, yet endoscopists inevitably suffer from variations in intra- and interobserver agreement.

AI systems have the potential to overcome these endoscopist-dependent limitations by serving as a second-reader using real-time image interpretation. In addition, new AI tools may improve and monitor endoscopic quality of endoscopists, which subsequently may result in higher neoplastic detection rates. However, the enthusiasm for the potential of AI should be tempered with caution by avoiding a hasty introduction of unvalidated AI tools in the endoscopy suite and promote proper validation, training, and quality assurances. New guidelines need to be formulated concerning ethical considerations, data ownership, and external validation of diagnostic performance before clinical implementation.

In the future, most neoplastic lesions will be detected by a combination of targeted biopsies guided by a combination of HD-WLE and optical chromoscopy. Algorithms will assist during the endoscopy by monitoring and improving the endoscopic quality and detect lesions that are initially missed by endoscopists. Subsequently, patients with nonvisible flat dysplasia will be identified by wide-field sampling techniques instead of random biopsies. In addition, noninvasive and low-cost screening tools supplemented by AI may even reduce the amount of unnecessary endoscopies and shift the screening and surveillance of BE toward a primary care, nonendoscopic, setting.

CLINICS CARE POINTS

- Endoscopic detection of early BE neoplasia can be improved via usage of high-definition endoscopes, structured BE surveillance protocols, and web-based teaching tools.
- Current guidelines do not recommend replacing the combination of HD-WLE with random biopsy analysis for optical chromoscopy examination with targeted biopsies only.
- AI systems have the potential to overcome the endoscopist-dependent limitations related to poor intra- and interobserver agreement.
- AI may be used for improving or monitoring endoscopic quality, for example, by indicating the amount of surface area that was not visualized during a colonoscopy or EGD.
- In the future, wide field sampling techniques with computer-assisted analysis may risk stratify patients to spare unnecessary endoscopies in low-risk patients and select the high-risk group for more patient-tailored surveillance strategies.

DISCLOSURE

M.R. Struyvenberg, A.J. de Groof, F. van der Sommen, W.L. Curvers, P.H.N. de With: none declared. V.J.A. Konda: Pentax (grant). J.J. Bergman: Fujifilm, NinePoint Medical (research support); Fujifilm (speaking fees).

REFERENCES

1. Schölvinck DW, van der Meulen K, Bergman JJGHM, et al. Detection of lesions in dysplastic Barrett's esophagus by community and expert endoscopists. Endoscopy 2017;49(2):113–20.
2. Sharma P, Savides TJ, Canto MI, et al. The American society for gastrointestinal endoscopy PIVI (preservation and incorporation of valuable endoscopic innovations) on imaging in Barrett's Esophagus. Gastrointest Endosc 2012;76(2):252–4.
3. Urban G, Tripathi P, Alkayali T, et al. Deep learning localizes and identifies polyps in real time with 96% accuracy in screening colonoscopy. Gastroenterology 2018; 155(4):1069–78.e8.
4. de Groof AJ, Struyvenberg MR, van der Putten J, et al. Deep-learning system detects neoplasia in patients with barrett's esophagus with higher accuracy than endoscopists in a multi-step training and validation study with benchmarking. Gastroenterology 2019;158(4):915–29.e4.
5. Lakhani P, Sundaram B. Deep learning at chest radiography: automated classification of pulmonary tuberculosis by using convolutional neural networks. Radiology 2017;284(2):574–82.
6. Ehteshami Bejnordi B, Veta M, Johannes van Diest P, et al. Diagnostic assessment of deep learning algorithms for detection of lymph node metastases in women with breast cancer. JAMA 2017;318(22):2199–210.
7. Esteva A, Kuprel B, Novoa RA, et al. Dermatologist-level classification of skin cancer with deep neural networks. Nature 2017;542(7639):115–8.
8. van der Sommen F, Curvers WL, Nagengast WB. Novel developments in endoscopic mucosal imaging. Gastroenterology 2018;154(7):1876–86.
9. Zhou J, Wu L, Wan X, et al. A novel artificial intelligence system for the assessment of bowel preparation (with video). Gastrointest Endosc 2019;91(2):428–35.e2.

10. Wu L, Zhang J, Zhou W, et al. Randomised controlled trial of WISENSE, a real-time quality improving system for monitoring blind spots during esophagogastroduodenoscopy. Gut 2019;68(12):2161–9.
11. Hvid-Jensen F, Pedersen L, Drewes AM, et al. Incidence of adenocarcinoma among patients with Barrett's esophagus. N Engl J Med 2011;365(15):1375–83.
12. Bergman JJGHM, de Groof AJ, Pech O, et al. An interactive web-based educational tool improves detection and delineation of barrett's esophagus-related neoplasia. Gastroenterology 2019;156(5):1299–308.e3.
13. Song J, Zhang J, Wang J, et al. Meta-analysis of the effects of endoscopy with narrow band imaging in detecting dysplasia in Barrett's esophagus. Dis Esophagus 2014;28(6):560–6.
14. ASGE Technology Committee, Thosani N, Abu Dayyeh BK, Sharma P, et al. ASGE technology committee systematic review and meta-analysis assessing the ASGE preservation and incorporation of valuable endoscopic innovations thresholds for adopting real-time imaging-assisted endoscopic targeted biopsy during endoscopic surveillance. Gastrointest Endosc 2016;83(4):684–98.e7.
15. De GJ, Van Der SF, Van Der PJ, et al. The Argos project : the development of a computer-aided detection system to improve detection of Barrett ' s neoplasia on white light endoscopy. United European Gastroenterol J 2019;7(4):538–47.
16. Ebigbo A, Mendel R, Probst A, et al. Computer-aided diagnosis using deep learning in the evaluation of early oesophageal adenocarcinoma. Gut 2018;68:1143–5.
17. de Groof AJ, Struyvenberg MR, Fockens KN, et al. Deep learning algorithm detection of Barrett's neoplasia with high accuracy during live endoscopic procedures: a pilot study (with video). Gastrointest Endosc 2020;91(6):1242–50.
18. Curvers WL, Bohmer CJ, Mallant-Hent RC, et al. Mucosal morphology in Barrett's esophagus: interobserver agreement and role of narrow band imaging. Endoscopy 2008;40(10):799–805.
19. Curvers W, Baak L, Kiesslich R, et al. Chromoendoscopy and narrow-band imaging compared with high-resolution magnification endoscopy in Barrett's esophagus. Gastroenterology 2008;134(3):670–9.
20. Sharma P, Bergman JJGHM, Goda K, et al. Development and validation of a classification system to identify high-grade dysplasia and esophageal adenocarcinoma in barrett's esophagus using narrow-band imaging. Gastroenterology 2016;150(3):591–8.
21. de Groof AJ, Swager A-F, Pouw RE, et al. Blue-light imaging has an additional value to white-light endoscopy in visualization of early Barrett's neoplasia: an international multicenter cohort study. Gastrointest Endosc 2019;89(4):749–58.
22. Leggett CL, Gorospe EC, Chan DK, et al. Comparative diagnostic performance of volumetric laser endomicroscopy and confocal laser endomicroscopy in the detection of dysplasia associated with Barrett's esophagus. Gastrointest Endosc 2016;83(5):880–8.e2.
23. Swager A-F, de Groof AJ, Meijer SL, et al. Feasibility of laser marking in Barrett's esophagus with volumetric laser endomicroscopy: first-in-man pilot study. Gastrointest Endosc 2017;86(3):464–72.
24. Evans JA, Poneros JM, Bouma BE, et al. Optical coherence tomography to identify intramucosal carcinoma and high-grade dysplasia in Barrett's esophagus. Clin Gastroenterol Hepatol 2006;4(1):38–43.
25. Swager A-F, Tearney GJ, Leggett CL, et al. Identification of volumetric laser endomicroscopy features predictive for early neoplasia in Barrett's esophagus using high-quality histological correlation. Gastrointest Endosc 2017;85(5):918–26.e7.

26. Kamboj AK, Kahn A, Wolfsen HC, et al. Volumetric laser endomicroscopy interpretation and feature analysis in dysplastic Barrett's esophagus. J Gastroenterol Hepatol 2018;33(10):1761–5.
27. Trindade AJ, Inamdar S, Smith MS, et al. Volumetric laser endomicroscopy in Barrett's esophagus: interobserver agreement for interpretation of Barrett's esophagus and associated neoplasia among high-frequency users. Gastrointest Endosc 2017;86(1):133–9.
28. Trindade AJ, McKinley MJ, Fan C, et al. Endoscopic surveillance of barrett's esophagus using volumetric laser endomicroscopy with artificial intelligence image enhancement. Gastroenterology 2019;157(2):303–5.
29. Katada C, Pai RK, Fukami N. Comparison of narrow-band imaging, volumetric laser endomicroscopy, and pathologic findings in Barrett's esophagus. VideoGIE 2019;4(7):319–22.
30. Struyvenberg MR, van der Sommen F, Swager AF, et al. Improved Barrett's neoplasia detection using computer-assisted multiframe analysis of volumetric laser endomicroscopy. Dis Esophagus 2019;33(2):1–6.
31. Fonollà R, Scheeve T, Struyvenberg MR, et al. Ensemble of deep convolutional neural networks for classification of early barrett's neoplasia using volumetric laser endomicroscopy. Appl Sci 2019;9(11):2183.
32. Levink IJM, Wolfsen HC, Siersema PD, et al. Measuring Barrett's epithelial thickness with volumetric laser endomicroscopy as a biomarker to guide treatment. Dig Dis Sci 2019;64(6):1579–87.
33. Gora MJ, Quénéhervé L, Carruth RW, et al. Tethered capsule endomicroscopy for microscopic imaging of the esophagus, stomach, and duodenum without sedation in humans (with video). Gastrointest Endosc 2018;88(5):830–40.e3.
34. Abela J-E, Going JJ, Mackenzie JF, et al. Systematic four-quadrant biopsy detects barrett's dysplasia in more patients than nonsystematic biopsy. Am J Gastroenterol 2008;103(4):850–5.
35. Johanson JF, Frakes J, Eisen D, et al. Computer-assisted analysis of abrasive transepithelial brush biopsies increases the effectiveness of esophageal screening: a multicenter prospective clinical trial by the EndoCDx collaborative group. Dig Dis Sci 2011;56(3):767–72.
36. Vennalaganti PR, Kaul V, Wang KK, et al. Increased detection of Barrett's esophagus–associated neoplasia using wide-area trans-epithelial sampling: a multicenter, prospective, randomized trial. Gastrointest Endosc 2018;87(2):348–55.
37. Smith MS, Ikonomi E, Bhuta R, et al. Wide-area transepithelial sampling with computer-assisted 3-dimensional analysis (WATS) markedly improves detection of esophageal dysplasia and Barrett's esophagus: analysis from a prospective multicenter community-based study. Dis Esophagus 2019;32(3):doy099.
38. Kadri SR, Lao-Sirieix P, O'Donovan M, et al. Acceptability and accuracy of a non-endoscopic screening test for Barrett's oesophagus in primary care: cohort study. BMJ 2010;341(sep10 1):c4372.
39. Ross-Innes CS, Debiram-Beecham I, O'Donovan M, et al. Evaluation of a minimally invasive cell sampling device coupled with assessment of trefoil factor 3 expression for diagnosing barrett's esophagus: a multi-center case–control study. PLOS Med 2015;12(1):e1001780. Franco EL, ed.
40. Ross-Innes CS, Chettouh H, Achilleos A, et al. Risk stratification of Barrett's oesophagus using a non-endoscopic sampling method coupled with a biomarker panel: a cohort study. Lancet Gastroenterol Hepatol 2017;2(1):23–31.

Advances in Biomarkers for Risk Stratification in Barrett's Esophagus

Rhonda F. Souza, MD*, Stuart Jon Spechler, MD

KEYWORDS

• Dysplasia • Esophageal adenocarcinoma • p53 • Systems biology • Mutational load

KEY POINTS

- The World Health Organization defines a biomarker as "any substance, structure, or process that can be measured in the body or its products and influence or predict the incidence of outcome or disease."
- Dysplasia currently is the primary biomarker used to risk stratify patients with Barrett's esophagus, but dysplasia has a number of considerable limitations in this regard.
- Biomarkers that presently appear most promising based on the availability of multiple published studies corroborating good results and on the commercial availability of the test include immunostaining for p53, TissueCypher, BarreGEN, and wide-area transepithelial sampling with computer-assisted 3-dimensional analysis (WATS^{3D}).
- Presently, only WATS^{3D} has received a conditional recommendation from an American gastrointestinal society as a biomarker for use in screening and surveillance for Barrett's esophagus.

During the past several decades in the United States, the primary strategy for preventing deaths from esophageal adenocarcinoma has been to use endoscopy to screen individuals with gastroesophageal reflux disease (GERD) symptoms for Barrett's esophagus, the metaplasia from which esophageal adenocarcinomas arise, and to enroll patients with Barrett's esophagus in a program of regular endoscopic surveillance in which 4-quadrant "Seattle protocol" biopsy sampling of the metaplastic esophageal mucosa is performed with the intent of detecting curable neoplasia, primarily in the form of dysplasia. The fact that the incidence of esophageal adenocarcinoma in this country has increased more than eightfold during this time period attests to the inadequacy of this strategy,[1] and has been the impetus for studies seeking to identify novel biomarkers that can be used for risk stratification in Barrett's esophagus.

Division of Gastroenterology, Center for Esophageal Diseases, Baylor University Medical Center at Dallas, Center for Esophageal Research, Baylor Scott & White Research Institute, 3500 Gaston Avenue, 2 Hoblitzelle, Suite 250, Dallas, TX 75246, USA
* Corresponding author.
E-mail address: Rhonda.Souza@BSWHealth.org

Gastrointest Endoscopy Clin N Am 31 (2021) 105–115
https://doi.org/10.1016/j.giec.2020.08.007

giendo.theclinics.com

DYSPLASIA AS A BIOMARKER FOR RISK STRATIFICATION

A number of definitions have been proposed for the term "biomarker," but the one perhaps most appropriate when applied to Barrett's esophagus is the World Health Organization's definition of a biomarker as "any substance, structure, or process that can be measured in the body or its products and influence or predict the incidence of outcome or disease."[2] Currently, dysplasia is the primary biomarker used to risk stratify patients with Barrett's esophagus. The rationale is the assumption that cancers in Barrett esophagus evolve through a gradual series of genetic and epigenetic alterations that give the cells growth advantages while also causing morphologic changes in the tissue recognizable as dysplasia, which progresses from low-grade dysplasia to high-grade dysplasia, to intramucosal carcinoma and, ultimately, to invasive adenocarcinoma.[3]

Unfortunately, dysplasia is far from a perfect biomarker for risk stratification in Barrett's esophagus for many reasons. Dysplasia is often patchy in extent and not always associated with visible abnormalities, and so biopsy sampling error can be a major problem when relying on random, Seattle protocol biopsies to identify this lesion. Furthermore, endoscopists frequently do not adhere to the Seattle protocol and take too few biopsy specimens during surveillance endoscopies, thus compounding the problem of biopsy sampling error.[4] Even when an appropriate number of biopsies are taken, technical or processing artifact of the tissue can hinder accurate identification of dysplasia.[5]

Inflammation can induce regenerative changes in the epithelium that can be difficult to distinguish from the histologic changes of low-grade dysplasia.[5] This issue of inflammation mimicking dysplasia is the rationale for the American College of Gastroenterology (ACG) guideline advising against taking biopsies in areas of erosive esophagitis until after intensive antisecretory therapy has healed any mucosal injury.[6] Even in the absence of inflammation, histologic interpretation of dysplasia is challenging. There are no scientifically validated morphologic features to distinguish low-grade dysplasia from high-grade dysplasia and, consequently, there can be substantial interobserver and intraobserver variability in the grading of dysplasia.[5,7,8] There is also substantial disagreement among pathologists in distinguishing high-grade dysplasia from intramucosal carcinoma.[5,9] In studies in which expert gastrointestinal pathologists reviewed histopathology slides of dysplastic and nondysplastic Barrett's esophagus, interobserver agreement for nondysplastic Barrett's was fair to moderate with a kappa statistic (κ) of 0.2.–0.58, better for high-grade dysplasia/carcinoma ($\kappa = 0.43–0.65$), and much poorer for low-grade dysplasia ($\kappa = 0.11–0.4$).[8–10]

Even if all these technical issues in biopsy sampling, processing, and grading of dysplasia could be resolved, the underlying premise that dysplasia in Barrett's esophagus progresses gradually to cancer might be fundamentally flawed. Recent data suggest that only a minority of cancers in Barrett's esophagus develop through the traditional pathway in which there is stepwise accumulation of genetic and epigenetic alterations that inactivate tumor suppressor genes and activate oncogenes to cause genomic instability. Rather, it appears that most Barrett's cancers develop via a genome-doubled pathway in which p53 mutation is followed by doubling of the whole genome, rapidly resulting in genomic instability, oncogene amplification, and malignancy.[11–13] This accelerated pathway to carcinogenesis might explain the many documented cases of failure of endoscopic surveillance to detect dysplasia before the development of invasive cancer in Barrett's esophagus.[14]

ALTERNATIVE BIOMARKERS FOR RISK STRATIFICATION IN BARRETT'S ESOPHAGUS

Noting the many limitations of dysplasia summarized previously, investigators have explored innumerable alternative molecular biomarkers for risk stratification in

Barrett's esophagus. Early studies often focused on individual molecular abnormalities in Barrett's metaplasia but, given the multiple possible molecular pathways to carcinogenesis in Barrett's esophagus, it is perhaps not surprising that individual biomarkers generally have performed poorly in risk stratification studies (immunohistochemical staining for p53 is the exception to this rule, see later in this article). More recent studies exploring panels of multiple biomarkers have had more promising results.

A recent study by Das and colleagues[15] used a Markov model involving a cohort of 50-year-old white men with nondysplastic Barrett's esophagus followed over a lifetime to assess how a biomarker panel indicating a high risk for cancer progression could guide the use of radiofrequency ablation (RFA), which presently is recommended only for patients with dysplasia. Four strategies were modeled in this cohort: (1) no surveillance or RFA, (2) adherence to current ACG surveillance and RFA guidelines, (3) RFA for *all* patients, and (4) a biomarker-guided strategy in which patients identified as high risk by biomarker panel underwent RFA, and patients identified as low or moderate risk had endoscopic surveillance intervals modified accordingly. The latter strategy was the dominant one predicted by this model, yielding the greatest number of quality-adjusted life years (QALY) at the lowest cost and with the fewest cancers.[15] Although the utility of the biomarker panel modeled in this study is not clear (mutational load as an index of cancer risk, see later in this article), the study demonstrates the potential benefit of using biomarker-based surveillance and treatment strategies for patients Barrett's esophagus. In this report we discuss only those biomarkers that appear most promising based on the availability of multiple published studies corroborating good results, and on the commercial availability of the test.

BIOMARKERS FROM THE LABORATORY TO CLINICAL PRACTICE: READY OR NOT HERE THEY COME

p53 Immunostaining: Utility in the Diagnosis of Dysplasia

The detection of p53 abnormalities in Barrett's esophagus by immunostaining has the largest body of evidence supporting its use as a biomarker that can be used as an adjunct to aid in the diagnosis of dysplasia, and as a biomarker to predict neoplastic progression. p53 is an important tumor suppressor gene whose inactivation appears to be a key event that occurs early and often during Barrett's carcinogenesis.[11] Wild-type p53 protein is rapidly degraded, resulting in relatively low levels of expression in nondysplastic Barrett's metaplasia. Mutations that inactivate the p53 gene can have 2 different effects on tissue p53 protein levels. Some p53 mutations render the altered protein stable so that its levels accumulate overexpression (**Fig. 1**), whereas other mutations lead to loss of p53 protein expression. Both of these types of abnormalities can be detected by p53 immunostaining of formalin-fixed, paraffin-embedded Barrett's biopsy specimens.

A number of studies have found that the use of p53 immunostaining (to detect either overexpression or absent staining) improves interobserver variability when the p53 results are incorporated into the morphologic criteria for the diagnosis of dysplasia.[16,17] In a study involving 10 pathologists from 4 institutions in the United Kingdom, slides of nondysplastic, indefinite for dysplasia, low-grade dysplasia and high-grade dysplasia Barrett's esophagus stained with hematoxylin and eosin (H&E) were reviewed and graded for histologic diagnoses, after which review and scoring of p53-stained slides was performed.[18] Finally, the pathologists reviewed both the H&E and the p53-stained slides and then rendered a final histologic diagnosis. Weighted kappa values varied from 0.27 to 0.69 with an average of 0.47 across all 4 histologic categories of Barrett's

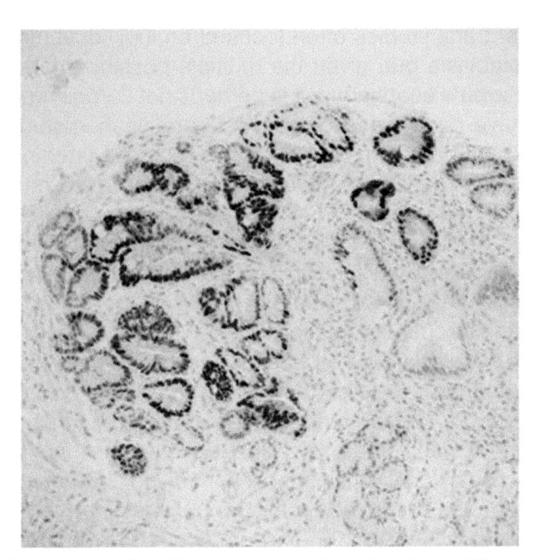

Fig. 1. Representative image of p53 immunostaining showing p53 overexpression in Barrett's patient who exhibited neoplastic progression. (*Adapted from* Stachler MD et al. Detection of Mutations in Barrett's Esophagus Before Progression to High-Grade Dysplasia or Adenocarcinoma. Gastroenterology 2018; 155:156-167, with permission.)

esophagus. For p53 scoring, unweighted kappa values ranged between 0.42 and 0.83, with an average of 0.6 (confidence interval [CI] 0.58–0.63). When p53 scoring was included with histologic grading, the weighted kappa values for final diagnosis improved from 0.47 to 0.55, demonstrating the utility of p53 immunostaining in improving reproducibility of dysplasia diagnoses.[18] The recent recommendation by the British Society of Gastroenterology that "the addition of p53 immunostaining to the histopathological assessment may improve the diagnostic reproducibility of a diagnosis of dysplasia in Barrett's esophagus, and should be considered as an adjunct to routine clinical diagnosis" stems from studies such as these.[19]

p53 Immunostaining: Utility as an Independent Risk Stratification Biomarker

P53 immunostaining has also been evaluated as an independent biomarker to risk stratify patients with Barrett's esophagus. Until recently, most of the studies that have addressed this role of p53 immunostaining focused primarily on p53 overexpression, largely because the importance of loss of its expression was not appreciated and thus was ignored. More recently, aberrant p53 expression including both overexpression and loss of expression has been studied to identify patients at high-risk for neoplastic progression. In a large, case-control study from the Netherlands, immunostaining for p53 protein expression was performed in biopsies from 49 patients with Barrett's esophagus that progressed to high-grade dysplasia or esophageal adenocarcinoma, and from 586 control patients who did not exhibit such neoplastic progression.[20] Aberrant p53 expression was identified in 49% of biopsies from the progressors, but in only 14% of controls who did not progress to high-grade dysplasia or cancer. With aberrant p53 expression, the overall relative risk of neoplastic progression increased by a factor of 6.2. After adjusting for age, sex, length of Barrett's esophagus, and esophagitis, aberrant p53 expression in nondysplastic Barrett's esophagus was associated with an increased relative risk (RR 4.3) of neoplastic progression, whereas an even higher RR (12.2) was seen for aberrant p53 expression in low-grade dysplasia.[20] Aberrant p53 expression had a sensitivity of 49% with a specificity of 86% for predicting neoplastic progression, and approximately 45% of patients had aberrant p53 expression detected in their biopsies up to 5 years before high-grade dysplasia or cancer was detected. Moreover, in nondysplastic Barrett's tissues, aberrant p53 immunostaining outperformed histology alone as a predictor of disease progression. A more recent case-control study also evaluated the ability of abnormal p53 immunostaining to predict progression to high-grade dysplasia or cancer in patients with nondysplastic Barrett's esophagus. An abnormal p53 expression pattern was found in 44.4% of the progressors, whereas only 8.5% of the nonprogressors exhibited abnormal p53 expression. In all these patients, p53 sequencing demonstrated a strong correlation between p53 DNA sequence mutations and p53 overexpression detected by immunostaining ($P<.001$).[21]

Aberrant p53 expression has also been prospectively evaluated as a predictor of neoplastic progression in a study of 91 patients with nondysplastic Barrett's esophagus enrolled in a surveillance program.[22] Over a median follow-up period of 71 months, progression to high-grade dysplasia or cancer occurred in 11 (12%) of the 91 patients.[22] Aberrant p53 expression was found significantly more often (63.6%) in progressors than in nonprogressors (7.5%).[22] Aberrant p53 expression detected by immunostaining was also found to be a significant (hazard ratio [HR] 17) and independent predictor of neoplastic progression in a multivariate analysis. Aberrant p53 expression had a sensitivity and specificity of 63.6% and 92.5%, respectively, with positive and negative predictive values of 53.8% and 94.9%, respectively for predicting neoplastic progression.[22]

A recent systematic review and meta-analysis reported an odds ratio of 46 for case-control studies and a relative risk of 14 to 17 for cohort studies evaluating progression to high-grade dysplasia or cancer among patients with Barrett's esophagus who had aberrant p53 immunostaining in their baseline biopsies.[23] Two of the studies included in this meta-analysis, one prospective and one retrospective, enrolled Barrett's patients with low-grade dysplasia exclusively. The prospective low-grade dysplasia cohort study found a relative risk for progression of 5.7, whereas the retrospective case-control study found an odds ratio for progression of 21.[23] The findings from this meta-analysis strongly suggest that p53 immunostaining can be useful as an adjunct to histology for risk stratification of patients with nondysplastic and low-grade dysplastic Barrett's esophagus.

A major limitation in using p53 immunostaining for clinical purposes is that interpretation of the p53 immunostain, like interpretation of the histologic features of dysplasia, also is subject to interobserver variability.[16] A group of prominent pathologists recently concluded that although p53 is a promising biomarker, it is not ready for routine clinical use until additional studies resolve a number of issues including stain interpretation.[24] The limitation of subjective interpretation is minimized in newer tests that incorporate computer imaging and algorithms to standardize biomarker analyses rather than relying solely on a pathologist's interpretation. The most promising of these newer tests are the molecular biomarker panels TissueCypher and BarreGEN, and the imaging biomarker Wide-Area Transepithelial Sampling (WATS) with computer-assisted 3D analysis.

TissueCypher: a Tissue Systems Pathology Assay

An innovative approach to biomarker studies uses systems biology, viewing tissue as a system comprising multiple compartments that can be analyzed quantitatively for genetic, immunologic, vascular, and morphologic features relevant to cancer progression.[25] In other words, systems biology uses a holistic approach rather than the reductionist approach used in more traditional studies of carcinogenesis. TissueCypher (Cernostics, Pittsburgh, PA) is a tissue systems pathology assay performed on formalin-fixed, paraffin-embedded Barrett's biopsy specimens. This automated assay uses immunofluorescence to label a panel of 9 biomarkers of epithelial and stromal cell abnormalities involved in Barrett's carcinogenesis while also assessing nuclear morphology.[26] The labeled slides are analyzed by computer to calculate an array of fluorescence intensity features in epithelial and stromal tissue compartments and within subcellular compartments, and these analyses can be displayed and quantitated using computer algorithms. A 15-feature assay eventually was developed and validated in a nested case-control study of patients with Barrett's esophagus enrolled in surveillance programs, including 79 who progressed to high-grade dysplasia or esophageal adenocarcinoma and 287 control patients who did not progress during a median follow-up of 5.9 years.[26] In a training cohort, the investigators developed a risk prediction model that stratified patients into low-, intermediate-, and high-risk categories based on performance of the 15-feature assay. The HR for the 5-year probability of progression to high-grade dysplasia or cancer was 4.19 for intermediate versus low-risk, and 14.73 for high risk versus low risk.[26] These risk categories provided stronger prognostic power than typically used clinical variables including age, sex, length of Barrett's metaplasia, histologic grading of dysplasia, and percentage of cells with p53 overexpression.[26] When the 15-feature assay was applied to a validation cohort, the HR for the 5-year probability of progression to high-grade dysplasia or cancer was 2.45 for intermediate versus low risk and 9.42 for high risk versus low risk, and the prevalence-adjusted positive and negative predictive values of the assay were 26% and 98%, respectively.[26] Thus, this assay was found to predict the probability of progression with a higher degree of accuracy than histology.

TissueCypher recently was validated in another independent case-control study of 268 patients with Barrett's esophagus (nondysplastic, indefinite for dysplasia, or low-grade dysplasia) enrolled in surveillance programs at 2 US institutions and followed for a median of 7 years.[27] Baseline biopsies taken at all esophageal levels were tested, and the risk prediction category was based on the highest scoring biopsy level. During follow-up, 58 patients progressed to high-grade dysplasia or cancer, with a median time to progression of 2.7 years; controls were 210 patients who did not exhibit neoplastic progression. In the entire patient group, the prevalence-adjusted proportions of patients scoring low, intermediate, and high risk were 84.2%, 9.4%, and 6.4%, respectively. The sensitivity and specificity of the test at 5 years were 29% and 86%, respectively, with prevalence-adjusted positive and negative predictive values for risk of neoplastic progression of 23% and 96.4%, respectively. For comparison, the sensitivity and specificity of the expert diagnosis of low-grade dysplasia for predicting risk of neoplastic progression were 19% and 88%, respectively. Moreover, risk stratification of the assay outperformed that of p53 alone (measured by the nuclear sum intensity of p53 staining, HR 4.7 vs 1.6, respectively). In the patients with nondysplastic Barrett's esophagus, those who were in the high-risk category were 5.1 times more likely to progress to neoplasia than those in the low-risk category, with an adjusted positive predictive value of 26%. Risk stratification by TissueCypher in patients with only nondysplastic Barrett's esophagus demonstrated an HR of 5.1 compared with an HR of 0.18 for p53 alone. Those with low-grade dysplasia only were at a 3.8-fold increased risk compared with patients with nondysplastic Barrett's esophagus, with an adjusted positive predictive value of 21.8%.[27] Thus, this tissue systems pathology assay appears to predict the risk of neoplastic progression better than p53 alone and better than a diagnosis of low-grade dysplasia made by an expert gastrointestinal pathologist. By multivariate analysis, the high-risk category was an independent predictor of neoplastic progression in a model that included clinical variables (histologic diagnosis, age, sex, length of Barrett's segment, hiatal hernia) with and without the addition of p53.[27] Moreover, evaluation of biopsies from multiple levels increased the sensitivity of the assay compared with the evaluation of only a single biopsy from a randomly selected level.[27]

This same 15-feature assay has been shown to detect a field effect in biopsies without neoplasia that can predict prevalent high-grade dysplasia or cancer in adjacent biopsy specimens. In one study, TissueCypher analyses of nondysplastic, indefinite, or low-grade dysplasia biopsy specimens from 30 patients with high-grade dysplasia or esophageal adenocarcinoma in biopsy specimens taken from elsewhere in the same esophagus were compared with TissueCypher analysis of nondysplastic, indefinite, or low-grade dysplasia biopsy specimens from 145 controls without high-grade dysplasia or cancer. Patients in the TissueCypher high-risk category had a 46-fold increased risk for prevalent high-grade dysplasia or cancer than those in the low-risk category.[28]

A Markov modeling study has suggested that the care of patients with Barrett's esophagus guided by the results of the TissueCypher assay might be more cost-effective than standard-of-care treatment.[29] In this 5-year modeling study, patients with nondysplastic, indefinite for dysplasia, or low-grade dysplasia Barrett's esophagus who had TissueCypher assays in the high-risk category underwent endoscopic eradication therapy followed by post-RFA endoscopic surveillance; those in the intermediate-risk category underwent standard-of-care surveillance and treatment, and those in the low-risk category underwent only endoscopic surveillance at 5 years. Compared with standard-of-care patients, patients in the assay-guided arm had a 16.6% reduction in endoscopies at 5 years (mostly driven by physician adherence to a 5-year surveillance interval for those in the low-risk category), but a 58.4% increase in endoscopic treatments. At year 5, assay-guided treatment resulted in a 51.7% reduction in the number of patients with high-grade dysplasia, a 47.1% reduction in those with esophageal adenocarcinoma, and a 37.6% reduction in cancer-related deaths. Assay-guided treatment also was cost-effective compared with standard-of-care treatment at 5 years, with an incremental cost-effectiveness ratio of $52,483/QALY.[29]

BarreGEN: mutational load

Esophageal adenocarcinomas often exhibit genomic instability, which is an increased tendency for genome alterations during cells divisions. Genomic instability in Barrett's cancers can be manifested both by small structural alterations such as base pair mutations and microsatellite instability, and by large structural alterations including changes in chromosome number and loss of heterozygosity (LOH). Mutational load is an index of genomic instability. The BarreGEN test (Interpace Diagnostics, Parsippany-Troy Hills, NJ) measures mutational load in Barrett's biopsy specimens from which a pathologist has micro-dissected the areas most worrisome for neoplasia. BarreGEN assays those micro-dissected targets to identify LOH mutations and microsatellite instability at 10 loci for tumor suppressor genes, and uses polymerase chain reaction and quantitative capillary electrophoresis of DNA to determine the mutational load, which then is quantitated on a scale of 0 to 10. In a case-control study, BarreGEN was used to compare mutational load in baseline biopsies of Barrett's esophagus from 23 patients (cases) who subsequently developed high-grade dysplasia or esophageal adenocarcinoma with baseline Barrett's biopsies from 46 similar control subjects who did not exhibit neoplastic progression.[30] At a mutational load of 1 or greater, the area under the receiver operating curve (AUC) for prediction of neoplastic progression was 0.95, indicating excellent sensitivity and specificity. Based on these impressive results, the authors concluded that mutational load in baseline biopsies of Barrett's esophagus could be used to predict progression to high-grade dysplasia and esophageal adenocarcinoma. In a subsequent study of similar design, however, the AUC was only 0.50, indicating that mutational load was a poor predictor of neoplastic progression.[31] The latter study used crude lysates prepared from archived tissue specimens, unlike the positive former study that used purified DNA for analysis. The authors of the latter study proposed this as a possible explanation for the disparities between the 2 studies. Further investigation is needed to resolve the discrepancies between these studies.

Wide-area Transepithelial Sampling with Computer-Assisted 3-Dimensional Analysis

Compared with forceps biopsy alone, wide-area transepithelial sampling with computer-assisted 3-dimensional analysis (WATS^{3D}) clearly enhances the identification of dysplasia in Barrett esophagus during screening and surveillance endoscopies. For WATS^{3D}, the endoscopist uses an abrasive cytology brush that is passed through the channel of the endoscope to scrape and so sample the entire segment of Barrett metaplasia. The brush sample is smeared on a microscope slide, yielding a tissue specimen that is, up to 150 μm in thickness. For comparison, on a typical forceps biopsy slide, a microtome is used to cut a tissue section that is, typically is only 3 to 5 μm thick. Analysis of the much thicker WATS^{3D} slide specimen is performed by a neural network computer system that captures up to 50 "optical slices" (each 3 μm in thickness) of the specimen that it reconstructs into 3-dimensional images of the Barrett's glands sampled. The computer then scans these images and flags areas it deems suspicious for dysplasia for final interpretation by a human pathologist. In one recent study, community endoscopists took both standard forceps biopsies and WATS^{3D} samples in 12,899 patients undergoing screening or surveillance endoscopies for Barrett's esophagus.[32] Forceps biopsies identified dysplasia in 88 patients, whereas WATS identified an additional 213 patients with dysplasia, increasing the dysplasia detection rate from 0.68% to 2.33%. In a similar, smaller study of 4203 patients undergoing screening or surveillance endoscopies for Barrett's esophagus, low-grade dysplasia was found by forceps biopsy alone in 26 patients, and 23 additional cases were detected by adding WATS^{3D}.[33] Recently, the use of WATS^{3D} has been sanctioned by the American Society for Gastrointestinal Endoscopy (ASGE). In its most recent guideline on screening and surveillance of Barrett esophagus, the ASGE suggests using WATS^{3D} in addition to Seattle protocol biopsy sampling for patients with known or suspected Barrett esophagus.[34] This is cited as a conditional recommendation based on low-quality evidence.

SUMMARY

The current, widely practiced cancer-preventive strategy of endoscopic screening and surveillance for Barrett's esophagus has failed to stem the rising tide of esophageal adenocarcinoma over the past several decades. The incidence of this deadly tumor continues to climb. Thus, there is an urgent need for a valid biomarker that can be used for appropriate risk stratification of patients at risk for esophageal adenocarcinoma. Ideally, such a biomarker would identify those high-risk patients who would benefit from an early cancer-preventive intervention such as endoscopic eradication therapy, and those low-risk patients who might not need intervention or surveillance.

The biomarkers discussed previously are those that we have identified as most promising based on multiple published studies corroborating good results, and on their commercial availability. Nevertheless, it remains unclear whether any of these biomarkers will fulfill the goals of an ideal biomarker for risk stratification in Barrett's esophagus. Among the biomarkers discussed, only WATS^{3D} has received a recommendation from the ASGE for use in screening and surveillance for Barrett's esophagus, and the ASGE considers this a conditional recommendation based on low-quality evidence. Although we are closer than ever to having a test that achieves the goals of an ideal biomarker, further studies are needed to validate the clinical utility of the tests discussed previously.

CLINICS CARE POINT

- Presently, only WATS^{3D} has received a conditional recommendation (low-quality evidence) from the ASGE as a biomarker for use in screening and surveillance for Barrett's esophagus.

DISCLOSURE

R.F. Souza has served as a consultant for Interpace Diagnostics, Cernostics, Phathom Pharmaceuticals, and Ironwood Pharmaceuticals. S.J. Spechler has served as a consultant for Interpace Diagnostics, Cernostics, Frazier Life Sciences, Phathom Pharmaceuticals, and Ironwood Pharmaceuticals, and receives royalties as an author for UpToDate.

REFERENCES

1. Vaughan TL, Fitzgerald RC. Precision prevention of oesophageal adenocarcinoma. Nat Rev Gastroenterol Hepatol 2015;12(4):243–8.
2. Strimbu K, Tavel JA. What are biomarkers? Curr Opin HIV AIDS 2010;5(6):463–6.
3. Spechler SJ. Dysplasia in Barrett's esophagus: limitations of current management strategies. Am J Gastroenterol 2005;100(4):927–35.
4. Roumans CAM, van der Bogt RD, Steyerberg EW, et al. Adherence to recommendations of Barrett's esophagus surveillance guidelines: a systematic review and meta-analysis. Endoscopy 2020;52(1):17–28.
5. Naini BV, Souza RF, Odze RD. Barrett's esophagus: a comprehensive and contemporary review for pathologists. Am J Surg Pathol 2016;40(5):e45–66.
6. Shaheen NJ, Falk GW, Iyer PG, et al. ACG clinical guideline: diagnosis and management of barrett's esophagus. Am J Gastroenterol 2016;111(1):30–50 [quiz: 51].
7. Curvers WL, ten Kate FJ, Krishnadath KK, et al. Low-grade dysplasia in Barrett's esophagus: overdiagnosed and underestimated. Am J Gastroenterol 2010; 105(7):1523–30.
8. Vennalaganti P, Kanakadandi V, Goldblum JR, et al. Discordance among pathologists in the United States and Europe in diagnosis of low-grade dysplasia for patients with Barrett's esophagus. Gastroenterology 2017;152(3):564–70.e4.
9. Montgomery E, Bronner MP, Goldblum JR, et al. Reproducibility of the diagnosis of dysplasia in Barrett esophagus: a reaffirmation. Hum Pathol 2001;32(4): 368–78.
10. Coco DP, Goldblum JR, Hornick JL, et al. Interobserver variability in the diagnosis of crypt dysplasia in Barrett esophagus. Am J Surg Pathol 2011;35(1):45–54.

11. Stachler MD, Taylor-Weiner A, Peng S, et al. Paired exome analysis of Barrett's esophagus and adenocarcinoma. Nat Genet 2015;47(9):1047–55.
12. Martinez P, Timmer MR, Lau CT, et al. Dynamic clonal equilibrium and predetermined cancer risk in Barrett's oesophagus. Nat Commun 2016;7:12158.
13. Nones K, Waddell N, Wayte N, et al. Genomic catastrophes frequently arise in esophageal adenocarcinoma and drive tumorigenesis. Nat Commun 2014;5:5224.
14. Corley DA, Mehtani K, Quesenberry C, et al. Impact of endoscopic surveillance on mortality from Barrett's esophagus-associated esophageal adenocarcinomas. Gastroenterology 2013;145(2):312–9.e1.
15. Das A, Callenberg KM, Styn MA, et al. Endoscopic ablation is a cost-effective cancer preventative therapy in patients with Barrett's esophagus who have elevated genomic instability. Endosc Int Open 2016;4(5):E549–59.
16. Kaye PV, Haider SA, Ilyas M, et al. Barrett's dysplasia and the Vienna classification: reproducibility, prediction of progression and impact of consensus reporting and p53 immunohistochemistry. Histopathology 2009;54(6):699–712.
17. Skacel M, Petras RE, Rybicki LA, et al. p53 expression in low grade dysplasia in Barrett's esophagus: correlation with interobserver agreement and disease progression. Am J Gastroenterol 2002;97(10):2508–13.
18. Kaye PV, Ilyas M, Soomro I, et al. Dysplasia in Barrett's oesophagus: p53 immunostaining is more reproducible than haematoxylin and eosin diagnosis and improves overall reliability, while grading is poorly reproducible. Histopathology 2016;69(3):431–40.
19. Fitzgerald RC, di Pietro M, Ragunath K, et al. British Society of Gastroenterology guidelines on the diagnosis and management of Barrett's oesophagus. Gut 2014;63(1):7–42.
20. Kastelein F, Biermann K, Steyerberg EW, et al. Aberrant p53 protein expression is associated with an increased risk of neoplastic progression in patients with Barrett's oesophagus. Gut 2013;62(12):1676–83.
21. Stachler MD, Camarda ND, Deitrick C, et al. Detection of mutations in barrett's esophagus before progression to high-grade dysplasia or adenocarcinoma. Gastroenterology 2018;155(1):156–67.
22. Davelaar AL, Calpe S, Lau L, et al. Aberrant TP53 detected by combining immunohistochemistry and DNA-FISH improves Barrett's esophagus progression prediction: a prospective follow-up study. Genes Chromosomes Cancer 2015;54(2):82–90.
23. Snyder P, Dunbar KB, Cipher DJ, et al. Aberrant p53 immunostaining in Barrett's esophagus predicts neoplastic progression: systematic review and meta-analyses. Dig Dis Sci 2019;64:1089–97.
24. Srivastava A, Appelman H, Goldsmith JD, et al. The use of ancillary stains in the diagnosis of barrett esophagus and barrett esophagus-associated dysplasia: recommendations from the Rodger C. Haggitt Gastrointestinal Pathology Society. Am J Surg Pathol 2017;41(5):e8–21.
25. Prichard JW, Davison JM, Campbell BB, et al. TissueCypher: A systems biology approach to anatomic pathology. J Pathol Inform 2015;6:48.
26. Critchley-Thorne RJ, Duits LC, Prichard JW, et al. A tissue systems pathology assay for high-risk barrett's esophagus. Cancer Epidemiol Biomarkers Prev 2016;25(6):958–68.
27. Davison JM, Goldblum J, Grewal US, et al. Independent blinded validation of a tissue systems pathology test to predict progression in patients with barrett's esophagus. Am J Gastroenterol 2020;115(6):843–52.

28. Critchley-Thorne RJ, Davison JM, Prichard JW, et al. A tissue systems pathology test detects abnormalities associated with prevalent high-grade dysplasia and esophageal cancer in Barrett's esophagus. Cancer Epidemiol Biomarkers Prev 2017;26(2):240–8.
29. Hao J, Critchley-Thorne R, Diehl DL, et al. A cost-effectiveness analysis of an adenocarcinoma risk prediction multi-biomarker assay for patients with Barrett's esophagus. Clinicoecon Outcomes Res 2019;11:623–35.
30. Eluri S, Brugge WR, Daglilar ES, et al. The presence of genetic mutations at key loci predicts progression to esophageal adenocarcinoma in Barrett's esophagus. Am J Gastroenterol 2015;110(6):828–34.
31. Eluri S, Klaver E, Duits LC, et al. Validation of a biomarker panel in Barrett's esophagus to predict progression to esophageal adenocarcinoma. Dis Esophagus 2018;31(11):doy026.
32. Smith MS, Ikonomi E, Bhuta R, et al. Wide-area transepithelial sampling with computer-assisted 3-dimensional analysis (WATS) markedly improves detection of esophageal dysplasia and Barrett's esophagus: analysis from a prospective multicenter community-based study. Dis Esophagus 2019;32(3):doy099.
33. Gross SA, Smith MS, Kaul V. Increased detection of Barrett's esophagus and esophageal dysplasia with adjunctive use of wide-area transepithelial sample with three-dimensional computer-assisted analysis (WATS). United European Gastroenterol J 2018;6(4):529–35.
34. Qumseya B, Sultan S, Bain P, et al. ASGE guideline on screening and surveillance of Barrett's esophagus. Gastrointest Endosc 2019;90(3):335–59.e2.

Current Status of Chemoprevention in Barrett's Esophagus

Paul Moayyedi, MD, PhD, MPH[a,*], Hashem B. El-Serag, MD, MPH[b]

KEYWORDS

- Barrett's esophagus • Esophageal adenocarcinoma • Chemoprevention
- Proton pump inhibitor • Aspirin • HRT • Metformin • Statins

KEY POINTS

- Chemoprevention is an attractive strategy for Barrett's esophagus as preventing esophageal adenocarcinoma from occurring is often more effective than identifying early disease.
- There are a number of promising candidates that may decrease progression to esophageal adenocarcinoma based on observational studies.
- There is insufficient evidence to recommend metformin or hormone replacement therapy for chemoprevention in Barrett's esophagus.
- There is insufficient evidence to recommend statins to decrease esophageal adenocarcinoma, but patients with Barrett's esophagus should be carefully evaluated to assess if there is a cardiovascular indication for statins.
- Twice daily proton pump inhibitor therapy combined with aspirin shows the most promise in preventing neoplastic progression in Barrett's esophagus and may decrease all-cause mortality.

INTRODUCTION

Esophageal cancer is the sixth leading cause of cancer death worldwide with more than 0.5 million cases annually.[1] The vast majority of global cases are squamous cell carcinoma but in developed countries esophageal adenocarcinoma (EA) has seen a rapid increase,[2] and now accounts for the majority of esophageal cancer cases in the United States and Northern Europe.[3] Indeed, in the United States the overall incidence of esophageal cancer remained relatively stable from 1975 to 2005,[4] but this apparent stability of cancer cases concealed the dramatic changes in histologic

[a] McMaster University, 1280 Main Street West, Hamilton, Ontario L8S 4K1, Canada; [b] Baylor College of Medicine Medical Center, McNair Campus (Clinic), 7200 Cambridge Street, 8th Floor, Suite 8B, Houston, TX 77030, USA
* Corresponding author.
E-mail address: moayyep@mcmaster.ca

Gastrointest Endoscopy Clin N Am 31 (2021) 117–130
https://doi.org/10.1016/j.giec.2020.08.008 giendo.theclinics.com

type of cancer that emerged over this time period. EA changed from being rare in the early 1970s to being twice as common as esophageal squamous carcinoma in men by 2005.[3] This rapid increase has been likely caused by an increase in gastroesophageal reflux disease (GERD)[5] and Barrett's esophagus (BE)[6] seen in developed nations. Patients with BE are offered surveillance[7] to detect dysplasia early because these patients are at a higher risk of developing EA. It is estimated that the annual risk of developing EA is 0.7% for low-grade dysplasia and 7% for high-grade dysplasia (HGD).[8] Ablation techniques can decrease this risk of progression of both low-grade dysplasia and HGD,[9] but in clinical practice this has only been partially successful, because patients with BE are still dying of EA.[10]

It is usually more effective to prevent a serious disease from occurring rather than to treat it when it is diagnosed. A classic example of this is aspirin for the secondary prevention of cardiovascular disease.[11] Aspirin can decrease cardiovascular events by approximately 30% in this setting[11] and is highly cost effective.[12] It is possible that similar prevention strategies can be offered to patients with BE, and this article evaluate options that might prevent EA and dysplasia from developing. There are a variety of risk factors for the development of EA in the setting of BE. *Helicobacter pylori* is associated with a decrease risk of EA,[13,14] and male sex confers a strong increased risk of developing EA in those with BE.[15] Obesity is associated with an increased risk,[13,16] as is tobacco smoking[13,17] with a possible protective effect of exercise[13,18] and dietary factors such as vegetable intake.[13,19] However, these factors are impossible or difficult to modify, so this article explores pharmacologic interventions that could reduce the risk of EA in BE. This review focuses on proton pump inhibitor (PPI) therapy,[20] nonsteroidal anti-inflammatory drugs (NSAIDs),[21] 3-hydroxy-3-methyl-glutaryl-coenzyme A reductase inhibitors,[22] metformin,[23] and hormone replacement therapy (HRT).

PROTON PUMP INHIBITOR THERAPY

Observational studies have shown that GERD symptoms are a strong risk factor for EA[24] and the risk of EA increases with increasing duration[24,25] and severity of GERD symptoms.[25] It is, however, unclear at what point along the causal pathway acid reflux may be acting to increase the risk of EA. GERD is also strongly associated with BE, so it is possible that acid reflux is acting to cause the precursor lesion BE, without having any impact on the subsequent development of adenocarcinoma. There are mechanistic data that would support acid reflux acting to increase the risk of neoplasia in BE. Acid reflux causes chronic inflammation and increased cell turnover, which can predispose to carcinogenesis.[26] Exposing metaplastic esophageal epithelium to acid also increases the production of reactive oxygen species and leads to greater genetic instability.[27] Increased reactive oxygen species activity is mediated through NADPH oxidase 5, and this agent is increased in the esophageal mucosa of patients with BE.[28] Microsomal prostaglandin E synthetase 1 and inducible nitric oxidase synthetase are also increased in the esophageal mucosa in BE, and these factors can promote carcinogenesis through promoting cell proliferation and angiogenesis.[28] Decreasing acid reflux should decrease inflammation and cell turnover and, therefore, decrease the possibility of genetic instability. Indeed, PPI therapy has been shown to decrease NADPH oxidase 5, microsomal prostaglandin E synthetase-1, and inducible nitric oxidase synthetase expression in biopsies from patients with BE[28] within 1 month. After 6 months of PPI therapy, patients with BE had a significant decrease in cell proliferation in those who had achieved normalization of esophageal pH.[29]

In contrast, there are concerns regarding the carcinogenic potential of PPI therapy. Acid suppression increases serum gastrin levels, and this trophic hormone can promote carcinogenesis.[30,31] One retrospective study evaluating patients with BE found those in the highest quartile of serum gastrin were more likely to have HGD or EA.[32] Confounding by indication[33] could explain these findings, because those with worse reflux may be more likely to develop dysplasia and may be prescribed higher dose PPI, which in turn could increase serum gastrin. Nevertheless, these data suggest that there is mechanistic equipoise as to whether PPI therapy may promote or prevent EA in BE.

Epidemiologic data may give clearer information on the impact of PPI therapy on risk of EA in BE. A UK primary care database study found an increased risk of EA in patients taking PPI therapy for a reflux indication.[34] Because reflux is a strong risk factor for developing EA, it is likely that such an association is due to confounding by indication.[33] This study also did not evaluate BE specifically, but all patients with reflux disease. When BE is evaluated specifically, there is evidence to support a significant decrease in the risk of EA among patients with BE taking PPIs. A systematic review[20] of cohort studies reported that PPI therapy significantly reduced the risk of progression to HGD or EA with an adjusted hazard ratio (HR) of 0.32 (95% confidence interval [CI], 0.15–0.67). In their meta-analysis of 7 observational studies, Singh and colleagues[20] found that patients with BE with a history of PPI use had 71% lower risk of progression to HGD or OAC compared with PPI nonusers (odds ratio [OR], 0.29; 95% CI, 0.12–0.79). There were insufficient data to evaluate HGD or EA alone in this meta-analysis and there was no information on whether taking PPI twice daily would provide any benefit over once daily administration in BE. Furthermore, another systematic review did not find a benefit of PPIs in decreasing the risk of neoplastic progression in BE.[35] This review combined different designs of observational studies, which is not recommended and therefore of questionable value, but still emphasizes that there is uncertainty around the impact of PPI on neoplastic progression in BE. Histamine type-2 receptor antagonists may also prevent progression of BE to EA; however, fewer studies have examined their use separate from PPIs.[36]

Whether PPIs may promote or inhibit the development of carcinogenesis is somewhat academic, because most patients with BE have reflux that significantly impacts their quality of life.[37] Patients require PPI therapy to control symptoms and improve their quality of life,[38] and this factor is likely to outweigh any putative carcinogenic potential of acid suppression. The main question around PPI therapy is whether it is appropriate to increase the dose beyond what is required in patients with BE to control reflux symptoms. Patients with BE may have continued acid reflux despite being asymptomatic[39,40] and the metaplastic change in the esophageal mucosa may decrease the symptom burden in patients with BE.[41] Inflammation and cell proliferation may therefore still be occurring in the esophageal mucosa of patients with BE, even in the absence of reflux symptoms. Increasing the dose of PPI from once to twice daily will decrease acid reflux[42] in patients with BE and may decrease the risk of EA. This approach has not been recommended in guidelines[8,9] given the lack of evidence around whether twice daily PPI therapy may have any impact on EA in BE. The Aspirin and Esomeprazole ChemoprevenTion in Barrett's metaplasia (AspECT) trial[43] addressed this question. This randomized controlled trial (RCT) was a partial factorial design conducted predominantly in the UK (with 1 center in Canada) that randomized 2557 patients to esomeprazole 20 mg once daily or 40 mg twice daily followed for a mean of 9 years translating to more than 20,000 patient-years of follow-up. Those not taking aspirin at baseline were randomized to aspirin 300 mg once daily (325 mg for Canadian patients) or no aspirin. The composite primary end point was time to HGD, EA, or all-cause mortality. Patients randomized to once daily PPI therapy had an increased risk of developing the primary end point (time ratio [TR], 1.27; 95% CI, 1.01–1.58). There was a trend for once daily PPI to have an increased all-cause mortality rate (TR, 1.25; 95% CI, 0.92–1.70) and HGD (TR, 1.51; 95% CI, 1.00–2.29) with no impact on EA (TR, 1.02; 95% CI, 0.64–1.64). These data are persuasive that twice daily PPI therapy may decrease progression to HGD and decrease all-cause mortality, and it is likely that the benefit of this approach outweighs any possible harm. Nevertheless, there are caveats to these data. The trial predominantly recruited men, as this group has the highest risk of developing the coprimary end point, so the impact of twice daily PPI in women is unclear. The RCT was also not double blind and the patient and clinicians looking after the patient were aware of which treatment allocation was given. The outcome assessor was masked and so objective outcomes such as EA and all-cause mortality are unlikely to be impacted by the open nature of the trial. The other issue with the trial is that the event rate was relatively low, so the 95% CIs are wide. Further follow-up of participants in this trial to accrue more events would be ideal, because this factor would make any findings more robust.

The other concern around increasing the dose of PPI therapy to twice daily in BE is the possible long-term harms of PPI therapy.[44] Acid suppression has been associated with risk of pneumonia,[45] fracture,[46] enteric infection,[47] *Clostridium difficile*–associated diarrhea,[48] cerebrovascular events,[49] chronic renal failure,[50] dementia,[51] and all-cause mortality[52] in observational studies. There is controversy around these possible risks of PPI therapy, because any association may relate to confounding and the bias that is inherent in observational studies,[53] in addition, studies consistently report that sicker patients tend to be taking PPI therapy, so some or all of these associations may relate to residual confounding.[54] The only approach that will resolve this possibility is to conduct an appropriately powered RCT.

The largest RCT[55] that evaluated the possible harms of PPIs enrolled 17,598 patients and followed them for a mean of 3 years. This study was a partial factorial RCT that randomized more than 25,000 patients to rivaroxaban and/or aspirin to evaluate whether these interventions could decrease cardiovascular events.[56] Those not taking a PPI were randomized to pantoprazole 40 mg once daily or placebo and the primary aim of the RCT was to evaluate whether acid suppression would prevent serious upper gastrointestinal events in patients taking anticoagulation.[57] A secondary aim was the safety of PPI therapy and harm data were collected every 6 months during the course of the RCT that had 53,000 patient-years of follow-up. The risk of all-cause mortality (HR, 1.03; 95% CI, 0.92–1.15), myocardial infarction (HR, 0.94; 95% CI, 0.79–1.12), and gastrointestinal cancers (HR, 1.04; 95% CI, 0.77–1.40) were similar in the PPI versus placebo groups.[55] The proportion of patients with fracture (OR, 0.96; 95% CI, 0.79–1.17), pneumonia (OR, 1.02; 95% CI, 0.87–1.19), chronic kidney disease (OR, 1.17; 95% CI, 0.94–1.45), and dementia (OR, 1.20; 95% CI, 0.81–1.78) were also similar in both arms of the trial.[55] Enteric infections did occur more frequently in the PPI group, but the number needed to harm for this event was more than 900 for each year of PPI therapy. This RCT did not collect serum on everyone at exit from the trial, so there were no data on anemia or vitamin B_{12} deficiency, which have also been raised as issues with long-term PPI therapy.[42] Data from 2 RCTs[58] comparing PPI therapy with antireflux surgery were, however, reassuring in this regard. These RCTs enrolled 812 GERD patients with 2842 patient-years of follow-up over a 5- to 12-year period. There was no difference in routine hematology, electrolytes, vitamin D, calcium, vitamin B_{12}, and alkaline phosphate between the 2 groups at baseline or during follow-up.[58] These studies cannot exclude a very small effect of PPIs in causing possible harm, but in general the RCT data are reassuring that PPIs are unlikely to cause major long-term harm.

NONSTEROIDAL ANTI-INFLAMMATORY DRUGS

The cyclo-oxygenase (COX) pathway is a key mediator of inflammation that upregulates a number of oncogenic factors[59] and has been implicated in many cancers,[60] including EA.[61,62] COX enzymes synthesize prostaglandins from arachidonic acid and prostaglandin E2, in particular, has been associated with both BE[63–65] and EA.[65] Any cause of inflammation will upregulate these pathways, including damage by acid and bile.[63–65] PPI therapy may, therefore, partially act through this pathway and this factor may explain the possible protective effect of PPI therapy in preventing neoplastic progression in BE.[20,58] There are more specific approaches to inhibiting the COX pathway, because NSAIDs mediate their anti-inflammatory activity by inhibiting both COX-1 and COX-2 and thereby inhibit prostaglandin E2 production. These drugs could therefore decrease the risk of EA developing in patients with BE, and animal models support this hypothesis.[66] Epidemiologic studies suggest that patients taking NSAIDs were less likely to develop EA compared with those not taking these drugs[21,67,68] with an OR of 0.68 (95% CI, 0.56–0.83).[21] The association was strongest for patients taking NSAIDs at least daily and had been taking these drugs for more than 10 years.[21] NSAIDs are also associated with upper gastrointestinal bleeding,[69] although this factor would be mitigated by PPI therapy,[70] which patients with BE will usually be taking. Most NSAIDs are also associated with an increased risk of cardiovascular events[71] so would not be suitable chemoprotective agents because the risk–benefit ratio is unlikely to be favorable.

The cardiovascular harms related to NSAIDs are thought to be COX-2 mediated and most NSAIDs exhibit significant COX-2 inhibitory activity.[72] Aspirin, in contrast, is COX-1 selective and has a major effect on platelet inhibition mediated through inhibition of platelet thromboxane B2.[73] This is why aspirin is a widely used cardioprotective agent,[11,74] whereas most other NSAIDs have the opposite effect.[71] Most guidelines do not recommend aspirin for primary prevention because all-cause mortality is not decreased, primarily because of an increase in gastrointestinal bleeding and hemorrhagic stroke deaths.[75] Indeed, the absolute reduction in fatal and nonfatal cardiovascular events is almost identical to the absolute increase in fatal and nonfatal gastrointestinal bleeding (0.4% in both cases). Patients with BE are taking long-term PPI therapy for their symptoms and so would be protected from some of the deleterious effects of aspirin on the upper gastrointestinal tract. Patients with BE may therefore have a net benefit from aspirin in terms of all-cause mortality. This outcome would relate to the decrease in cardiovascular events in patients with BE taking aspirin, but also possibly from an effect in reducing progression to EA.

The effect of NSAIDs in decreasing EA is seen equally for aspirin as well as other NSAIDs.[21,68] Data were predominantly from case control studies.[21] A pooled analysis[21] of individual-level participant data from 5 population-based case-control studies and one cohort study in the Barrett's and Esophageal Adenocarcinoma Consortium (BEACON; http://beacon.tlvnet.net) found a 32% lower risk of EA associated with any NSAID use (OR, 0.68, 95%CI 0.56–0.83); the magnitude of the inverse association was similar for aspirin (OR, 0.77, 95%CI 0.60–0.97) and nonaspirin NSAID (OR, 0.81, 95%CI 0.67–0.96) users (vs nonusers of these classes of medication). The strength of the inverse association was greatest for current users, and the risk was shown to decrease linearly with both increased frequency and duration of use. In contrast, an analysis of data from studies in BEACON[76] (involving 1474 BE cases and 2256 population-based controls) found no association between use of any NSAIDs and the risk of BE (OR, 1.00; 95% CI, 0.76–1.32). Therefore, it is likely that the most, if not all, of the protective effect of NSAIDs on risk of EA occurs after the development of BE.[77] Analogous to colon cancer and polyps, NSAIDs may stop progression from BE to EAC,[77] but not the development of BE. These data are observational and, as stated elsewhere in this article, are open to bias and confounding,[53] so it would be important to evaluate whether there is any RCT evidence that supports the use of aspirin in BE.

A post hoc meta-analysis of a subgroup of RCTs[78] evaluating the effect of aspirin in preventing cardiovascular disease found that aspirin also decreases the risk of EA by approximately 33%. The trials in this meta-analysis were not designed to specifically evaluate cancer as an outcome and there could be diagnostic bias because patients on aspirin will have more upper gastrointestinal symptoms and may have more endoscopies.[79] The number of EA in these trials were modest[79] and this was in healthy patients whose BE status was unknown. Nevertheless, the use of aspirin in BE is appealing[80] and is supported by a mechanistic phase II RCT.[81] This trial[81] evaluated 114 patients with BE taking esomeprazole 40 mg twice daily and randomized participants to aspirin 325 mg versus aspirin 81 mg or placebo with 298 days of follow-up. There was a statistically significant decrease in tissue prostaglandin E2 levels in the esophageal biopsies of patients allocated to the high-dose aspirin arm.

The AspECT trial[43] evaluated the impact of aspirin 300 to 325 mg once daily as well as PPI therapy on the combined end point of HGD, EA, and all-cause mortality. The numbers randomized to the aspirin group were slightly lower; 255 of the 2557 patients in the trial were not randomized to aspirin or no aspirin. The power of this arm of the trial was therefore slightly lower than for the PPI arms and, although the magnitude of effect on the primary end point was similar to PPI (TR, 1.24; 95% CI, 0.98–1.57; $P = .68$), this difference was not statistically significant.[58] If patients using other NSAIDs were censored at the time of first use, then the effect of aspirin was statistically significant (TR, 1.29; 95% CI, 1.01–1.66). Interestingly, the effect was greatest in the twice daily PPI and aspirin group where the TR was 1.59 (95% CI, 1.14–2.23), suggesting that the combination of aspirin and PPI have at least an additive effect in decreasing HGD, EA, and all-cause mortality.

HORMONE REPLACEMENT THERAPY

A possible explanation for the strong male predominance of EA, with an average 3- to 6-fold higher incidence among men,[82] is differences in levels of endogenous protective exposure to female sex hormones. If this hypothesis is true, preventive effects of exogenous HRT might be evident. HRT consists of estrogen or estrogen combined with progestin and is administered mainly for climacteric symptoms in postmenopausal women.[83] HRT has also been shown to be effective for treating vasomotor symptoms, vaginal atrophy, and sexual problems, as well as in preventing osteoporosis and bone fractures.[84,85] Systematic reviews[86–89] comparing ever users of HRT with nonusers have shown statistically significantly decreased relative risk estimates of EA and gastric adenocarcinoma, as well as of esophageal squamous cell carcinoma, irrespective of the mostly unknown BE status in these studies. Among patients with BE, a meta-analysis[86] including 5 studies (2 population-based cohort studies, 2 case-control studies, and 1 pooled analysis of 4 case-control studies) found a decreased likelihood of EA among users of HRT, compared with never users (OR, 0.75; 95% CI, 0.58–0.98). However, no subanalyses based on the dosage, type, or duration were possible owing to the few and small studies available. In contrast, a case-control study[90] found a modest increase in the risk of GERD symptoms (HR, 1.57; 95% CI, 1.45–1.70) when comparing ever users of HRT with never users, but no increased risk of BE (HR, 1.15; 95% CI, 0.81–1.63) or EA (HR, 0.89; 95% CI, 0.28–2.82) was found. Thus, the available literature[84–92] addressing HRT in relation to the risk of EA to date is limited, but might suggest a preventive effect.

STATINS

Statins are usually prescribed as prevention of cardiovascular disease but may also have cancer preventive effects. Statins have antiproliferative, proapoptotic, anti-invasive, and radiosensitizing properties in preclinical studies.[93–95] Statin use was inversely associated[96] with a person's risk of developing BE in an observational study. A number of observational studies[97,98] have examined the role of statins in EA in the general population regardless of whether they are known to have BE. For example, Alexandre and colleagues[99] in a population-based nested case-control study using data from individuals in the UK General Practice Research Database (581 cases and 2167 controls) showed a 42% decrease in the risk of EA among statin users as compared with nonusers (OR, 0.58, 95% CI, 0.39–0.87). The risk of EA decreased linearly with increased dose and duration of use. A systematic review[22] of 13 observational studies (5 cohort studies, of which 2 were population based; 7 case-control studies, of which 6 were population based; and 1 post hoc analysis of 22 RCTs) of individuals without known BE found an adjusted OR of 0.72 for developing esophageal cancer (95% CI, 0.60–0.86). This possible benefit was also shown in a subanalysis of patients with known BE (5 studies: 3 cohort and 2 case-control studies, of which 1 was population based) found a 43% decrease in the risk of EA (adjusted OR, 0.59; 95% CI, 0.45–0.78) among users of statins compared with never users.[22] Subsequently, a nested case-control study[100] within a large BE cohort in the Veterans Administration health care system compared 311 EAC cases with 856 BE controls and found that statin use was inversely associated with development of EAC (adjusted OR, 0.65; 95% CI 0.47–0.91). This protective effect was strongest against advanced stage EA and increased with statin dose; there was no association between EA and nonstatin lipid-lowering medications.[100]

These data are based on case-control and cohort studies; however, the results form RCTs are less clear. A systematic review[101] of RCTs, none of which was conducted primarily for cancer prevention, failed to show significant decrease in EA risk. The main limitation of this systematic review was that there were a small number of esophageal cancer cases (total 164 cases), and the main analyses were for cancer in general with no separate analysis of EA alone. A recent systematic review[102] identified 11 studies including 5 cohort studies, 2 case-control studies, and 4 nested case-control studies with a total sample of 1057 cancer or HGD cases and 17,741 BE controls without neoplasia. The pooled unadjusted data showed a significant inverse association between statin use and the incidence of EA in BE cohorts (OR ,0.54; 95% CI 0.46–0.63). Both case-control and cohort studies produced similar results. Information on statin type, dose, and duration could not be pooled but individual studies showed a tendency to a dose- and duration-dependent decrease in EA incidence.[103]

Thus, most available observational studies indicate a preventive effect on the development of EA of treatment with statins in BE, but this needs further study in large RCTs with sufficient length of follow-up. Given the relatively low rate of neoplastic progression in BE, it may not be cost effective to use statins as chemopreventative agents if the patient does not have an indication for these drugs. However, given that the main cause of death in patients with BE is vascular diseases, it may be prudent to ensure that statins that are prescribed to patients with BE were indicated by vascular risk.

METFORMIN

Metformin decreases serum insulin levels and is one of the most commonly used drugs to treat diabetes mellitus. It activates AMP-activated protein kinase, which has downstream effects of reduced cellular proliferation and protein synthesis.[103,104] Studies[23,105,106] have shown a potential for metformin to be a chemopreventive agent in obesity-associated cancers. Given that central obesity is believed to play an important role in the neoplastic progression of BE,[107] the association between metformin use and progression in BE was examined in a retrospective cohort study of BE progression to EA. Although a protective trend for metformin was observed, this difference was not statistically significant.[108] A recent RCT[109] also did not find metformin to decrease any markers of inflammation in BE. Therefore, there is insufficient evidence to recommend metformin for chemoprevention in BE.

SUMMARY

Candidates for chemoprevention in BE have been suggested for decades and there has been observational data to support many of these drugs.[80] The evidence base for statins remains insufficient to recommend in clinical practice, although it would be sensible to ensure all patients with BE that have appropriate cardiovascular risk factors are taking these drugs. HRT also shows promise, but this treatment would only be appropriate for women and EA is not a major concern in this group. The evidence for metformin is weak and conflicting, and this agent needs further study before consideration as a chemotherapeutic agent. The most likely candidates for chemoprevention are PPI therapy and aspirin. Recently, evidence from RCTs[43] has emerged that provides greater evidence that these agents might be effective. Data suggest that both aspirin and twice daily PPI therapy can decrease the risk of neoplastic progression in BE. Aspirin has the added advantage that it can prevent cardiovascular disease[75] and ischemic heart disease is the leading cause of mortality in BE.[110] Indeed, the combination of aspirin and twice daily PPI reduced all-cause mortality in patients with BE by approximately 33%.[43] Future guideline groups need to evaluate the evidence rigorously, but the combination of PPI twice daily and aspirin is a promising approach for patients with BE.

CLINICS CARE POINTS

- There is insufficient information to recommend most approaches to chemoprevention in Barrett's esophagus.
- Carefully discuss reflux symptoms with your Barrett's patients. If there are any symptoms it is sensible to increase their PPI to twice daily. Discuss with the patient the risks and benefits of increasing PPI even if they do not have symptoms.
- Discuss any cardiovascular risks with the patient and have a low threshold for recommending aspirin.

REFERENCES

1. Available at: https://gco.iarc.fr/today/data/factsheets/cancers/6-Oesophagus-fact-sheet.pdf. Accessed May 1, 2020.
2. Pohl H, Sirovich B, Welch HG. Esophageal adenocarcinoma incidence: are we reaching the peak? Cancer Epidemiol Biomarkers Prev 2010;19:1468–70.
3. Wong MCS, Hamilton W, Whiteman DC, et al. Global Incidence and mortality of oesophageal cancer and their correlation with socioeconomic indicators temporal patterns and trends in 41 countries. Sci Rep 2018;8:4522.

4. Available at: https://seer.cancer.gov/statfacts/html/esoph.html. Accessed May 1, 2020.
5. El-Serag H. Time trends of gastroesophageal reflux disease: a systematic review. Clin Gastroenterol Hepatol 2007;5:17–26.
6. Van Soest EM, Dieleman JP, Siersema PD, et al. Increasing incidence of Barrett's oesophagus in the general population. Gut 2005;54:1062–6.
7. Bennett C, Moayyedi P, Corley DA, et al. BOB CAT: a large-scale review and Delphi consensus for management of Barrett's esophagus with no dysplasia, indefinite for, or low-grade dysplasia. Am J Gastroenterol 2015;110:662–82.
8. Shaheen NJ, Falk GW, Iyer PG, et al. ACG clinical guideline: diagnosis and management of Barrett's esophagus. Am J Gastroenterol 2016;111:30–50.
9. Wani S, Qumseya B, Sultan S, et al. Endoscopic eradication therapy for patients with Barrett's esophagus–associated dysplasia and intramucosal cancer. Gastrointest Endosc 2018;87:907–31.
10. Shaheen NJ, Overholt BF, Sampliner RE, et al. Durability of radiofrequency ablation in Barrett's esophagus with dysplasia. Gastroenterology 2011;141:460–8.
11. Antiplatelet Trialists' Collaboration. Collaborative overview of randomised trials of antiplatelet therapy. I. Prevention of death, myocardial infarction, and stroke by prolonged antiplatelet therapy in various categories of patients. BMJ 1994; 308:81–106.
12. Gaspoz J-M, Coxson PG, Goldman PA, et al. Cost effectiveness of aspirin, clopidogrel, or both for secondary prevention of coronary heart disease. N Engl J Med 2002;346:1800–6.
13. Coleman HG, Xie S-H, Lagergren J. Epidemiology of esophageal adenocarcinoma. Gastroenterology 2018;154:390–405.
14. Wang Z, Shaheen NJ, Whiteman DC, et al. *Helicobacter pylori* infection is associated with reduced risk of Barrett's esophagus: an analysis of the Barrett's and esophageal adenocarcinoma consortium. Am J Gastroenterol 2018;113: 1148–55.
15. Ford AC, Forman D, Reynolds PD, et al. Ethnicity, gender, and socioeconomic status as risk factors for esophagitis and Barrett's esophagus. Am J Epidemiol 2005;162:454–60.
16. Thrift AP, Shaheen NJ, Gammon MD, et al. Obesity and risk of esophageal adenocarcinoma and Barrett's esophagus: a Mendelian randomization study. J Natl Cancer Inst 2014;106(11):dju252.
17. Coleman HG, Bhat S, Johnston BT, et al. Tobacco smoking increases the risk of high-grade dysplasia and cancer among patients with Barrett's esophagus. Gastroenterology 2012;142:233–40.
18. Moore SC, Lee IM, Weiderpass E, et al. Association of leisure-time physical activity with risk of 26 types of cancer in 1.44 million adults. JAMA Intern Med 2016;176:816–25.
19. Murphy SJ, Anderson LA, Ferguson HR, et al. Dietary antioxidant and mineral intake in humans is associated with reduced risk of esophageal adenocarcinoma but not reflux esophagitis or Barrett's esophagus. J Nutr 2010;140: 1757–63.
20. Singh S, Garg SK, Singh PP, et al. Acid suppressive medications and risk of oesophageal adenocarcinoma in patients with Barrett's oesophagus: a systematic review and meta-analysis. Gut 2014;63:1229–37.
21. Liao LM, Vaughan TL, Corley DA, et al. Nonsteroidal anti-inflammatory drug use reduces the risk of adenocarcinomas of the esophagus and esophagogastric junction in a pooled analysis. Gastroenterology 2012;142:442–52.

22. Singh S, Singh AG, Singh PP, et al. Statins associated with reduced risk of esophageal cancer, particularly in patients with Barrett's esophagus: a systematic review and meta-analysis. Clin Gastroenterol Hepatol 2013;11:620–9.
23. Joo MK, Park JJ, Chun HJ. Additional benefits of routine drugs on gastrointestinal cancer: statin, metformin, and proton pump inhibitors. Dig Dis 2018; 36:1–14.
24. Cook MB, Corley DA, Murray LJ, et al. Gastroesophageal reflux in relation to adenocarcinomas of the esophagus: a pooled analysis from the Barrett's and esophageal adenocarcinoma consortium (BEACON). PLoS One 2014;9(7): e103508.
25. Lagergren J, Bergstrom R, Lindgren A, et al. Symptomatic gastroesophageal reflux as a risk factor for esophageal adenocarcinoma. N Engl J Med 1999;340: 825–31.
26. Souza RF, Shewmake K, Terada LS, et al. Acid exposure activates the mitogen-activated protein kinase pathways in Barrett's esophagus. Gastroenterology 2002;122:299–307.
27. Zhang HY, Hormi-Carver K, Zhang X, et al. In benign Barrett's epithelial cells, acid exposure generates reactive oxygen species that cause DNA double-strand breaks. Cancer Res 2009;69:9083–9.
28. Li D, Deconda D, Li A, et al. Effect of proton pump inhibitor therapy on NOX-5, mPEGS-1, and iNOS expression in Barrett's esophagus. Sci Rep 2019;9:16242.
29. Ouatu-Lascar R, Fitzgerald RC, Triadafilopoulos G. Differentiation and proliferation in Barrett's esophagus and the effects of acid suppression. Gastroenterology 1999;117:327–35.
30. Chueca E, Lanas A, Piazuelo E. Role of gastrin-peptides in Barrett's and colorectal carcinogenesis. World J Gastroenterol 2012;18:6560–70.
31. Haigh CR, Attwood SE, Thompson DG, et al. Gastrin induces proliferation in Barrett's metaplasia through activation of the CCK2 receptor. Gastroenterology 2003;124:615–25.
32. Wang JS, Varro A, Lightdale CJ, et al. Elevated serum gastrin is associated with a history of advanced neoplasia in Barrett's esophagus. Am J Gastroenterol 2010;105:1039–45.
33. Dunbar KB, Souza RF, Spechler SJ. The effect of proton pump inhibitors on Barrett's esophagus. Gastroenterol Clin North Am 2015;44:415–24.
34. Garcia Rodriguez LA, Lagergren J, Lindblad M. Gastric acid suppression and risk of oesophageal and gastric adenocarcinoma: a nested case control study in the UK. Gut 2006;55:1538–44.
35. Hu Q, Sun TT, Hong J, et al. Proton pump inhibitors do not reduce the risk of esophageal adenocarcinoma in patients with Barrett's esophagus: a systematic review and meta-analysis. PLoS One 2017;12:e0169691.
36. Tan MC, El-Serag HB, Yu X, et al. Acid suppression medications reduce risk of oesophageal adenocarcinoma in Barrett's oesophagus: a nested case-control study in US male veterans. Aliment Pharmacol Ther 2018;48:469–77.
37. Crockett SD, Lippmann QK, Dellon ES, et al. Health related quality of life in patients with Barrett's esophagus: a systematic review. Clin Gastroenterol Hepatol 2009;7:613–23.
38. Moayyedi P, Armstrong D, Hunt RH, et al. The gain in quality-adjusted life months by switching to esomeprazole in those with continued reflux symptoms in primary care: EncomPASS-A cluster-randomized trial. Am J Gastroenterol 2010;105:2341–6.

39. Katzka DA, Castell DO. Successful elimination of reflux symptoms does not insure adequate control of acid reflux in patients with Barrett's esophagus. Am J Gastroenterol 1994;89:989–91.
40. Gerson LB, Boparai V, Ullah N, et al. Oesophageal and gastric pH profiles in patients with gastro-oesophageal reflux disease and Barrett's oesophagus treated with proton pump inhibitors. Aliment Pharmacol Ther 2004;20:637–43.
41. Weijenborg PW, Smout AJPM, Krishnadath KK, et al. Esophageal sensitivity to acid in patients with Barrett's esophagus is not related to preserved esophageal mucosal integrity. Neurogastroenterol Motil 2017;29:e13066.
42. Basu KK, Bale R, West KP, et al. Persistent acid reflux and symptoms in patients with Barrett's oesophagus on proton-pump inhibitor therapy. Eur J Gastroenterol Hepatol 2002;14:1187–92.
43. Jankowski JA, de Caestecker J, Love SB, et al. Esomeprazole and aspirin in Barrett's oesophagus (AspECT): a randomised factorial trial. Lancet 2018;392: 400–8.
44. Vaezi M, Yang Y-X, Howden CW. Complications of proton pump inhibitor therapy. Gastroenterology 2017;153:35–48.
45. Laheij RJ, Sturkenboom MC, Hassing RJ, et al. Risk of community-acquired pneumonia and use of gastric acid suppressive drugs. JAMA 2004;292: 1955–60.
46. Yang YX, Lewis JD, Epstein S, et al. Long-term proton pump inhibitor therapy and risk of hip fracture. JAMA 2006;296:2947–53.
47. Leonard J, Marshall JK, Moayyedi P. Systematic review of the risk of enteric infection in patients taking acid suppression. Am J Gastroenterol 2007;102: 2047–56.
48. Dial S, Delaney JAC, Barkun AN, et al. Use of gastric acid-suppressive agents and the risk of community-acquired Clostridium difficile-associated disease. JAMA 2005;294:2989–95.
49. Charlot M, Grove EL, Hansen PR, et al. Proton pump inhibitor use and risk of adverse cardiovascular events in aspirin treated patient with first time myocardial infarction: a nationwide propensity score matched analysis. BMJ 2011; 342:d2690.
50. Lazarus B, Chen Y, Wilson FP, et al. Proton pump inhibitor use and risk of chronic kidney disease. JAMA Intern Med 2016;176:238–46.
51. Gomm W, von Holt K, Thome F, et al. Association of proton pump inhibitors with risk of dementia: a pharmacoepidemiological claims data analysis. JAMA Neurol 2016;73:410–6.
52. Xie Y, Bowe B, Li T, et al. Risk of death among users of proton pump inhibitors: a longitudinal observational cohort study of United States veterans. BMJ Open 2017;7(6):e015735.
53. Altman N, Krzywinski M. Association, correlation and causation. Nat Methods 2015;12:899–900.
54. Moayyedi P, Leontiadis GI. The risks of PPI therapy. Nat Rev Gastroenterol Hepatol 2012;9:132–9.
55. Moayyedi P, Eikelboom JW, Bosch J, et al. Safety of proton pump inhibitors based on a large, multi-year, randomized trial of patients receiving rivaroxaban or aspirin. Gastroenterology 2019;157:682–91.
56. Eikelboom JW, Connolly SJ, Bosch J, et al. Rivaroxaban with or without aspirin in stable cardiovascular disease. N Engl J Med 2017;377:1319–30.

57. Moayyedi P, Eikelboom JW, Bosch J, et al. Pantoprazole to prevent gastroduodenal events in patients receiving rivaroxaban and/or aspirin in a randomized, double-blind, placebo-controlled trial. Gastroenterology 2019;157:403–12.
58. Attwood SE, Ell C, Galmiche JP, et al. Long-term safety of proton pump inhibitor therapy assessed under controlled, randomised clinical trial conditions: data from the SOPRAN and LOTUS studies. Aliment Pharmacol Ther 2015;41: 1162–74.
59. Hashemi Goradel N, Najafi M, Salehi E, et al. Cyclooxgenase-2 in cancer: a review. J Cell Physiol 2019;234:5683–99.
60. Roos J, Grosch S, Werz O, et al. Regulation of tumorigenic Wnt signaling by cyclooxygenase-2, 5-lipoxygenase and their pharmacological inhibitors: a basis for novel drugs targeting cancer cells? Pharmacol Ther 2016;157:43–64.
61. Buas MF, He Q, Johnson LG, et al. Germline variation in inflammation-related pathways and risk of Barrett's oesophagus and oesophageal adenocarcinoma. Gut 2017;66:1739–47.
62. Zhang T, Wang Q, Ma WY, et al. Targeting the COX1/2-Driven thromboxane A2 pathway suppresses Barrett's esophagus and esophageal adenocarcinoma development. EBioMedicine 2019;49:145–56.
63. Jang T, Min S, Bae J, et al. Expression of cyclooxygenase-2, microsomal prostaglandin e synthetase 1, and EP receptors is increased in rat oesophageal squamous cell dysplasia and Barrett's metaplasia induced by duodenal contents reflux. Gut 2004;53:27–33.
64. Kaur B, Triadafilopoulos G. Acid-and bile-induced PGE2 release and hyperproliferation in Barrett's esophagus are COX-2 and PKC-ε dependent. Am J Physiol 2002;283:G327–34.
65. Shrivani VN, Ouatu-Lascar R, Kaur BS, et al. Cyclooxygenase 2 expression in Barrett's esophagus and adenocarcinoma: ex vivo induction by bile salts and acid exposure. Gastroenterology 2000;118:487–96.
66. Buttar NS, Wang KK, Leontovich O, et al. Chemoprevention of esophageal adenocarcinoma by COX-2 inhibitors in an animal model of Barrett's esophagus. Gastroenterology 2002;122:1101–12.
67. Corley DA, Kerlikowske K, Verma R, et al. Protective association of aspirin/ NSAIDs and esophageal cancer: a systematic review and meta-analysis. Gastroenterology 2003;124:47–56.
68. Wang F, Lv ZS, Fu YK. Nonsteroidal anti-inflammatory drugs and esophageal inflammation – Barrett's esophagus – adenocarcinoma sequence. Dis Esophagus 2011;24:318–24.
69. Castellsague J, Riera-Guardia N, Calingaert B, et al. Safety of Non-Steroidal Anti-Inflammatory Drugs (SOS) Project Individual NSAIDs and upper gastrointestinal complications: a systematic review and meta-analysis of observational studies (the SOS project). Drug Saf 2012;35:1127–46.
70. Scally B, Emberson JR, Spata E, et al. Effects of gastroprotectant drugs for the prevention and treatment of peptic ulcer disease and its complications: meta-analysis of randomised trials. Lancet Gastroenterol Hepatol 2018;3:231–41.
71. Coxib and traditional NSAID Trialists' (CNT) Collaboration. Vascular and upper gastrointestinal effects of non-steroidal anti-inflammatory drugs: meta-analyses of individual participant data from randomised trials. Lancet 2013; 382:769–79.
72. Hawkey CJ. COX-2 chronology. Gut 2005;54:1509–14.

73. Capone ML, Tacconelli S, Sciulli MG, et al. Clinical Pharmacology of Platelet, Monocyte, and Vascular Cyclooxygenase Inhibition by Naproxen and Low-Dose Aspirin in Healthy Subjects. Circulation 2004;109:1468–71.
74. Williams CD, Chan AT, Elman MR, et al. Aspirin use among adults in the U.S.: results of a national survey. Am J Prev Med 2015;48:501–8.
75. Zheng SL, Roddick AJ. Association of aspirin use for primary prevention with cardiovascular events and bleeding events. a systematic review and meta-analysis. JAMA 2019;321(3):277–87.
76. Thrift AP, Anderson LA, Murray LJ, et al. Nonsteroidal anti-inflammatory drug use is not associated with reduced risk of Barrett's esophagus. Am J Gastroenterol 2016;111:1528–35.
77. Vaughan TL, Dong LM, Blount PL, et al. Non-steroidal anti-inflammatory drugs and risk of neoplastic progression in Barrett's oesophagus: a prospective study. Lancet Oncol 2005;6:945–52.
78. Rothwell PM, Fowkes FGR, Belch JFF, et al. Effect of daily aspirin on long-term risk of death due to cancer: analysis of individual patient data from randomised trials. Lancet 2011;377:31–41.
79. Jankowski J, Barr H, deCastecker J, et al. Aspirin in the prevention of cancer. Lancet 2011;377:1649–50.
80. Zeb MH, Baruah A, Kossak SK, et al. Chemoprevention in Barrett's esophagus. Current status. Gastroenterol Clin North Am 2015;44:391–413.
81. Falk GW, Buttar NS, Foster NR, et al. A combination of esomeprazole and aspirin reduces tissue concentrations of prostaglandin E (2) in patients with Barrett's esophagus. Gastroenterology 2012;143:917–26.
82. Thrift AP, El-Serag HB. Sex and racial disparity in incidence of esophageal adenocarcinoma: observations and explanations. Clin Gastroenterol Hepatol 2016;14:330–2.
83. Maclennan AH, Broadbent JL, Lester S, et al. Oral oestrogen and combined oestrogen/progestogen therapy versus placebo for hot flushes. Cochrane Database Syst Rev 2004;(4):CD002978.
84. North American Menopause Society. The 2012 hormone therapy position statement of: the North American Menopause Society. Menopause 2012;19:257–71.
85. Santen RJ, Allred DC, Ardoin SP, et al. Postmenopausal hormone therapy: an Endocrine Society scientific statement. J Clin Endocrinol Metab 2010;95:s1–66.
86. Lagergren K, Lagergern J, Brusselaers N. Hormone replacement therapy and oral contraceptives and risk of oesophageal adenocarcinoma: a systematic review and meta- analysis. Int J Cancer 2014;135:2183–90.
87. Brusselaers N, Maret-Ouda J, Konings P, et al. Menopausal hormone therapy and the risk of esophageal and gastric cancer. Int J Cancer 2017;14o:1693–9.
88. Camargo MC, Goto Y, Zabaleta J, et al. Sex hormones, hormonal interventions, and gastric cancer risk: a meta-analysis. Cancer Epidemiol Biomarkers Prev 2012;21:20–38.
89. Wang BJ, Zhang B, Yan SS, et al. Hormonal and reproductive factors and risk of esophageal cancer in women: a meta-analysis. Dis Esophagus 2016;29: 448–54.
90. Menon S, Nightingale P, Trudgill N. Is hormone replacement therapy in post-menopausal women associated with a reduced risk of oesophageal cancer? United European Gastroenterol J 2014;2:374–82.
91. Edgren G, Adami HO, Weiderpass E, et al. A global assessment of the oesophageal adenocarcinoma epidemic. Gut 2013;62:1406–14.

92. Warren MP. Hormone therapy for menopausal symptoms: putting benefits and risks into perspective. J Fam Pract 2010;59:E1–7.
93. Chan KK, Oza AM, Siu LL. The statins as anticancer agents. Clin Cancer Res 2003;9:10–9.
94. Ogunwobi OO, Beales IL. Statins inhibit proliferation and induce apoptosis in Barrett's esophageal adenocarcinoma cells. Am J Gastroenterol 2008;103: 825–37.
95. Sadaria MR, Reppert AE, Yu JA, et al. Statin therapy attenuates growth and malignant potential of human esophageal adenocarcinoma cells. J Thorac Cardiovasc Surg 2011;142:1152–60.
96. Nguyen T, Khalaf N, Ramsey D, et al. Statin use is associated with a decreased risk of Barrett's esophagus. Gastroenterology 2014;147:314–23.
97. Maret-Ouda J, El-Serag HB, Lagergren J. Opportunities for preventing esophageal adenocarcinoma. Cancer Prev Res 2016;9:828–34.
98. Thomas T, Loke Y, Beales ILP. Systematic review and meta-analysis: use of statins is associated with a reduced incidence of oesophageal adenocarcinoma. J Gastrointest Cancer 2018;49:442–54.
99. Alexandre L, Clark AB, Bhutta HY, et al. Statin use is associated with reduced risk of histologic subtypes of esophageal cancer: a nested case-control analysis. Gastroenterology 2014;146(3):661–8.
100. Nguyen T, Duan Z, Naik AD, et al. Statin use reduces risk of esophageal adenocarcinoma in US veterans with Barrett's esophagus: a nested case-control study. Gastroenterology 2015;149:1392–8.
101. Emberson JR, Kearney PM, Blackwell L, et al. Lack of effect of lowering LDL cholesterol on cancer: meta-analysis of individual data from 175,000 people in 27 randomised trials of statin therapy. PLoS One 2012;7:e29849.
102. Krishnamoorthi R, Singh S, Ragunathan K, et al. Factors associated with progression of Barrett's esophagus: a systematic review and meta-analysis. Clin Gastroenterol Hepatol 2018;16:1046–55.
103. Zhou G, Myers R, Li Y, et al. Role of AMP-activated protein kinase in mechanism of metformin action. J Clin Invest 2001;108:1167–74.
104. Kobayashi M, Kato K, Iwama H, et al. Antitumor effect of metformin in esophageal cancer: in vitro study. Int J Oncol 2013;42:517–24.
105. Evans JM, Donnelly LA, Emslie-Smith AM, et al. Metformin and reduced risk of cancer in diabetic patients. BMJ 2005;330:1304–5.
106. Landman GW, Kleefstra N, van Hateren KJ, et al. Metformin associated with lower cancer mortality in type 2 diabetes ZODIAC-16. Diabetes care 2010;33: 322–6.
107. Singh S, Sharma AN, Murad MH, et al. Central adiposity is associated with increased risk of esophageal inflammation, metaplasia, and adenocarcinoma: a systematic review and meta-analysis. Clin Gastroenterol Hepatol 2013;11: 1399–412.
108. Krishnamoorthi R, Borah B, Heien H, et al. Rates and predictors of progression to esophageal carcinoma in a large population-based Barrett's esophagus cohort. Gastrointest Endosc 2016;84:40–6.
109. Chak A, Buttar NS, Foster NR, et al. Metformin does not reduce markers of cell proliferation in esophageal tissues of patients with Barrett's esophagus. Clin Gastroenterol Hepatol 2015;13:665–72.
110. Solaymani-Dodaran M, Card TR, West J. Cause-specific mortality of people with Barrett's esophagus compared with the general population: a population-based cohort study. Gastroenterology 2013;144:1375–83.

Optimizing Outcomes with Radiofrequency Ablation of Barrett's Esophagus

Candidates, Efficacy and Durability

Philippe Leclercq, MD, Raf Bisschops, MD, PhD*

KEYWORDS

- Barrett's esophagus • Radiofrequency ablation • Outcomes

KEY POINTS

- Barrett's esophagus (BE) is the precursor for esophageal adenocarcinoma (EAC). The risk of progression from non-dysplastic BE to EAC increases progressively with stages of dysplasia.
- If early-stage cancer or high-grade dysplasia is diagnosed, endoscopic therapy is the treatment of choice with better safety profile and similar efficacy compared with esophagectomy.
- Endoscopic therapy is based on a "2-step concept": visible lesions are endoscopically removed and the remaining flat BE is ablated to prevent metachronous neoplasia.
- Radiofrequency ablation (RFA) effectively eradicates dysplastic Barrett esophagus (BE) and reduces the metachronous risk of esophageal adenocarcinoma (EAC), with an acceptable low complication rate.
- After achieving complete eradication of intestinal metaplasia (CE-IM) by RFA, dysplasia recurrence rate is approximately 2% per patient year of follow-up time, justifying post-ablation surveillance.

INTRODUCTION

Barrett's esophagus (BE) is the precursor for esophageal adenocarcinoma (EAC). The risk of progression from nondysplastic BE (NDBE) to EAC is 30-fold to 125-fold greater than in the general population, increasing progressively with different stages of dysplasia.[1,2] Progression occurs stepwise from nondysplastic intestinal metaplasia to low-grade to high-grade dysplasia and ultimately to adenocarcinoma.[3]

Gastroenterology and Hepatology, University Hospital Leuven, 49 Herestraat, Leuven 3000, Belgium
* Corresponding author.
E-mail address: raf.bisschops@uzleuven.be

Gastrointest Endoscopy Clin N Am 31 (2021) 131–154
https://doi.org/10.1016/j.giec.2020.09.004

The risk of EAC for patients with NDBE ranges between 0.12% and 0.5% per year.[4–6] Patients with NDBE have a reported lifetime EAC risk of 5% to 6% increasing to 30% at 5 years if high-grade dysplasia (HGD) is present.[7,8]

Endoscopic resection (ER) for BE early neoplasia was introduced more than 10 years ago, showing to be an effective and safe treatment strategy with up to 5 years of follow-up.[9–12] If early-stage cancer or HGD (early Barrett neoplasia) is diagnosed, endoscopic therapy is the treatment of choice with better safety profile and similar efficacy compared with esophagectomy.[13–18] Endoscopic therapy is based on a "2-step concept": visible lesions are endoscopically removed and sent for histopathological evaluation. Afterward, the remaining flat BE is eradicated by ablation therapy to prevent metachronous neoplasia.[19] BE ablation is also indicated for flat HGD and confirmed flat low-grade dysplasia (LGD).[20] Focusing only on eradication of visible dysplasia while leaving residual (apparently nondysplastic) BE untreated will lead to recurrent neoplasia in 20% to 30% of patients within 3 years of follow-up.[10,21]

During the past decades, numerous BE ablative modalities have been proposed (laser, multipolar electrocoagulation, heater probe, photodynamic therapy, ultrasonic intraluminal ablation, argon plasma coagulation, cryoablation, radiofrequency ablation).[22–28] The rationale was to induce superficial ablation of the metaplastic mucosa which in combination with sufficient acid suppression should lead to neosquamous reepithelialization of the ablated area.[29] Nowadays, radiofrequency ablation (RFA) is still the strongest evidence-based ablation technique for BE.

CANDIDATES

Nondysplastic Barrett's Esophagus

Endoscopic ablation was initially proposed as an alternative to surveillance for NDBE. A multicenter study of RFA of NDBE achieved complete eradication of BE in 98.4% of patients at 2.5 years and 92% at 5 years, without progression during follow-up.[30] The average risk of cancer progression in patients with NDBE is now better estimated, at approximately 0.3% per year.[4,31–33] This low risk level renders the cost-effectiveness analysis unfavorable for preventive RFA in NDBE, especially when the stricture rate and procedural costs are taken into consideration.[34,35] Furthermore, long-term follow-up after ablation in patients with NDBE cannot be abandoned because of a recurrence of intestinal metaplasia in approximately 20% of cases after ablation.[32] Even if RFA cannot be recommended in patients with NDBE, its place in high-lifetime risk of cancer (familial history of EAC, young patients with long segments of BE) or biomarker-driven risk stratification is still debated and can be considered.[20,32,36–39]

Low-Grade Dysplasia

There were controversies about the natural history of LGD during the early previous decade due to a variable reported risk of progression to EAC/HGD, ranging between a risk similar to NDBE and HGD.[33,40–42] Later on, LGD was shown to be widely overestimated because a single LGD diagnosis is often not reproduced on further endoscopies in almost 30% of patients and will be downstaged in 50% to 85% of the cases after expert/panel pathologic review.[42–44] Several studies showed a significant increased risk of progression when the histopathological diagnosis of LGD is confirmed by a second expert pathologist, if possible, at an external institution with a consensus diagnosis from an expert panel.[42,43,45–49] Confirmed LGD diagnosis over time (on at least 2 subsequent endoscopies in 6 months) and/or at multiple esophageal levels are risk factors for progression to HGD/EAC.[49–51] A confirmed diagnosis of LGD correlates with a higher risk of progression to cancer, but it is unclear yet whether this warrants therapeutic intervention. Pathologic, temporal, and spatial LGD confirmation are cornerstones before considering ablation for LGD-BE, to balance the risk of progression against the complications of bleeding and stenosis to RFA.[52] Especially, RFA in LGD-BE should be balanced against surveillance (or even absence of surveillance) in patients with major comorbidities and limited life-expectancy.

On the other hand, the finding of LGD in a BE may be an indicator of more severe prevalent disease. Careful endoscopic inspection of the BE mucosa under proton pump inhibitor (PPI) regimen is therefore crucial to detect and resect any visible lesion before considering RFA. The UK RFA registry nicely showed that early recognition and resection of any visible lesion before RFA is key for adequate staging of invasive disease and to improve the long-term success rate of RFA in terms of complete remission for intestinal metaplasia and dysplasia.[53]

High-Grade Dysplasia and Superficial Esophageal Adenocarcinoma

Patients with HGD-BE and intramucosal EAC have a low risk of lymph node metastasis (HGD: 0%; intramucosal EAC: up to 2%).[54] Endoscopic treatment with ER and RFA of HGD-BE and intramucosal EAC is more effective and cost-effective than endoscopic follow-up and surgery in case of disease progression. In addition, the strategy is oncologically equal but significantly safer than surgery.[27,55,56] ER is the first-choice treatment for T1a EAC, followed by complete RFA of all remaining Barrett's mucosa. Because the vast majority of the patients with confirmed HGD-intramucosal EAC harbor endoscopically visible lesions, patients should be carefully endoscopically inspected to detect and resect any suspicious lesion before considering RFA.[57,58] It has been shown that experienced endoscopists in BE may detect overlooked lesions in up to 75% of patients during workup, supporting the need for referral to expert BE centers.[59,60] Confirmation of histopathology by expert review is also required, especially in case of flat HGD to avoid overstaging and subsequent overtreatment.

Even if in case of T1b EAC (especially sm2-3), esophagectomy (with discussion of neoadjuvant therapy) is recommended in patients fit for surgery, there are still conflicting data around the lymph node invasion risk in T1b sm1 EAC.[20,61–63] For these T1b sm1 patients, ER followed by surveillance is under evaluation in subjects at high complication risk with surgery, especially for those with best prognosis: well-differentiated tumors, no lymphovascular invasion (Prefer study ongoing, AMC Amsterdam, NL ClinicalTrials.gov Identifier: NCT03222635). The optimal timing of ablation of the residual Barrett's in these particular patients is still undefined. In our practice, we usually wait 6 to 12 months and only perform RFA of the remaining Barrett epithelium if staging with endoscopic ultrasound and PET–computed tomography are negative for metastasis.

Pretreatment Workup to Improve Selection of Patients and Efficacy of Radiofrequency Ablation

The informed consent process is of crucial importance to guarantee treatment success. First, clinicians should duly inform patients about the natural history of BE-associated dysplasia and balance this against the risk of the procedure and comorbidity status of the patient. Patients should be made aware about the RFA treatment track that comprises a long time span with multiple sessions and intervals and they need to agree that this is necessary to achieve successful eradication. Indeed, in most trials, up to 5 treatment sessions of RFA were allowed to obtain complete remission of dysplasia (CE-D) and intestinal metaplasia (CE-IM).[27,46,57,64] To improve compliance with the RFA treatment program, patients should be warned about the side effects (pain) and the need for a soft diet after each session to avoid these. Complications (stricture, bleeding) need to be explained. The alternatives of surgery and endoscopic surveillance need to be discussed, especially in case poor compliance is anticipated. Finally, the patient should be informed about the efficacy of the treatment and about the need for pursuing endoscopic surveillance program after complete eradication of intestinal metaplasia because of risk of recurrence. The patient should also be aware of the need for compliance with acid-suppression therapy during and after eradication.

Uncontrolled ongoing reflux disease may compromise the success rate of RFA. In this situation, tailoring acid suppression and patient's compliance (PPI, health and diet advice) is the key to avoid poor responders/poor healers to RFA. In case of persistent esophageal reflux under high-dose PPI, antireflux surgery before RFA could be discussed after impedance pH-monitoring. Squamous reepithelialization of the ER wound and presence of numerous squamous islands in the Barrett's area after Seattle biopsies is a good predictor for a good responder to RFA.[65] Esophageal stenosis is also a predictor of poor response to RFA treatment, probably due to more severe reflux disease and poorer contact of the RFA probe with the target tissue with less effective ablation.[65]

EFFICACY

Clinical Trials: Assurance for Safe Oncological Outcome

A meta-analysis of 2013, reported pooled CE-IM and CE-D in 78% (95% confidence interval [CI], 70%–86%) and 91% (95% CI, 87%–95%) in data from 18 studies (3802 patients).[66] In 2016, Desai and colleagues[67] reported the pooled analysis of 9 studies (774 patients) using focal-endoscopic mucosal resection (EMR) in combination with RFA for BE-related HGD/EAC, reaching CE-D in 93.4% and CE-IM in 73.1%.

The most recent meta-analysis from 2018 by Pandey and colleagues,[68] showed overall pooled rates of CE-IM and CE-D of 88.2% (95% CI, 88.1% and 88.2%) and 96.7% (95% CI, 96.67%–96.71%) in 8 studies including 619 patients with LGD-BE treated by RFA.

It is clear from the earliest clinical trials that the success rate of RFA to obtain CE-IM and CE-D depends largely on 2 factors: first a combination of circumferential and focal ablation and second a low threshold for performing EMR before RFA. The efficacy outcomes of prospective trials registries are summarized in **Table 1**.

In 2007, Sharma and colleagues[69] reported the early results of the prospective multicenter AIM-trial, initially only using the circumferential ablation device in 70 patients with NDBE patients. At 1-year follow-up, CE-IM was achieved in only 70%

Table 1
Energy setting for Barrett's esophagus ablation

RFA device	Classic Protocol	Simplified Protocol
HALO express	1 × 10 J/cm^2-clean-1 × 10 J/cm^2	Not recommended[78,102]
HALO 90	EU: 2 × 15 J/cm^2-clean-2 × 15 J/cm^2 [94,95] US: 2 × 12 J/cm^2-Clean-2 × 12 J/cm^2 [27]	3 × 12 J/cm^2-no clean[75]
HALO 60	EU: 2 × 15 J/cm^2-clean-2 × 15 J/cm^2 US: 2 × 12 J/cm^2-clean-2 × 12 J/cm^2	3 × 12 J/cm^2-no clean
HALO TTS	EU: 2 × 15 J/cm^2-clean-2 × 15 J/cm^2 US: 2 × 12 J/cm^2-clean-2 × 12 J/cm	3 × 12 J/cm^2-no clean

with a maximum of 2 balloon-based circumferential RFA sessions (2 × 10J No Clean/session) per patient.

However after add-on therapy with the focal ablation device, CE-IM was achieved in 98% of the patients without any stricture.[70] Similarly, Ganz and colleagues[71] reported efficacy of balloon-based circumferential RFA in 142 HGD-BE, reaching 54.3% CE-IM and 80.4% CE-D at 1-year follow-up. A focal device was not available in this study and the protocol was not standardized (10J-Clean-10J vs 2 × 10J No clean).

The efficacy of combination of EMR of visible lesions to achieve CE-IM and CE-D is demonstrated in several prospective controlled trials, as well as in prospective registries. In the 3 major prospective trials, AIM dysplasia, EURO-II trial and the SURF trial CE-D ranges between 81% and 95%. For CE-IM, the efficacy ranged between 77% and 87%[27,57,72]

These high success rates were subsequently confirmed outside of the stringent selection criteria of prospective trials in real-life prospective registries. CE-D ranges between 77% and 100% and CE-IM is achieved between 56% and 85% (see **Table 1**). One may wonder that there is indeed a huge variation in success, and this probably depends on the correct selection of patients for RFA.

In 2013, Haidry and colleagues[73] reported the results of the UK National Halo RFA Multicenter Registry (508 patients), achieving only CE-IM in 62% and CE-D in 81% at 12 months. A secondary analysis by period showed a significant improvement over time of CE-D and CE-IM from 77% and 56% to 92% and 83% that coincided with an increase in EMR before RFA therapy from 48% to 60%. This also led to a significant reduction in the need of rescue EMR after RFA from 13% to 2%.[53] In another trial, the use of EMR before RFA also significantly reduced the risk of treatment failure.[74]

This indicates that thorough inspection by an experienced endoscopist before commencing endotherapy in dysplastic BE is the most important and crucial step for success. This may appear trivial but is in real-life quite challenging. Indeed, a study looking at patients referred for endoluminal therapy for neoplastic BE, showed that expert endoscopists can find a suspicious lesion in 75% of cases that was missed or not mentioned by the referring physician.[59]

Optimizing the Energy Settings and Treatment Protocol: from Here to There and Back Again

Acid-suppression therapy is of crucial importance to achieve optimal outcomes. All trials included 2 × 40-mg PPIs that is usually continued after reaching the endpoint of CE-IM. Noncompliance to PPI therapy is therefore one of the first differentials to exclude in case of poor response after RFA. Other predictive factors for a poor response include active reflux esophagitis at baseline, EMR scar regeneration with BE epithelium, esophageal narrowing before RFA and the duration of neoplasia presence before RFA.[65]

Efficacy of RFA is also determined by the energy settings and treatment protocols. For both circumferential and focal RFA devices, energy settings can be adapted manually. The very first AIM trial[69] indicated that energy settings less than 10 J/cm^2 were inefficient and that in NDBE 2 × 10 J ought to be use without compromising safety in terms of stricture rate. However, in case of dysplasia, it seemed that there was an apparent difference in efficacy between the AIM dysplasia and EURO II trial.[57] The Amsterdam group adapted the protocol by increasing energy settings to 2 × 12 J/cm^2 for circumferential ablation with an extensive cleaning step in between the ablations. For focal ablations, the settings of the AIM dysplasia trial were increased from 12 J/cm^2 to 15 J/cm^2, applied as 2 × 15 J/cm^2 with an extensive cleaning step in between. The systematic ablation of the neo-z-line on each occasion a focal ablation was

Table 2
RFA efficacy in BE ablation

Authors	Patients	RFA Protocol	Follow-up	Definition of CE	RFA Sessions	Escape Treatment	CE-IM (%)	CE-D (%)	AE (Number of Patients)
Sharma et al,[69] 2007 *AIM-trial*	70 (70 NDBE)	HALO 360: 10 J/cm² (2 hits no clean) Max sessions: 2	At 12 mo	4Q/1-2 cm Bx negative for IM (cardia excluded), from neosquamous mucosa	• Mean 360: 1.5	NS	70	NS	Stricture: 0 (0%) Bleeding: 0 (0%)
Ganz et al,[71] 2008 *US registry*	142 (142 HGD)	HALO 360: 12 J/cm² (2 hits no clean or 1 hit-clean-1hit) Max sessions: 2	MED 12 mo	4Q/1-2 cm Bx negative for IM and/or D, from neosquamous epithelium	• MED 360: 1	NS	54.3	80.4	Stricture: 1 (0.7%) Bleeding: 0 (0%)
Fleischer et al,[70] 2008 *AIM-trial extension*	70 (70 NDBE)	HALO 360: 10 J/cm² (2 hits no clean) Max sessions: 2 + *12 mo:* HALO 90: 12 J/cm² (2 hits-clean-2 hits) Max sessions: 3	At 30 mo	4Q/1-2 cm Bx negative for IM (cardia excluded), from neosquamous mucosa	• Mean 360: 1.5 • Mean focal: 1.9	NS	98	NS	Stricture: 0 (0%) Bleeding:1 (1.4%)
Gondrie et al,[94] 2008 AMC-I trial	11 (2 LGD, 9 HGD)	HALO 360: 12 J/cm² (1 hit-clean-1hit) Max sessions: 2 HALO 90: 12–15 J/cm² (2 hits-clean-2 hits) Max sessions: 3	At 14 mo	4Q/1 cm Bx negative for IM and/or D (CE-IM/CE-D), from neosquamous epithelium + neo-Z-line	• MED 360: 2 • MED focal: 2	0	100	100	Stricture: 0 (0%) Bleeding:0 (0%)

Gondrie et al,[95] 2008 AMC-II trial	12 (1 LGD, 11 HGD)	HALO 360: 12 J/cm^2 (1 hit-clean-1hit) Max sessions: 2 HALO 90: 12 J/cm^2 (2 hits-clean-2 hits) Max sessions: 3	At 14 mo	4Q/1 cm Bx negative for IM and/or D (CE-IM/CE-D), from neosquamous epithelium + neo-Z-line	• MED 360: 1 • MED focal: 2	1 (EMR)	100	100	Stricture: 1 (8%) Bleeding: 0 (0%)
Sharma et al,[96] 2009 *Mayo Clinic cohort*	63 (39 LGD, 24 HGD)	1st session: HALO 360: 12 J/cm^2 (1hit-clean-1hit) Max session: 1 Following sessions: HALO 90: 12 J/cm^2 (2hits-clean-2hits) Max sessions: NS	MED 24 mo	• 4Q/1 cm Bx negative for IM and/or D (CE-IM/CE-D), from neosquamous epithelium (4Q/1 cm) Rem: IM distal to GEJ not considered as failure.	• MED 360: 1 • MED focal: 1	3 (EMR)	79	89	Stricture: 1 (1.6%) Bleeding: 1 (1.6%)
Shaheen et al,[27] 2009 AIM-dysplasia trial *US RCT*	84 (42 LGD, 42 HGD) *vs* 43 sham	1st session: HALO 360: 12 J/cm^2 (1hit-clean-1hit) Max session: 1 Following sessions: HALO 90: Energy NS (2 hits-clean-2 hits) Max sessions: 3	At 12 mo	4Q/1 cm Bx negative for IM and/or D (CE-IM/CE-D), from neosquamous epithelium	• Mean total: 3.5	NS	77	86	Stricture: 5 (6%) Bleeding:1 (1.2%)

(*continued on next page*)

Table 2
(continued)

Authors	Patients	RFA Protocol	Follow-up	Definition of CE	RFA Sessions	Escape Treatment	CE-IM (%)	CE-D (%)	AE (Number of Patients)
Lyday et al,[97] 2010 *US registry*	429 (safety cohort, 326 NDBE,12 IND, 52 LGD, 39 HGD) −338 (efficacy cohort, 255 NDBE, 10 IND, 42 LGD,31 HGD)	HALO 360: 10 or 12 J/cm^2 (1hit-clean-1hit) Focal ablation: 12 J/cm^2 (2 hits-clean-2hits) Max sessions: NS	MED: 20 mo	4Q/1-2 cm Bx negative for IM and/or D (CE-IM/CE-D), from neosquamous epithelium	• Mean total: 2.1	NS	77	100	Stricture: 9 (2.1%) Bleeding: 4 (0.9%)
Pouw et al,[98] 2010 *EURO-I trial*	23 (7 HGIN, 16 early EAC)	HALO 360: 12 J/cm^2 (1hit-clean-1hit) Max sessions: 2 HALO 90: 12 J/cm^2 (2hits-clean-2hits) Max sessions: 3	MED: 22 mo	4Q/1 cm Bx negative for IM and/or D (CE-IM/CE-D), from neosquamous epithelium	• MED 360: 1 • MED focal: 1	2 (EMR)	96	100	Stricture: 1 (4%) Bleeding: 1 (4%)
Van Vilsteren et al,[99] 2011 *AMC-IV trial*	22 (15 EAC, 7 HGD) vs 25 SRER	1st session: HALO 360: 12 J/cm^2 (1hit-clean-1hit) Max sessions: 2 HALO 90: 15 J/cm^2 (2hits-clean-2 hits) Max sessions: 3	MED 24 mo	4Q/1 cm Bx negative for IM and/or D (CE-IM/CE-D), from neosquamous epithelium	• MED total: 3	4 (2 hot biopsy forceps, 1 EMR + APC, 1 EMR)	95.4	95.4	Stricture: 3 (14%) Bleeding: 3 (14%) *vs* *Stricture:* 88% in SRER group

Okoro et al,[100] 2012 *Mayo Clinic cohort* *Retrospective comparison EMR + RFA - RFA alone group*	44 (RFA after EMR: 2 NDBE, 3 LGD, 35 HGD, 4 IMC) - 46 (RFA alone: 25 NDBE, 13 LGD, 8 HGD)	HALO 360: 12 J/cm² (1hit-clean-1hit) Max session: NS HALO 90: Energy NS (2hits-clean-2hits) Max sessions: 5	MED 20.5 mo - MED 32 mo	4Q/1-2 cm Bx negative for IM and/or D (CE-IM/CE-D), from neosquamous epithelium + neo-Z-line	• MED total: 2, in 2 groups	NS	43–74	76–71	Stricture: 6–4 (13.6%-8.7%) Bleeding: 0–0 (0%)
Gupta et al,[84] 2013 *US registry - BETRNet Consortium*	592 (safety cohort) 448 (efficacy cohort, 63 NDBE, 68 LGD, 268 HGD, 49 EAC)	NS (NDBE: 10 J/cm², LGD/HGD/EAC: 12 J/cm²)	MED 24 mo	4Q/1-2 cm Bx negative for IM and/or D (CE-IM/CE-D), from neosquamous epithelium + neo-Z-line	RFA sessions 1 session: 29% 2 sessions: 35% 3–10 sessions: 36%	NS	56	NS	Stricture: 27 (4.6%) Bleeding: 8 (13.5%)
Haidry et al,[53] 2015 UK registry	508 (14 LGD, 369 HGD, 125 IMC)	HALO 360: 12 J/cm² (1hit-clean-1hit) Focal: 15 J/cm² (2hits-clean-2hits) Max sessions: 4 (in 12 mo) + 1 escape RFA	At 12 mo	• 4Q/1-2 cm Bx negative for IM and/or D (CE-IM/CE-D), from neosquamous epithelium + neo-Z-line Rem: IM distal to GEJ not considered as failure	*2008–2010:* Mean total: 2.6 *2011–2013:* Mean total: 2.5	*2008–2010:* 13% (EMR) *2011–2013:* 2% (EMR)	*total* 70 *2008–10* 56 *2011–13* 83	*total* 84 *2008–10* 77 *2011–13* 92	*2008–2010* Stricture: 25 (9.4%) Perforation: 1 Bleeding: <1% *2011–2013* Stricture: 15 (6.2%) Bleeding<1%

(*continued on next page*)

Table 2
(continued)

Authors	Patients	RFA Protocol	Follow-up	Definition of CE	RFA Sessions	Escape Treatment	CE-IM (%)	CE-D (%)	AE (Number of Patients)
Pasricha et al,[83] 2014 US Registry	1634 (668 NDBE, 114 IND, 323 LGD, 416 HGD, 113 EAC)	HALO 360: 12 J/cm^2 (1hit-clean-1hit) HALO 90: Energy NS (2 hits-clean-2hits) Max sessions: NS	At 12 mo	4Q/1 cm Bx negative for IM (CE-IM), from neosquamous epithelium	• MED 360: 0.7 • MED 90: 2.2	2% (RFA)	85	NS	NS
Phoa et al,[72] 2014 SURF trial EU RCT	68 (68 LGD) *vs* 68 surveillance	HALO 360: 12 J/cm^2 (1 hit-clean-1hit) Max sessions: 2 Focal: 12 J/cm^2 (2hits-clean-2hits) Max sessions: 3	At the end of EET	4Q/2 cm Bx negative for IM and/or D (CE-IM/CE-D), from neosquamous epithelium + neo-Z-line	MED total: 3	5 EMR 12 APC	88.2	92.6	Stricture 8 (11.8%) Bleeding:1 (1.5%)
Phoa et al,[57] 2016 EURO-II trial	132 (51 NDBE, 45 LGD, 36 HGD)	HALO 360: 12 J/cm^2 (1hit-clean-1hit) Max sessions: 2 Focal: 12 J/cm^2 (2hits-clean-2hits) Max sessions: 3	MED 12 mo	4Q/2 cm Bx negative for IM and/or D (CE-IM/CE-D), from neosquamous epithelium + neo-Z-line	• MED 360: 1 • MED focal: 2	9 EMR 15 APC	87	92	Stricture: 8 (6.1%) Bleeding: 1 (<1%)

Li et al,[101] 2016 US Registry *comparison ER + RFA - RFA alone*	994 (efficacy cohort, 832 HGD, 162 IMC) 1263 (safety cohort, 1054 HGD, 209 IMC)	HALO 360: 12 J/cm² (1hit-clean-1hit) HALO 90: Energy NS (2hits-clean-2 hits) Max sessions: NS	ER before RFA: mean 2.86 mo RFA alone: mean 2.76 mo	4Q/1-2 cm Bx negative for IM and/or D (CE-IM/CE-D), from neosquamous epithelium + neo-Z-line	ER + RFA: Mean 360: 0.7 Mean focal: 2.1 RFA alone: Mean 360: 0.9 Mean focal: 2.4	NS	ER + RFA: 84 RFA alone: 84	ER + RFA: 94 RFA alone: 92	ER + RFA: Stricture: 29 Bleeding: 0 RFA alone: Stricture: 52 Bleeding: 0
Vliebergh et al,[64] 2019 Belgian registry	295 (efficacy cohort) 342 (safety cohort, NS 4, NDBE 3, LGD 23, HGD 186, EAC 126)	NS	At 12 mo	4Q/1-2 cm Bx negative for IM and/or D (CE-IM/CE-D), from neosquamous epithelium + neo-Z-line	• MED total: 2	13%	82	87	Stenosis: 18 (5.3%) Bleeding: 3 (<1%)

Abbreviations: 100PY, percent patient-year; 4Q, 4 quadrants; APC, argon plasma coagulation; BE, Barrett's esophagus; Bx, biopsies; CE, complete eradication; CE-D, complete eradication of dysplasia; CE-IM, complete eradication of intestinal metaplasia; D, dysplasia; EAC, esophageal adenocarcinoma; EMR, endoscopic mucosal resection; ER, endoscopic resection; EU, European; HGD, high-grade dysplasia; IM, intestinal metaplasia; IMC, intramucosal cancer; IND, indefinite for dysplasia; LGD, low-grade dysplasia; MED, median; mo, month; ND, nondysplastic; NS, not-specified; RCT, randomized controlled trial; RFA, radiofrequency ablation; SRER, stepwise radical endoscopic resection; UK, United Kingdom; US, Unites States; y, year.

performed for residual islands, most likely contributed also to a higher CE-IM rate in the EURO II trial.

Although highly effective, the EURO II protocol was perceived often as cumbersome due to the cleaning step between the 2 ablations. The Amsterdam group assessed in a multicenter trial setting whether this cleaning step could be omitted.[75] Recently, it was shown that focal ablation with 3×12 J/cm^2 without cleaning was noninferior in comparison with a classic 2×15 J/cm^2 -clean-2×15 J/cm^2 protocol, without an increased risk of strictures and with a reduction of 7 minutes on average in procedure time.[75] For circumferential ablation they also showed that a simplified 2×12 J/cm^2 ablation was equally safe and effective as the classic 12 J/cm^2 -clean-12 J/cm^2 protocol.[76] However, it needs to be emphasized that for the new-generation circumferential ablation device that integrates esophageal sizing and ablation in one catheter, this no longer applies. First, energy settings need to be decreased to 10 J/cm^2: because of the better apposition of this device to the esophageal mucosa, energy delivery is likely to be more efficient and resulted in more scarring in 23% of the patients after a single session with a classic ablation protocol.[77] It was therefore decided to use 10 J/cm^2 as a standard setting for the new generation circumferential ablation device. In addition, a recent trial showed that with this new generation device a simplified procedure cannot be used safely due to an increased risk of stenosis. A simplified protocol using only a single hit with 10 J/cm^2 had inferior efficacy.[78] So, after a journey using different treatment energy setting, we are since the introduction of the HALO 360 express back to the original energy and treatment settings of 10 J/cm^2 -clean-10 J/cm^2 (**Table 2**: energy setting for ablation).

Finally, it needs to be emphasized that the patient should be informed about the long time span of the endoluminal treatment to enhance compliance. Indeed, the high success rates in EURO-II and AIM dysplasia were obtained after a median of 1

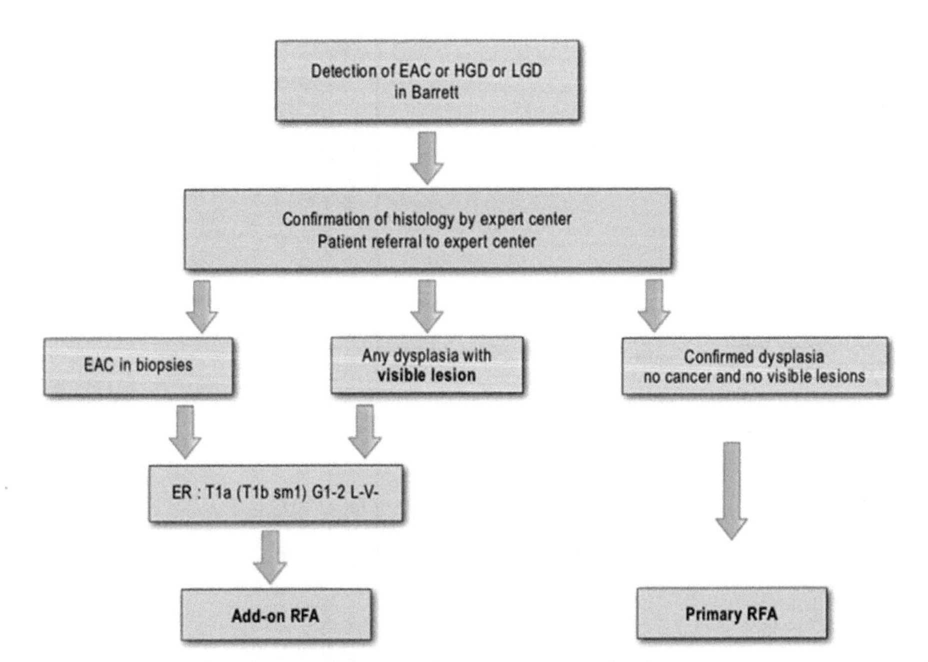

Fig. 1. Flowchart for patient selection and treatment optimization.

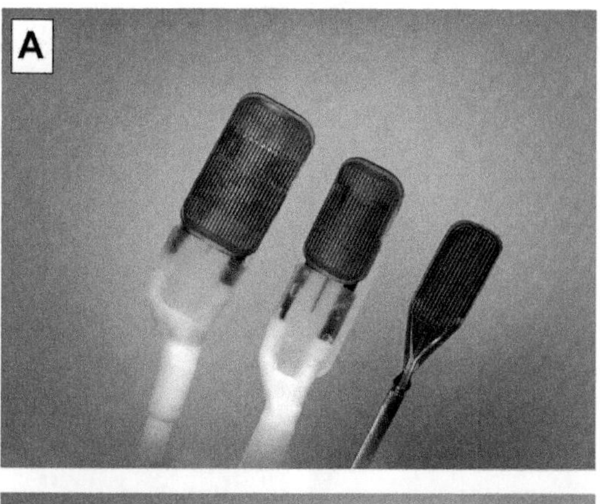

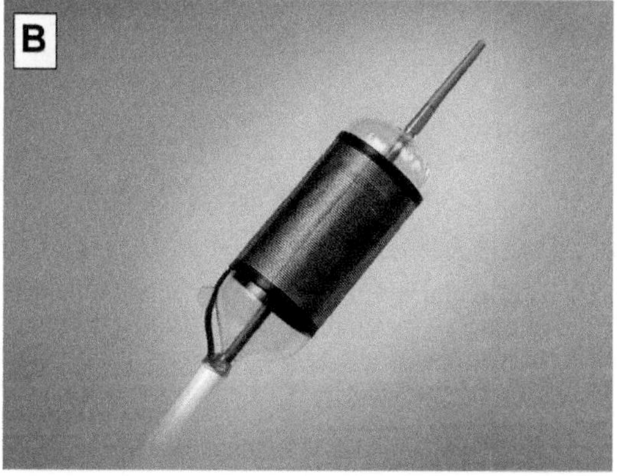

Fig. 2. RFA devices. (*A*) Focal RFA device. The bipolar electrode array is positioned at the upper orange and black surface. (*B*) Circumferential RFA balloon, inflated.

circumferential ablation and 2 focal ablation sessions, with 2 to 3 months interval and with a maximum of 5 RFA sessions in total. In our experience, we leave 3 months between each RFA session, because the 8-week interval we adhered to in the beginning resulted in too many postponed treatments and unnecessary endoscopies due to residual inflammation after the previous RFA session.

One final question to optimize treatment is when one needs to stop and decide that the patient is entirely treated. Indeed, often the neo-Z-line is still irregular and small projections may contain residual BE. From a practical viewpoint, if no residual islands are identified and no clear residual BE is present endoscopically (<1 cm), we take 4 to 6 random biopsies under the neo-Z-line. In case of residual IM, the patient will be scheduled for one more final focal ablation. If residual IM is found during the subsequent endoscopy with biopsies, we accept this situation and perform further follow-up (**Figs. 1–3**).

Efficacy Conclusion

Pooled remission rates range from 54% to 100% for IM and from 80% to 100% for dysplasia. Optimizing efficacy is obtained by (1) proper esophageal inspection before RFA to resect all visible abnormalities, (2) using correct energy settings depending on each ablation device, (3) adhering to the treatment protocols with

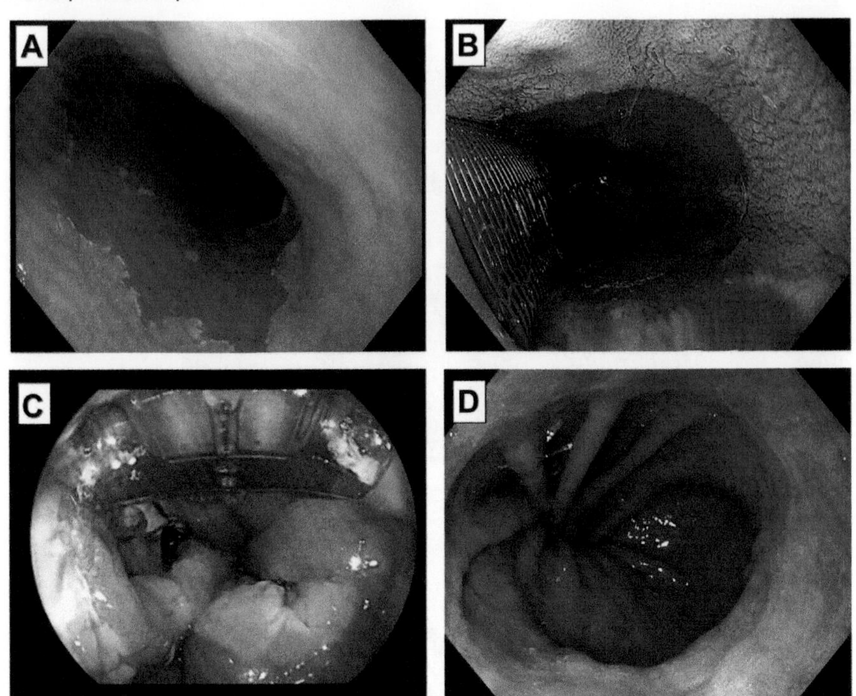

Fig. 3. Endoscopic view from patients with confirmed, persistent and multistage LGD BE from diagnosis to CE-IM through RFA treatment. (*A*) Endoscopic view showing proximal extent of Barrett mucosa before eradication. (*B*) Deflated circumferential ablation device re-positioning after first proximal hit (see whitish coagulum). (*C*) Focal radiofrequency ablation device used for targeting smaller area. (*D*) Endoscopic view after reaching CE-IM of Barrett mucosa.

(4) allowing an interval of 3 months between RFA sessions, and (5) emphasizing the importance of reflux control by compliance to high-dose PPI in between RFA sessions.

DURABILITY

Optimal endoscopic treatment of dysplastic BE should result in long-lasting durability, defined by the maintenance of neosquamous epithelium after reaching CE-IM. Dysplastic BE and EAC following RFA based CE-IM are rare, recurring most often within the first year after finalization of treatment. There is some variability in the literature regarding the definition and consensus of the exact definition of CE-IM as well as recurrence. In our opinion, to assess RFA efficacy and durability, the only clinically hard endpoint is complete endoscopic and histologic eradication of all BE, documented on 2 successive biopsy sessions to reduce sampling error due to random biopsies. According to the study setting (registries, RCT) and the durability definitions, recurrent IM ranges between 8% to 32% of patients at a rate of 6% to 11% patient-year of follow-up (**Table 3**). Recurrence of dysplasia is less frequent, arising at a rate ranging between 1% to 5% patient-year. Emergence of EAC after CE-IM is very uncommon in post-RFA surveillance studies, occurring in up to 0.4% to 2.0%. In a recent meta-analysis of 21 RFA studies of 3186 patients with 5741 patient-years of follow-up, there were 603 recurrences.[79] The pooled incident ratios of recurrent IM, dysplasia, and HGD/EAC after RFA were 9.5%, 2.0%, and 1.2% patient-years, respectively.[79] In a pooled analysis, Fujii-Lau and colleagues[80] reported an

Table 3
RFA durability in BE ablation

Study	Sample Size	Follow-up, Mean or Median, mo	Recurrence of IM, % (Incidence Rate)	Recurrence of Dysplasia, % (Incidence Rate)	Recurrence of EAC, % (Incidence Rate)
AIM extension trial Fleischer et al,[30] 2010 US prospective cohort	50 (NDBE)	51	8	0	0
AIM-dysplasia trial Cotton et al,[81] 2017 US prospective cohort	119 (LGD-HGD)	43 (401 PY)	32 (10.8/100PY)	17 (5.2/100PY)	1.7
AMC-I/II/IV + EURO-I Phoa et al,[89] 2013 EU prospective cohort	54 (LGD, HGD, EAC)	61	10	5.5	1.8
BETRNet consortium Gupta et al,[84] 2013 US prospective cohort	229 (NDBE, LGD, HGD, EAC)	24	16	3.5	0.4
Meta-analysis Orman et al,[66] 2013	540 (NDBE, LGD, HGD, IMC)	18	13	0.9	0.7 (0.1/100PY)
US RFA registry Pasricha et al,[83] 2014	1634 (31% NDBE)	28.8	20	2.9	
Wolf et al,[90] 2015 US prospective cohort	4982 (NDBE, IND, LGD, HGD, IMC)	32.4 (13,835 PY)			2 (0.8/10OPY)
UK RFA registry Haidry et al,[53] 2015 UK prospective registry	508 (LGD, HGD, IMC)	NR (At 5y)	32% at 5 y	19% at 5 y	2.1% at 1y 3% at 34 mo
Meta-analysis Krishnamoorthi et al,[79] 2016	3186 (NDBE, LGD, HGD, EAC)	NR (5741 PY)	NR (9.5/100PY)	NR (2.0/100PY)	1.2/100PY
North Carolina Hospital Guthikonda et al,[82] 2017 US retrospective cohort	218 (LGD, HGD, EAC)	NS (540.6 PY)	24 (9.6/100PY)	NR	1.8 (0.65/100PY)
Meta-analysis Fujii-Lau et al,[80] 2017	4042 (NDBE, IND, LGD, HGD, EAC)	NR	NR (5.8/100PY)	NR (1.9/100PY)	NR

(*continued on next page*)

Table 3
(*continued*)

Study	Sample Size	Follow-up, Mean or Median, mo	Recurrence of IM, % (Incidence Rate)	Recurrence of Dysplasia, % (Incidence Rate)	Recurrence of EAC, % (Incidence Rate)
VA Corporate Date Warehouse Tan et al,[93] 2019 US retrospective cohort	337 (34% NDBE)	22.8 (906 PY)	29.1 (10.8/100PY)	5.9 (2.2/100PY)	0.9 (0.3/100PY)
Netherland Nationwide cohort Van Munster et al,[87] 2020 NL prospective cohort	1154 (LGD, HGD, EAC)	30	NS	3 (0.8/100PY)	0.4

Abbreviations: 100PY, percent patient-year of follow-up; BE, Barrett's esophagus; D, dysplasia; EAC, esophageal adenocarcinoma; EU, European; HGD, high-grade dysplasia; IM, intestinal metaplasia; IND, indefinite for dysplasia; LGD, low-grade dysplasia; mo, month; NDBE, nondysplastic Barrett's esophagus; NL, Netherlands; NR, not-reported; RCT, randomized controlled trial; RFA, radiofrequency ablation; UK, United Kingdom; US, Unites States; y, year.

IM recurrence rate of 5.8% and dysplasia recurrence rate of 1.9% per patient-year. Because most recurrences occur within the first year of surveillance, intensive surveillance is required within the first year after CE-IM followed by spacing of the surveillance interval.[53,81] Nevertheless, others investigators observed that recurrence risk remained stable over time, suggesting that endoscopic surveillance is necessary.[82] Recurrence is often small (<10 mm), close to the gastroesophageal junction, especially for dysplastic recurrence, and visible lesion in only 25% of case.[82–86] This supports the need of systematic random biopsies at the cardia during post-RFA surveillance. Even if presence of IM at the cardia is not considered as recurrence by all studies, presence of recurrent dysplasia at the cardia after EET is widely regarded as recurrent disease. Furthermore, even if buried BE glands rate after RFA is rare (estimated at <1%), carcinoma developing from these subsquamous BE glands have been described, justifying careful inspection of neosquamous esophagus within the previous territory of BE, seeking subtle relief or discoloration change preferably with advanced imaging techniques like Narrow-Band imaging. Targeted and random biopsies according to initial Prague C&M classification are still recommended by some guidelines; however, recent data do not show a great benefit in favor of these systematic biopsies when performed randomly in the neosquamous esophagus in absence of visible lesion.[87,88] We have also abandoned this practice of Seattle protocol of the neosquamous epithelium. The yield of random biopsies from the tubular esophagus, in the absence of visible lesions, range from 0% to 0.2% for dysplasia detection rate and random biopsies of the gastroesophageal junction detect dysplasia in only 0.8% while IM is detected in 11% with limited clinical relevance.[87,88] Whether recurrence at the cardia represents incident or prevalent lesions that preexisted before ablation and are missed due to sampling error in the early post-RFA surveillance, is unclear.[82] We do not generally recommend treating the neo-Z-line in case of recurrence of IM at the cardia during the first year of follow-up because in 50% of the cases recurrence of IM at the cardia cannot be reproduced during subsequent follow-up endoscopies.[89]

Recurrent disease is mostly NDBE without dysplasia with favorable outcome. Recurrent disease with histologic progression has been reported to occur in 2% to 6% of cases with recurrent disease.[83,84] Data coming from the US RFA Registry, on 4698 patients treated by RFA, showed 2% of EAC during average follow-up of 2.7 years and very low EAC-related death calculated to 0.6%.[90] The vast majority of dysplastic or EAC recurrences are amenable to repeat endoscopic "touch-up" treatment, requiring esophagectomy in less than 1%.[90]

Several studies have reported on predictors of recurrence. Non-Caucasian race, Increased age, longer circumferential and maximal length of BE, increasing number of RFA sessions were predictive of recurrence.[79,82–84,91] Higher grade of dysplasia at baseline histology was not associated with recurrence in a meta-analysis[79] while predictive for recurrence for others.[83,92] Sex was not associated with recurrence prediction.[79] High-volume RFA centers are associated with reduced risk of BE recurrence.[93]

SUMMARY

Endoscopic management of neoplastic BE encompasses a multimodality treatment approach. This treatment has revolutionized the management of early neoplasia for patients with BE by replacing esophagectomy. The treatment has now been optimized through several studies over the past decades and sets an example of how new devices should be used in clinical practice using a scientifically sound approach. We have obtained insight in the factors that provide optimal outcomes for our patients. Now that this technique becomes more widely available, it is important to emphasize the crucial elements in the recipe for success: (1) thorough inspection and low threshold for EMR before ablation, (2) correct patient selection, (3) correct application of ablation protocols, and (4) adequate surveillance.

CLINICS CARE POINTS

- Before any treatment, always confirm any degree of dysplasia by an experience pathologist.
- All endoscopic visible lesions with dysplasia need to be resected prior to ablation to safeguard a good onlogical outcome.
- Acid suppression during and after RFA treatment is crucial to obtain and maintain remission of dysplasia and Barrett Endoscopic surveillance is essential to prevent long term recurrence.

DISCLOSURE

P. Leclercq has received honorarium for speaker assignments from Medtronic. R. Bischops has received honorarium for consultancy and speaker assignments and a research grant from Medtronic. (Belgium)

REFERENCES

1. Stein HJ, Siewert JR. Barrett's esophagus: Pathogenesis, epidemiology, functional abnormalities, malignant degeneration, and surgical management. Dysphagia 1993;8(3):276–88.

2. Coletta M, Sami SS, Nachiappan A, et al. Acetic acid chromoendoscopy for the diagnosis of early neoplasia and specialized intestinal metaplasia in Barrett's esophagus: a meta-analysis. Gastrointest Endosc 2016;83(1):57–67.e1.
3. Otaki F, Iyer PG. Point-counterpoint: screening and surveillance for Barrett's esophagus, is it worthwhile? Dig Dis Sci 2018;63(8):2081–93.
4. Hvid-Jensen F, Pedersen L, Drewes AM, et al. Incidence of adenocarcinoma among patients with Barrett's esophagus. N Engl J Med 2011;365(15):1375–83.
5. Desai TK, Krishnan K, Samala N, et al. The incidence of oesophageal adenocarcinoma in non-dysplastic Barrett's oesophagus: a meta-analysis. Gut 2012; 61(7):970LP–976. http://gut.bmj.com/content/61/7/970.abstract.
6. Dunbar KB, Souza RF. Beyond dysplasia grade. Gastrointest Endosc Clin 2017; 27(3):447–59.
7. Shaheen NJ, Crosby MA, Bozymski EM, et al. Is there publication bias in the reporting of cancer risk in Barrett's esophagus? Gastroenterology 2000;119(2): 333–8.
8. Wani S, Puli SR, Shaheen NJ, et al. Esophageal adenocarcinoma in Barrett's esophagus after endoscopic ablative therapy: a meta-analysis and systematic review. Am J Gastroenterol 2009;104(2):502–13.
9. Ell C, May A, Pech O, et al. Curative endoscopic resection of early esophageal adenocarcinomas (Barrett's cancer). Gastrointest Endosc 2007;65(1):3–10.
10. Pech O, Behrens A, May A, et al. Long-term results and risk factor analysis for recurrence after curative endoscopic therapy in 349 patients with high-grade intraepithelial neoplasia and mucosal adenocarcinoma in Barrett's oesophagus. Gut 2008;57(9):1200–6.
11. Chennat J, Ross AS, Konda VJA, et al. Advanced pathology under squamous epithelium on initial EMR specimens in patients with Barrett's esophagus and high-grade dysplasia or intramucosal carcinoma: implications for surveillance and endotherapy management. Gastrointest Endosc 2009;70(3):417–21.
12. Moss A, Bourke MJ, Hourigan LF, et al. Endoscopic resection for Barrett's high-grade dysplasia and early esophageal adenocarcinoma: an essential staging procedure with long-term therapeutic benefit. Am J Gastroenterol 2010; 105(6):1276–83.
13. Wijnhoven BP, Siersema PD, Hop WC, et al. Adenocarcinomas of the distal oesophagus and gastric cardia are one clinical entity. Rotterdam Oesophageal Tumour Study Group. Br J Surg 1999;86(4):529–35.
14. Stein HJ, Feith M, Bruecher BLDM, et al. Early esophageal cancer: pattern of lymphatic spread and prognostic factors for long-term survival after surgical resection. Ann Surg 2005;242(4):565–6.
15. Oh DS, Hagen JA, Chandrasoma PT, et al. Clinical biology and surgical therapy of intramucosal adenocarcinoma of the esophagus. J Am Coll Surg 2006;203(2): 152–61.
16. Das A, Singh V, Fleischer DE, et al. A comparison of endoscopic treatment and surgery in early esophageal cancer: an analysis of surveillance epidemiology and end results data. Am J Gastroenterol 2008;103(6):1340–5.
17. Prasad GA, Wu TT, Wigle DA, et al. Endoscopic and surgical treatment of mucosal (T1a) esophageal adenocarcinoma in Barrett's esophagus. Gastroenterology 2009;137(3):815–23.
18. Pech O, Bollschweiler E, Manner H, et al. Comparison between endoscopic and surgical resection of mucosal esophageal adenocarcinoma in Barrett's esophagus at two high-volume centers. Ann Surg 2011;254(1):67–72.

19. May A, Gossner L, Pech O, et al. Local endoscopic therapy for intraepithelial high-grade neoplasia and early adenocarcinoma in Barrett's oesophagus: acute-phase and intermediate results of a new treatment approach. Eur J Gastroenterol Hepatol 2002;14(10):1085–91.
20. Weusten B, Bisschops R, Coron E, et al. Endoscopic management of Barrett's esophagus: European Society of Gastrointestinal Endoscopy (ESGE) Position Statement. Endoscopy 2017;49(2):191–8.
21. Peters FP, Kara MA, Rosmolen WD, et al. Endoscopic treatment of high-grade dysplasia and early stage cancer in Barrett's esophagus. Gastrointest Endosc 2005;61(4):506–14.
22. Brandt LJ, Kauvar DR. Laser-induced transient regression of Barrett's epithelium. Gastrointest Endosc 1992;38(5):619–22.
23. Berenson MM, Johnson TD, Markowitz NR, et al. Restoration of squamous mucosa after ablation of Barrett's esophageal epithelium. Gastroenterology 1993; 104(6):1686–91.
24. Laukka MA, Wang KK. Initial results using low-dose photodynamic therapy in the treatment of Barrett's esophagus. Gastrointest Endosc 1995;42(1):59–63.
25. Sampliner RE, Fennerty B, Garewal HS. Reversal of Barrett's esophagus with acid suppression and multipolar electrocoagulation: preliminary results. Gastrointest Endosc 1996;44(5):532–5.
26. Wahab PJ, Mulder CJ, den Hartog G, et al. Argon plasma coagulation in flexible gastrointestinal endoscopy: pilot experiences. Endoscopy 1997;29(3):176–81.
27. Shaheen NJ, Sharma P, Overholt BF, et al. Radiofrequency ablation in Barrett's esophagus with dysplasia. N Engl J Med 2009;360(22):2277–88.
28. Ganz RA, Utley DS, Stern RA, et al. Complete ablation of esophageal epithelium with a balloon-based bipolar electrode: a phased evaluation in the porcine and in the human esophagus. Gastrointest Endosc 2004;60(6):1002–10.
29. Kahaleh M, Van Laethem J-L, Nagy N, et al. Long-term follow-up and factors predictive of recurrence in Barrett's esophagus treated by argon plasma coagulation and acid suppression. Endoscopy 2002;34(12):950–5.
30. Fleischer DE, Overholt BF, Sharma VK, et al. Endoscopic radiofrequency ablation for Barrett's esophagus: 5-year outcomes from a prospective multicenter trial. Endoscopy 2010;42(10):781–9.
31. Bhat S, Coleman HG, Yousef F, et al. Risk of malignant progression in Barrett's esophagus patients: results from a large population-based study. J Natl Cancer Inst 2011;103(13):1049–57.
32. Shaheen NJ, Falk GW, Iyer PG, et al. ACG Clinical Guideline: diagnosis and management of Barrett's Esophagus. Am J Gastroenterol 2016;111(1):30–50. https://journals.lww.com/ajg/Fulltext/2016/01000/ACG_Clinical_Guideline__Diagnosis_and_Management.17.aspx.
33. Wani S, Falk G, Hall M, et al. Patients with nondysplastic Barrett's esophagus have low risks for developing dysplasia or esophageal adenocarcinoma. Clin Gastroenterol Hepatol 2011;9(3):220–7 [quiz: e26].
34. Hur C, Choi SE, Rubenstein JH, et al. The cost effectiveness of radiofrequency ablation for Barrett's esophagus. Gastroenterology 2012;143(3):567–75.
35. Bulsiewicz WJ, Kim HP, Dellon ES, et al. Safety and efficacy of endoscopic mucosal therapy with radiofrequency ablation for patients with neoplastic Barrett's esophagus. Clin Gastroenterol Hepatol 2013;11(6):636–42.
36. Anaparthy R, Gaddam S, Kanakadandi V, et al. Association between length of Barrett's esophagus and risk of high-grade dysplasia or adenocarcinoma in patients without dysplasia. Clin Gastroenterol Hepatol 2013;11(11):1430–6.

37. Pohl H, Wrobel K, Bojarski C, et al. Risk factors in the development of esophageal adenocarcinoma. Am J Gastroenterol 2013;108(2):200–7.
38. Sikkema M, Looman CWN, Steyerberg EW, et al. Predictors for neoplastic progression in patients with Barrett's Esophagus: a prospective cohort study. Am J Gastroenterol 2011;106(7):1231–8.
39. Fitzgerald RC, di Pietro M, Ragunath K, et al. British Society of Gastroenterology guidelines on the diagnosis and management of Barrett's oesophagus. Gut 2014;63(1):7LP–42. http://gut.bmj.com/content/63/1/7.abstract.
40. Kerkhof M, van Dekken H, Steyerberg EW, et al. Grading of dysplasia in Barrett's oesophagus: substantial interobserver variation between general and gastrointestinal pathologists. Histopathology 2007;50(7):920–7.
41. Montgomery E, Bronner MP, Goldblum JR, et al. Reproducibility of the diagnosis of dysplasia in Barrett esophagus: a reaffirmation. Hum Pathol 2001;32(4):368–78.
42. Curvers WL, ten Kate FJ, Krishnadath KK, et al. Low-grade dysplasia in Barrett's esophagus: overdiagnosed and underestimated. Am J Gastroenterol 2010;105(7):1523–30.
43. Duits LC, Phoa KN, Curvers WL, et al. Barrett's oesophagus patients with low-grade dysplasia can be accurately risk-stratified after histological review by an expert pathology panel. Gut 2015;64(5):700LP–706.
44. Pech O, Vieth M, Schmitz D, et al. Conclusions from the histological diagnosis of low-grade intraepithelial neoplasia in Barrett's oesophagus. Scand J Gastroenterol 2007;42(6):682–8.
45. Skacel M, Petras RE, Gramlich TL, et al. The diagnosis of low-grade dysplasia in Barrett's esophagus and its implications for disease progression. Am J Gastroenterol 2000;95(12):3383–7.
46. Duits LC, van der Wel MJ, Cotton CC, et al. Patients with Barrett's esophagus and confirmed persistent low-grade dysplasia are at increased risk for progression to neoplasia. Gastroenterology 2017;152(5):993–1001.e1.
47. Krishnamoorthi R, Lewis JT, Krishna M, et al. Predictors of progression in Barrett's esophagus with low-grade dysplasia: results from a multicenter prospective BE Registry. Am J Gastroenterol 2017;112(6):867–73.
48. Kestens C, Offerhaus GJA, van Baal JWPM, et al. Patients with Barrett's esophagus and persistent low-grade dysplasia have an increased risk for high-grade dysplasia and cancer. Clin Gastroenterol Hepatol 2016;14(7):956–62.e1.
49. Song KY, Henn AJ, Gravely AA, et al. Persistent confirmed low-grade dysplasia in Barrett's esophagus is a risk factor for progression to high-grade dysplasia and adenocarcinoma in a US Veterans cohort. Dis Esophagus 2020;33(2). https://doi.org/10.1093/dote/doz061.
50. Qumseya BJ, Wani S, Gendy S, et al. Disease progression in Barrett's low-grade dysplasia with radiofrequency ablation compared with surveillance: systematic review and meta-analysis. Am J Gastroenterol 2017;112(6):849–65.
51. Srivastava A, Hornick JL, Li X, et al. Extent of low-grade dysplasia is a risk factor for the development of esophageal adenocarcinoma in Barrett's esophagus. Am J Gastroenterol 2007;102(3):483–93 [quiz: 694].
52. Parasa S, Sharma P. Barrett's Esophagus with low-grade dysplasia: ablate or wait? Am J Gastroenterol 2017;112(2):195–6.
53. Haidry RJ, Butt MA, Dunn JM, et al. Improvement over time in outcomes for patients undergoing endoscopic therapy for Barrett's oesophagus-related neoplasia: 6-year experience from the first 500 patients treated in the UK patient registry. Gut 2015;64(8):1192–9.

54. Dunbar KB, Spechler SJ. The risk of lymph-node metastases in patients with high-grade dysplasia or intramucosal carcinoma in Barrett's esophagus: a systematic review. Am J Gastroenterol 2012;107(6):850–62 [quiz 863].
55. Wu J, Pan Y, Wang T, et al. Endotherapy versus surgery for early neoplasia in Barrett's esophagus: a meta-analysis. Gastrointest Endosc 2014;79(2): 233–41.e2.
56. Wani S, Drahos J, Cook MB, et al. Comparison of endoscopic therapies and surgical resection in patients with early esophageal cancer: a population-based study. Gastrointest Endosc 2014;79(2):224–32.e1.
57. Phoa KN, Pouw RE, Bisschops R, et al. Multimodality endoscopic eradication for neoplastic Barrett oesophagus: results of an European multicentre study (EURO-II). Gut 2016;65(4):555–62.
58. Wani S, Abrams J, Edmundowicz SA, et al. Endoscopic mucosal resection results in change of histologic diagnosis in Barrett's esophagus patients with visible and flat neoplasia: a multicenter cohort study. Dig Dis Sci 2013;58(6): 1703–9.
59. Schölvinck DW, van der Meulen K, Bergman JJGHM, et al. Detection of lesions in dysplastic Barrett's esophagus by community and expert endoscopists. Endoscopy 2017;49(2):113–20.
60. Cameron GR, Jayasekera CS, Williams R, et al. Detection and staging of esophageal cancers within Barrett's esophagus is improved by assessment in specialized Barrett's units. Gastrointest Endosc 2014;80(6):971–83.e1.
61. Scholvinck D, Kunzli H, Meijer S, et al. Management of patients with T1b esophageal adenocarcinoma: a retrospective cohort study on patient management and risk of metastatic disease. Surg Endosc 2016;30(9):4102–13.
62. Manner H, Pech O, Heldmann Y, et al. The frequency of lymph node metastasis in early-stage adenocarcinoma of the esophagus with incipient submucosal invasion (pT1b sm1) depending on histological risk patterns. Surg Endosc 2015; 29(7):1888–96.
63. Wani S, Qumseya B, Sultan S, et al. Endoscopic eradication therapy for patients with Barrett's esophagus–associated dysplasia and intramucosal cancer. Gastrointest Endosc 2018;87(4):907–31.e9.
64. Vliebergh JH, Deprez PH, de Looze D, et al. Efficacy and safety of radiofrequency ablation of Barrett's esophagus in the absence of reimbursement: a multicenter prospective Belgian registry. Endoscopy 2019;51(4):317–25.
65. van Vilsteren FGI, Alvarez Herrero L, Pouw RE, et al. Predictive factors for initial treatment response after circumferential radiofrequency ablation for Barrett's esophagus with early neoplasia: a prospective multicenter study. Endoscopy 2013;45(7):516–25.
66. Orman ES, Li N, Shaheen NJ. Efficacy and durability of radiofrequency ablation for Barrett's Esophagus: systematic review and meta-analysis. Clin Gastroenterol Hepatol 2013;11(10):1245–55.
67. Desai M, Saligram S, Gupta N, et al. Efficacy and safety outcomes of multimodal endoscopic eradication therapy in Barrett's esophagus-related neoplasia: a systematic review and pooled analysis. Gastrointest Endosc 2017;85(3):482–95.e4.
68. Pandey G, Mulla M, Lewis WG, et al. Systematic review and meta-analysis of the effectiveness of radiofrequency ablation in low grade dysplastic Barrett's esophagus. Endoscopy 2018;50(10):953–60.
69. Sharma VK, Wang KK, Overholt BF, et al. Balloon-based, circumferential, endoscopic radiofrequency ablation of Barrett's esophagus: 1-year follow-up of 100 patients. Gastrointest Endosc 2007;65(2):185–95.

70. Fleischer DE, Overholt BF, Sharma VK, et al. Endoscopic ablation of Barrett's esophagus: a multicenter study with 2.5-year follow-up. Gastrointest Endosc 2008;68(5):867–76.
71. Ganz RA, Overholt BF, Sharma VK, et al. Circumferential ablation of Barrett's esophagus that contains high-grade dysplasia: a U.S. Multicenter Registry. Gastrointest Endosc 2008;68(1):35–40.
72. Phoa KN, van Vilsteren FGI, Weusten BLAM, et al. Radiofrequency ablation vs endoscopic surveillance for patients with Barrett esophagus and low-grade dysplasia: a randomized clinical trial. JAMA 2014;311(12):1209–17.
73. Haidry RJ, Dunn JM, Butt MA, et al. Radiofrequency ablation and endoscopic mucosal resection for dysplastic Barrett's esophagus and early esophageal adenocarcinoma: outcomes of the UK National Halo RFA Registry. Gastroenterology 2013;145(1):87–95.
74. Agoston AT, Strauss AC, Dulai PS, et al. Predictors of treatment failure after radiofrequency ablation for intramucosal adenocarcinoma in Barrett esophagus: a multi-institutional retrospective cohort study. Am J Surg Pathol 2016;40(4):554–62.
75. Pouw RE, Künzli HT, Bisschops R, et al. Simplified versus standard regimen for focal radiofrequency ablation of dysplastic Barrett's oesophagus: a multicentre randomised controlled trial. Lancet Gastroenterol Hepatol 2018;3(8):566–74.
76. van Vilsteren FGI, Phoa KN, Alvarez Herrero L, et al. Circumferential balloon-based radiofrequency ablation of Barrett's esophagus with dysplasia can be simplified, yet efficacy maintained, by omitting the cleaning phase. Clin Gastroenterol Hepatol 2013;11(5):491–8.e1.
77. Belghazi K, Pouw RE, Sondermeijer CMT, et al. A single-step sizing and radiofrequency ablation catheter for circumferential ablation of Barrett's esophagus: results of a pilot study. United Eur Gastroenterol J 2018;6(7):990–9.
78. Belghazi K, Pouw RE, Koch AD, et al. Self-sizing radiofrequency ablation balloon for eradication of Barrett's esophagus: results of an international multicenter randomized trial comparing 3 different treatment regimens. Gastrointest Endosc 2019;90(3):415–23.
79. Krishnamoorthi R, Singh S, Ragunathan K, et al. Risk of recurrence of Barrett's esophagus after successful endoscopic therapy. Gastrointest Endosc 2016;83(6):1090–106.e3.
80. Fujii-Lau LL, Cinnor B, Shaheen N, et al. Recurrence of intestinal metaplasia and early neoplasia after endoscopic eradication therapy for Barrett's esophagus: a systematic review and meta-analysis. Endosc Int Open 2017;5(6):E430–49.
81. Cotton CC, Wolf WA, Overholt BF, et al. Late recurrence of Barrett's esophagus after complete eradication of intestinal metaplasia is rare: final report from ablation in intestinal metaplasia containing dysplasia trial. Gastroenterology 2017;153(3):681–8.e2.
82. Guthikonda A, Cotton CC, Madanick RD, et al. Clinical outcomes following recurrence of intestinal metaplasia after successful treatment of Barrett's esophagus with radiofrequency ablation. Am J Gastroenterol 2017;112(1):87–94.
83. Pasricha S, Bulsiewicz WJ, Hathorn KE, et al. Durability and predictors of successful radiofrequency ablation for Barrett's esophagus. Clin Gastroenterol Hepatol 2014;12(11):1840–7.e1.
84. Gupta M, Iyer PG, Lutzke L, et al. Recurrence of esophageal intestinal metaplasia after endoscopic mucosal resection and radiofrequency ablation of Barrett's esophagus: results from a US Multicenter Consortium. Gastroenterology 2013;145(1):79–86.e1.

85. Vaccaro BJ, Gonzalez S, Poneros JM, et al. Detection of intestinal metaplasia after successful eradication of Barrett's Esophagus with radiofrequency ablation. Dig Dis Sci 2011;56(7):1996–2000.
86. Korst RJ, Santana-Joseph S, Rutledge JR, et al. Patterns of recurrent and persistent intestinal metaplasia after successful radiofrequency ablation of Barrett's esophagus. J Thorac Cardiovasc Surg 2013;145(6):1529–34.
87. van Munster S, Nieuwenhuis EA, Weusten B, et al. Recurrent neoplasia after endoscopic treatment for Barrett's neoplasia is rare: results from a nationwide cohort including all 1,154 patients treated in the netherlands from 2008-2018. Endoscopy 2020;52(S 01):OP12.
88. Sami SS, Ravindran A, Kahn A, et al. Timeline and location of recurrence following successful ablation in Barrett's oesophagus: an international multicentre study. Gut 2019. https://doi.org/10.1136/gutjnl-2018-317513. gutjnl-2018-317513.
89. Phoa KN, Pouw RE, van Vilsteren FGI, et al. Remission of Barrett's esophagus with early neoplasia 5 years after radiofrequency ablation with endoscopic resection: a Netherlands cohort study. Gastroenterology 2013;145(1):96–104.
90. Wolf WA, Pasricha S, Cotton C, et al. Incidence of Esophageal Adenocarcinoma and Causes of Mortality After Radiofrequency Ablation of Barrett's Esophagus. Gastroenterology 2015;149(7):1752–61.e1.
91. Tan WK, Rattan A, O'Donovan M, et al. Comparative outcomes of radiofrequency ablation for Barrett's oesophagus with different baseline histology. United Eur Gastroenterol J 2018;6(5):662–8.
92. Orman ES, Kim HP, Bulsiewicz WJ, et al. Intestinal metaplasia recurs infrequently in patients successfully treated for Barrett's esophagus with radiofrequency ablation. Am J Gastroenterol 2013;108(2):187–95 [quiz: 196].
93. Tan MC, Kanthasamy KA, Yeh AG, et al. Factors associated with recurrence of Barrett's esophagus after radiofrequency ablation. Clin Gastroenterol Hepatol 2019;17(1):65–72.e5.
94. Gondrie JJ, Pouw RE, Sondermeijer CMT, et al. Stepwise circumferential and focal ablation of Barrett's esophagus with high-grade dysplasia: results of the first prospective series of 11 patients. Endoscopy 2008;40(5):359–69.
95. Gondrie JJ, Pouw RE, Sondermeijer CMT, et al. Effective treatment of early Barrett's neoplasia with stepwise circumferential and focal ablation using the HALO system. Endoscopy 2008;40(5):370–9.
96. Sharma VK, Jae Kim H, Das A, et al. Circumferential and focal ablation of Barrett's esophagus containing dysplasia. Am J Gastroenterol 2009;104(2):310–7.
97. Lyday WD, Corbett FS, Kuperman DA, et al. Radiofrequency ablation of Barrett's esophagus: outcomes of 429 patients from a multicenter community practice registry. Endoscopy 2010;42(4):272–8.
98. Pouw RE, Wirths K, Eisendrath P, et al. Efficacy of radiofrequency ablation combined with endoscopic resection for Barrett's esophagus with early neoplasia. Clin Gastroenterol Hepatol 2010;8(1):23–9.
99. van Vilsteren FGI, Pouw RE, Seewald S, et al. Stepwise radical endoscopic resection versus radiofrequency ablation for Barrett's oesophagus with high-grade dysplasia or early cancer: a multicentre randomised trial. Gut 2011; 60(6):765–73.
100. Okoro NI, Tomizawa Y, Dunagan KT, et al. Safety of prior endoscopic mucosal resection in patients receiving radiofrequency ablation of Barrett's esophagus. Clin Gastroenterol Hepatol 2012;10(2):150–4.

101. Li N, Pasricha S, Bulsiewicz WJ, et al. Effects of preceding endoscopic mucosal resection on the efficacy and safety of radiofrequency ablation for treatment of Barrett's esophagus: results from the United States Radiofrequency Ablation Registry. Dis Esophagus 2016;29(6). https://doi.org/10.1111/dote.12386.
102. Pouw RE, Bergman JJ. Safety signal for the simple double ablation regimen when using the Barrx 360 express radiofrequency ablation balloon catheter. Gastroenterology 2017;153(2):614.

Updates in Cryotherapy for Barrett's Esophagus

Charlotte N. Frederiks, MD[a,b], Marcia Irene Canto, MD, MHS[c], Bas L.A.M. Weusten, MD, PHD[a,b,*]

KEYWORDS

- Barrett's esophagus • Barrett's dysplasia • Barrett's neoplasia • Ablation therapy
- Cryotherapy • Cryoablation

KEY POINTS

- Cryotherapy is an ablative modality for the treatment of Barrett's esophagus, involving cycles of freezing and thawing to induce cell death.
- Cryotherapy potentially enables deeper tissue ablation with less post-procedural pain by its anesthetic effect, and possibly less stricture formation by preserving the extracellular matrix.
- The current available systems for esophageal application are cryospray ablation using liquid nitrogen, and cryoballoon ablation using liquid nitrous oxide.
- Although cryotherapy is safe and effective, the exact role for cryotherapy in the management of Barrett's esophagus still needs to be established.

INTRODUCTION

Cryotherapy, the therapeutic use of cold temperature, dates back to Egyptian time in 3000 BC.[1] In ancient times, cryotherapy was mainly used for its anti-inflammatory and anesthetic properties.[2] In 1850 James Arnott was the first physician to advocate the local application of cold for the treatment and palliation of malignant diseases.[1,3] Since then, cryotherapy has been widely used for the treatment of oncological conditions across a variety of medical specialties including dermatology, gynecology, orthopedics and urology.[1,2]

Cryotherapy has also been extensively studied in esophageal neoplasia, in particular Barrett's esophagus (BE). First, a solid cryoprobe was investigated that involved

[a] Department of Gastroenterology and Hepatology, University Medical Center Utrecht, PO Box 85500, 3508 GA Utrecht, the Netherlands; [b] Department of Gastroenterology and Hepatology, St. Antonius Hospital, Koekoekslaan 1, PO Box 2500, 3430 EM Nieuwegein, the Netherlands; [c] Division of Gastroenterology and Hepatology, The Johns Hopkins Medical Institutions, Johns Hopkins Hospital, 1800 Orleans Street, Blalock 407, Baltimore, MD 21287, USA
* Corresponding author. Department of Gastroenterology and Hepatology, St. Antonius Hospital, Koekoekslaan 1, PO Box 2500, 3430 EM Nieuwegein, the Netherlands.
E-mail address: b.weusten@antoniusziekenhuis.nl

Gastrointest Endoscopy Clin N Am 31 (2021) 155–170
https://doi.org/10.1016/j.giec.2020.09.005
1052-5157/21/

direct mucosal contact of the probe with the esophagus. The main drawback of this technique was the inability to control the extent and depth of the tissue ablation resulting in esophageal perforation in some cases.[4] Thereafter, a cryogenic spraying system was developed enabling endoscopic application of cryogen without direct mucosal contact. This alternative approach allowed more accurate mucosal ablation and potentially reduced the risk of complications.[5]

In the past decades, various cryogenic agents have been investigated. The pursuit of achieving lower tissue temperatures led to the liquefaction of gases, such as air, oxygen, carbon dioxide (CO_2), and nitrogen. Liquid nitrogen (LN) is currently the most acceptable cryogen mainly due to its predictable effect and ability to refrigerate to extreme low temperature (−197°C).[2]

In this review, we aim to provide an overview on the recent state of knowledge on the use of cryotherapy for the treatment of BE, and to formulate directions for future research.

BACKGROUND AND PRINCIPLES OF CRYOTHERAPY

Cryotherapy is an ablative modality triggering tissue destruction through the repetition of rapid cooling and slow thawing (freeze-thaw cycle).[6] Three major mechanisms of action are involved in the destructive changes caused by cryotherapy.

The first mechanism of action comprises direct cell injury mediated by ice crystal formation. Initially, extracellular ice crystal formation generates a hyperosmotic environment, resulting in cell dehydration through water extraction from the cells. Subsequently, intracellular ice crystals are formed which disrupt organelles and cell membranes. During thawing disturbances in the osmotic gradient cause water to reenter the damaged cells promoting membrane rupture.[7] This deleterious cascade eventually leads to cell death within hours to days.[6]

Cell death is further affected within hours to days by the induction of apoptosis, the second mechanism of action.[8] Apoptosis results from the activation of an extrinsic rapid membrane-related apoptotic pathway in the core of the cryogenic lesion, and intrinsic delayed mitochondrial damage in the peripheral zone of the cryogenic lesion, partly due to severe oxidative stress.[6]

The third mechanism of action consists of the failure of microcirculation and vascular stasis, over days to weeks.[6] At first freezing of tissue induces vasoconstriction and stagnation of the blood flow. After thawing of the tissue the circulation is restored with vasodilation propagating endothelial damage.[7] This endothelial damage facilitates edema, platelet aggregation and microthrombus formation, ultimately leading to tissue ischemia and secondary necrosis.[8]

Multiple factors contribute to the degree of cell injury, including the number of the freeze-thaw cycles, the duration of freezing, and the achieved nadir tissue temperature.[6,8,9] Although it has been demonstrated that a temperature below −50°C sufficiently induces cell death in a single freeze-thaw cycle, cycles are typically repeated to enhance the lethal effect.[8,9] Nevertheless, the exact dosimetry of cryotherapy remains challenging due to the heterogeneity in application techniques and device types, and variability within the target tissue.[6]

Cryotherapy holds several potential advantages over heat-based ablation techniques, such as radiofrequency ablation (RFA) and argon plasma coagulation (APC). In contrast to cryotherapy, heat-based techniques induce denaturation of (extracellular) structural proteins leading to irreversible changes in protein structure. With cryotherapy, the extracellular matrix architecture is believed to be preserved.[6] Specifically for the esophagus, this preservation might enable deeper ablation without increasing the risk of stricture formation. Furthermore, cryotherapy might have a favorable tolerability due to direct effects of the cold. For example, in patients with renal tumors less sedation and analgesia medication were required during cryotherapy compared to RFA.[10,11] Likewise, lower pain levels were associated with cryotherapy in patients treated for atrioventricular reentrant tachycardia.[12] Potential underlying mechanisms previously described include an anesthetic effect on the tissue, and the inactivation of nerve conduction.[13]

CRYOTHERAPY DEVICES FOR ESOPHAGEAL USE

Currently, 2 different techniques are available for esophageal application of cryotherapy. The first is cryospray ablation, a noncontact method performed with either CO_2 or LN. The second is cryoballoon ablation, in which the cryogenic agent nitrous oxide (NO) is contained within a balloon that is mounted on a catheter, thereby cooling the balloon and subsequently the esophageal wall.

Cryospray Ablation

The most widely used cryospray ablation system (truFreeze, STERIS, Mentor, OH; https://www.steris.com/healthcare/products/endoscopy-equipment/trufreeze-spray-cryotherapy-system) delivers liquid nitrogen (LN) at −196°C using a flexible spray catheter that is passed through the working channel of an endoscope. During application, the LN rapidly expands from liquid into gas, therefore the concomitant placement of an oro-gastric decompression tube is required in order to prevent barotrauma.[14] Typically, 2 to 4 freeze-thaw-cycles are used when performing cryoablation with this technology; the most frequently reported dosages are either 2 applications of 20 seconds or 4 applications of 10 seconds (**Fig. 1**). The truFreeze system is approved by the US Food and Drug Administration and commercially available in the United States for endoscopic cryotherapy.

The Polar Wand (GI Supply, Camphill, PA) consists of a generator connected to a through-the-scope spray catheter delivering liquid CO_2 at −78°C. The system has been shown in detail elsewhere.[15] Compared with LN, liquid CO_2 has a lower flow volume thereby reducing the risk of overextension of the stomach. To achieve a

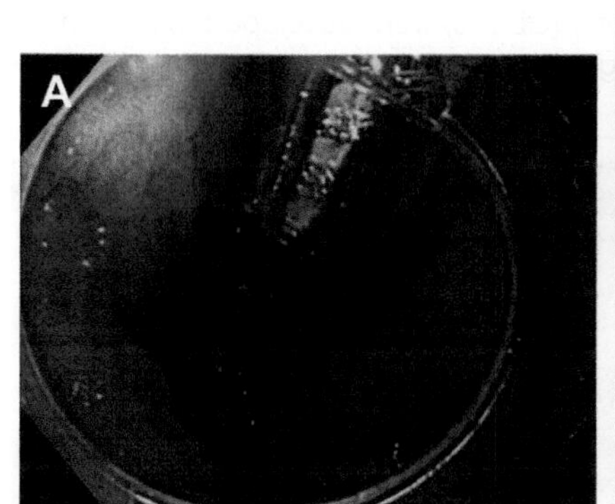

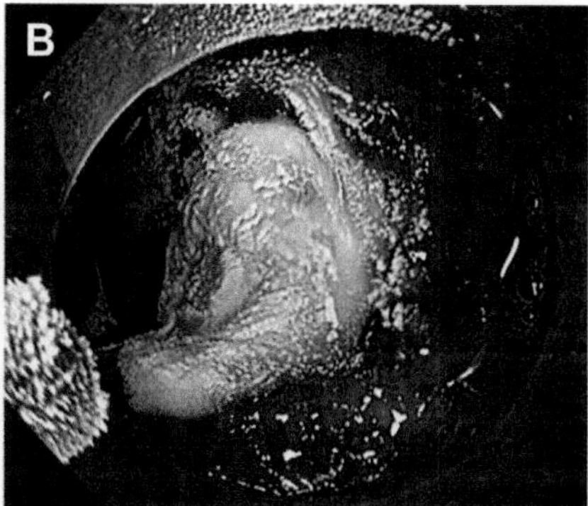

Fig. 1. Liquid nitrogen cryospray ablation of Barrett's esophagus. (*A*) Decompression tube as seen through the endoscope with a cap before therapy. (*B*) During therapy. (*Adapted from:* Shaheen NJ, Greenwald BD, Peery AF, et al. (2010) Safety and efficacy of endoscopic spray cryotherapy for Barrett's esophagus with high-grade dysplasia. Gastrointest Endosc. 71(4):680-685; with permission.)

temperature of less than −70°C, a flow of 6 to 8 L/min CO_2 is required.[14] A slim suction catheter is directly connected to the tip of the endoscope to prevent barotrauma. Using the system, cryospray is generally applied during 15 seconds followed by thaw, after which this freeze-thaw cycle is typically repeated 6 to 8 times resulting in a distinctive red mucosal color (**Fig. 2**).[16] However, this system is no longer commercially available because the catheters were suspended from production by the manufacturer in 2016.[17]

Cryoballoon Ablation

The more novel technique for intra-esophageal cryotherapy is C2 CryoBalloon Ablation (PENTAX Medical, Redwood City, CA). The cryoballoon ablation system consists of a hand-held controller, a cartridge containing liquid NO, a foot pedal, and a through-the-scope catheter with a rotatable spray diffuser covered by an inflatable, low-pressure transparent balloon (**Fig. 3**). The highly compliant balloon, which is 3 cm in length, adapts to the esophageal diameter, and makes contact with the esophageal wall on inflation (maximum diameter of 3.6 cm).[18] After inflation, pressurized liquid NO is emitted through the diffuser in the center of the cryoballoon, which cools the balloon to a temperature of −85°C without direct contact of the cryogen with the target tissue. When applying cryotherapy, the liquid NO expands to gas inside the balloon. This gas instantly exits the balloon through the catheter where it condenses into a sponge in the controller. Using the foot pedal, the spray diffuser can be rotated clockwise and counter clockwise, in addition to up-down movements in the axial direction, while keeping the inflated balloon in place in the esophagus.

So far, 3 different cryoballoon catheters have been developed. The C2 CryoBalloon Focal Catheter (CBF) allows ablation of smaller surfaces, covering approximately 2 cm^2 per application. For this focal system, 2 distinctive balloon shapes are available: a standard oval-shaped balloon and a pear-shaped balloon (see **Fig. 3**). The pear-shaped balloon seems more suitable for application of cryotherapy at the gastroesophageal junction, because this design enables a more stable balloon positioning, especially in patients with large hiatal hernias. It also seems useful in treating across or within esophageal strictures as the nitrous gas collects in the balloon above and below the luminal narrowing. The most frequently used cryogen dosimetry for the CBF is 10 seconds for each ablation site (**Fig. 4**). Recently, the C2 CryoBalloon 90° Catheter (CB90) and the C2 Cryoballoon 180° Catheter (CB180) were developed to treat larger and wider esophageal surfaces, covering respectively a quarter and half of the

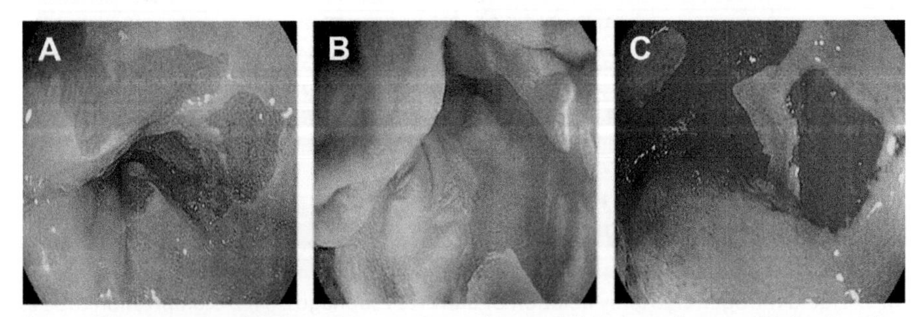

Fig. 2. CO_2 cryospray ablation of Barrett's esophagus. (*A*) Before therapy. (*B*) During therapy. (*C*) Immediately after therapy. (*Adapted from:* Canto MI, Shin EJ, Khashab MA, et al. (2015) Safety and efficacy of carbon dioxide cryotherapy for treatment of neoplastic Barrett's esophagus. Endoscopy. 47(7):591; with permission.)

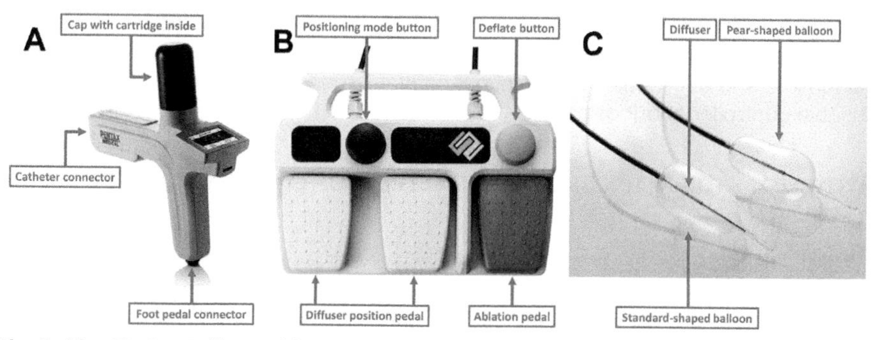

Fig. 3. The C2 CryoBalloon Ablation system consisting of (*A*) a controller, (*B*) a foot pedal and (*C*) a catheter with a compliant balloon, which is available in different shapes. (*Courtesy of* PENTAX Medical, Redwood City, CA; with permission.)

esophageal circumference.[19,20] In the latter 2, the diffuser traverses along the 3 cm length of the balloon starting at the distal end and moving in proximal direction, while the balloon remains stationary during delivery of NO. Therefore, the dose of both systems is based on the pullback rate at which the diffuser travels along the 3-cm-long axis of the balloon (see **Fig. 4**). Currently, the most efficient and safe dosages for these 2 systems are being investigated in clinical studies (Swipe 180 study, Netherlands Trial Register NL6495).

Cryoballoon ablation was developed to overcome some of the limitations of the spraying technique. Cryospray therapy suffers from possible unequal dosing and operator dependency, in addition to the need for a decompression tube to prevent overinflation of the stomach during treatment. Moreover, using cryospray technology, typically multiple freeze-thaw cycles are needed for an effective ablation of the esophageal lining. Using cryoballoon technology, the depth of ablation is believed to be more uniform and less operator dependent: the inflated balloon stabilizes the position of the diffuser in relation to the esophageal wall, whereas in cryospray the ablation effect is influenced by the distance of the catheter tip to the esophageal wall and the ability of the operator to keep the probe in a stable position. In addition, as the NO gas is contained within the balloon and directly vented back through the catheter there is no risk of overinflation, thereby obviating the need of a venting tube. In cryoballoon ablation, typically only one freeze-thaw cycle is delivered during treatment instead of multiple cycles. Furthermore, the cryogen for cryoballoon ablation is contained in small portable disposable capsules, while LN used for cryospray is stored in large

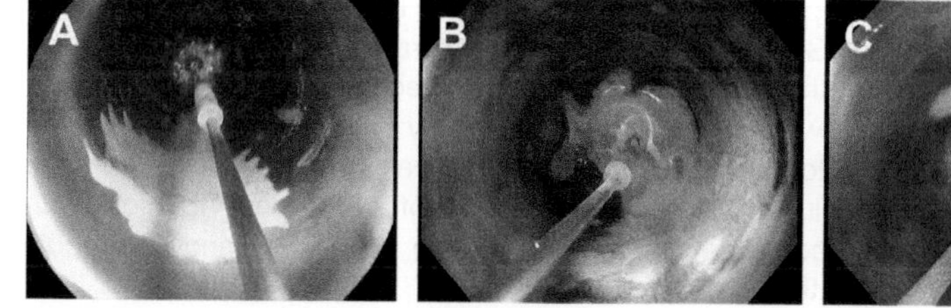

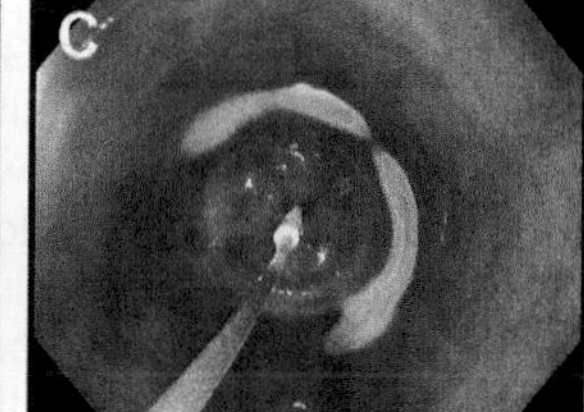

Fig. 4. Liquid nitrous oxide cryoballoon ablation of Barrett's esophagus using (*A*) a CryoBalloon Focal Catheter, (*B*) a CryoBalloon 90° Catheter, and (*C*) a Cryoballoon 180° Catheter. (*Courtesy of* PENTAX Medical, Redwood City, CA; with permission.)

heavy tanks. This obviates the need for tank storage and changing, and contributes to the former system's ease of use. Finally, the cryoballoon ablation system is more economical and affordable, with minimal capital expense for the current generation reusable controller and foot pedal.

CRYOTHERAPY FOR ERADICATION OF BARRETT'S ESOPHAGUS AND RELATED DYSPLASIA

Efficacy

The first study reporting on the efficacy of CO_2 cryospray ablation enrolled 22 patients of whom a total of 20 patients (90.9%) reached complete eradication of intestinal metaplasia (CE-IM).[21] In a retrospective, single-center study using the same technique, 67% achieved CE-IM after 3 years or at the last follow-up. More importantly, most of the 64 patients had undergone previous treatment: 28 patients with prior ablative therapy (RFA and/or photodynamic therapy) and 19 patients with prior endoscopic mucosal resection (EMR) for visible lesions.[16] In contrast to the other studies using the same technique, a surprisingly low effect (CE-IM 11% and CE-D 44%) was observed in a recent prospective study resulting in premature termination.[15] No clear explanation could be found for the lack of efficacy in this trial. Hereafter, CO_2 cryospray ablation has no longer been subject of research as a result of the unavailability of the system.

Most studies on cryotherapy for BE have focused on cryospray ablation with LN. For this application technique, rates for complete eradication of dysplasia (CE-D) and CE-IM were 87% to 88% and 53% to 57%, respectively, in large retrospective cohorts.[22,23] Comparable results were seen in the largest prospective cohort thus far, comprising 96 patients with either low-grade dysplasia (n = 32) or high-grade dysplasia (n = 64). In this cohort CE-D and CE-IM was obtained in 81% and 61%, respectively.[24] Recently, a retrospective single-center study demonstrated higher rates of CE-D (98.1%) and CE-IM (75%) after a mean follow-up of 4.8 years. These higher rates might be due to the multimodality treatment approach that was allowed in this study. During the course of treatment, 68.4% (39/57) of patients underwent prior EMR for nodular lesions, and 43.9% (25/57) underwent additional RFA for residual or recurrent IM after cryotherapy.[25]

The durability of cryospray ablation with LN is still largely unknown, partly due to insufficient follow-up in the majority of studies. The longest follow-up thus far has been reported in a retrospective cohort consisting of 40 patients undergoing endoscopic surveillance after LN cryospray ablation. The initial response was 90% (36/40) and 65% (26/40) for CE-D and CE-IM, respectively. After 5 years of follow-up, 81% (21/26) of the patients with initial CE-IM had persistent CE-IM. In the group with initial CE-IM the incidence rates for recurrent IM and dysplasia were 12.2% and 4.0%, respectively, per person-year of follow-up.[26] However, in a retrospective cohort of 36 patients with HGD the reported recurrence rate for IM was 72% after a median follow-up of 37 months. Of the 23 patients with recurrent IM, 12 patients underwent repeat cryotherapy which was successful in only 5 patients (CE-IM 42%).[27] Furthermore, the wide variation in the reported recurrence rates (0%–40%) makes it difficult to draw any conclusions on the durability of cryospray ablation with LN.[26,28–33] The large differences in definition of recurrence, and surveillance protocols might contribute to this variation.

The most recently published articles relate to the different cryoballoon devices. First, the feasibility and safety of CBF was investigated in 39 patients by treating only 1 or 2 focal areas within a flat segment BE. In this dose-finding study, 56 of 62 ablations (90.3%) were successfully performed with a median procedure time of 7 minutes. Full squamous regeneration was seen in 100% of the ablation sites targeted with a dose of 10sec.[18] Subsequently, the efficacy of CBF was investigated for the treatment of BE islands. Most BE islands (44/47, 94%) were adequately targeted, achieving CE-IM in 100% of the completely ablated areas.[34] It should be emphasized that in both these studies only 1 or 2 areas of 2 cm^2 were ablated instead of the complete BE segment. Canto and colleagues[35] were the first to apply side-by-side multiple ablations for treatment of all visible BE of any length until CE-IM was achieved. A median of 3 ablation procedures were performed per patient with an overall technical success rate of 98%. After a median follow-up of 20.9 months overall rates of CE-D and CE-IM were 95% and 88%, respectively. An ongoing multicenter American trial (Coldplay-3 study, Clinical Trial NCT02514525) reported similar but preliminary results, with CE-D and CE-IM rates of 100% and 91%, respectively, in 120 BE patients.[36] However, while these 2 clinical trials provide encouraging reports on the efficacy of multifocal cryoballoon ablation in neoplastic BE, more research is needed. Importantly, it should be noted that the cryoballoon ablation system has been upgraded meanwhile. Therefore, it is uncertain if the dosing used in these 2 studies (ie, 10sec per ablation) can be converted easily for cryogen dosing for the next (current) generation of the device. Currently, a large multicenter European trial is enrolling and treating BE patients using the new version of the device (EURO-Coldplay study, Netherlands Trial Register NL7253). This study will provide additional information on the efficacy, safety, and optimal dosing of the CBF.

Recently, the feasibility and efficacy of CB90, which targets a quarter of the esophageal circumference over a length of 3 cm, was assessed in the first-in-human study including 25 patients with ablation naive dysplastic flat BE. In the dose-finding phase, 13 patients underwent semi-circumferential treatment during a single endoscopy resulting in an effective dose of 0.7 mm/s. Next, 12 patients were subjected to circumferential treatment using the effective dose in 2 consecutive endoscopies with an 8-week interval. The median BE surface regression after circumferential treatment was 93%. Although the first efficacy results on CB90 are promising, 2 of 12 patients (17%) developed esophageal stricture after circumferential treatment with cryoballoon ablation. Therefore, the authors stated that larger clinical studies are warranted in order to establish the optimal dosage for CB90 that balances efficacy and safety.[19]

Safety

Cryotherapy is generally considered to be safe. The most common post-procedural adverse events include retrosternal pain and dysphagia. Pain requiring analgesics is reported in up to 9.7% of patients treated with cryotherapy.[16,18,22,23,35,37,38] Esophageal stricture rates range from 1% to 9.8%,[16,22–24,27,32,35,38,39] therefore being comparable with stricture rates for RFA (6%–11.8%).[40–42] One study showed a higher stricture rate (14.3%), although this was observed in patients who previously underwent RFA (median of 3 sessions).[29] In most cases, esophageal stricture can be treated successfully with endoscopic dilation.

Perforation rarely occurs after cryotherapy and is reported in 3 cases. One patient, previously treated with RFA, developed a small esophageal perforation after cryospray ablation with LN, which could be managed conservatively.[29] In 2 patients undergoing cryospray ablation, one with LN and one with CO_2, a gastric perforation was detected requiring surgical intervention.[15,38] One of these patients had Marfan syndrome. As a consequence, it is recommended to avoid cryospray ablation in patients with the limited ability to distend the stomach such as patients with connective tissue diseases or altered gastric anatomy after surgery.[23,38] For cryoballoon ablation, the risk of perforation is presumably negligible. In a porcine model, profound ablation effects were seen in the deeper esophageal wall layers after supratherapeutic doses, surprisingly without causing perforation.[20,43]

Buried Barrett's Esophagus Glands

A possible risk after ablative therapy is the persistence of Barrett's epithelium under an overlying layer of neosquamous epithelium, so called buried BE or subsquamous Barrett's glands. Subsquamous metaplastic glands may have neoplastic potential,[44] although the risk of malignant progression is believed to be lower compared with unablated epithelium because these glands are not exposed to acid reflux.[45] The prevalence of buried BE after RFA is demonstrated to be 0.1%,[46] whereas for cryospray ablation a prevalence ranging from 0% to 9.1% is reported.[15,18,21,22,28,37] An explanation for these higher percentages after cryospray ablation might be the unequal distribution of this technique. Since the cryoballoon systems theoretically generate a more homogenous ablation effect, the risk of buried BE might be lower with these devices. So far, no buried BE was observed in 2 studies using the CB90 and CBF.[19,34] Nevertheless, the number of patients included in these 2 studies is insufficient to draw any conclusions on the risk of buried BE after cryoballoon ablation.

Cryoablation for Radiofrequency Ablation–Refractory Barrett's Esophagus

Several articles address the possibility of cryotherapy as salvage therapy in RFA-refractory cases. In the study of Sengupta and colleagues[29] 21 patients with failed eradication of dysplasia or recurrent dysplasia after ≥3 RFA sessions were offered cryotherapy. LN cryospray ablation was applied to all visible Barrett's epithelium for 2 cycles of 20 seconds. After a median of 3 cryotherapy sessions, 12 of the 16 evaluable patients (75%) achieved CE-D and 5 patients (31%) achieved CE-IM. None of the patients with CE-D had recurrence of dysplasia after a median follow-up of 7.5 months. The same cryoablation protocol was carried out in another study including patients with persistent dysplasia (n = 11) or persistent intestinal metaplasia (n = 7) after RFA. In this cohort overall rates of CE-D and CE-IM were 72% (13/18) and 50% (9/18), respectively, after a median follow-up of 4.3 months. More importantly, 3 of the 7 patients (43%) with persistent IM after RFA reached CE-IM with cryotherapy.[30] In a retrospective cohort of 46 patients receiving either LN cryospray or cryoballoon ablation as salvage therapy, 38 patients (83%) achieved CE-D after a median of 2 cryotherapy sessions. CE-IM was reached in 21 patients (46%).[32] Although cryotherapy might be a valid option for RFA-refractory cases, the results of these studies must be interpreted with caution. Applying multiple treatment modalities consecutively, logically results in a larger number of patients achieving complete eradication. Nevertheless, the persistence of IM in 50% to 69% of the included patients disputes the effectiveness of cryotherapy. A possible explanation might be that the selected cases are not truly RFA-refractory. In our experience, true RFA unresponsiveness is very uncommon. In all 3 studies the rates of endoscopic resection (ER) before ablative therapy are low.[29,30,32] This possibly indicates underuse of EMR for visible lesions, which might have contributed to the reported failure rates of RFA considering visible lesions are thicker making them less susceptible to RFA. In addition, mucosal thickening as a result of inflammation due to poorly controlled reflux might contribute to failure of or incomplete response to RFA. In these cases, optimizing reflux control might eliminate the inflammatory changes that limited the maximal effect of RFA.[47]

Efficacy Compared with Heat-Based Ablation

Data on the efficacy of cryotherapy in comparison with heat-based ablation such as RFA or APC are very limited. A retrospective study reviewed data on patients with Barrett's dysplasia or intramucosal adenocarcinoma who underwent either RFA (n = 73) or cryospray ablation with LN (n = 81).[31] The rate for CE-IM was higher in the RFA group compared to the cryotherapy group (66.7% vs 41.3% respectively, $P = .002$), whereas the rate for CE-D was similar between the 2 groups (87.5% vs 78.8% respectively, $P = .15$). There were no significant differences in progression rates (12.5% vs 12.5%) or disease recurrence (11.1% vs 14.3%). Patients who underwent RFA were more likely to achieve CE-IM than those who underwent cryotherapy (odds ratio [OR] 2.9, 95% confidence interval [CI] 1.4–6.0, $P = .004$), but not CE-D (OR 1.7, 95% CI 0.7–4.3, $P = .28$). It must be highlighted that the CE-IM achieved in the RFA group of this study is low in contrast to other large prospective series. In a prospective UK registry on RFA including 508 patients CE-IM was reached in 83%.[48] In prospective studies including only patients in expert centers reported CE-IM was even higher (88%–93%), partly due to the very strict RFA protocol that was endorsed.[40,49] The 2 largest series on cryospray ablation including 96 and 98 patients show much lower CE-IM rates, varying from 57% to 61%.[22,24] These data suggest that in terms of efficacy of cryospray therapy, there is room for improvement, and RFA should still be considered the standard of care. For cryoballoon ablation, large prospective series on the effectiveness are still lacking, as are direct prospective comparisons with RFA.

Tolerability

Compared to heat-based ablation, cryotherapy appears to be associated with better patient tolerance. In a retrospective cohort including 20 patients treated with CBF and 26 patients with focal RFA, BE surface regression was equal in both groups after a single treatment session (88% vs 90% respectively, $P = .62$). Median peak pain, however, was consistently lower after cryotherapy (visual analog scale 2 vs 4, $P<.01$) and the duration of pain was shorter (2 vs 4 days, $P<.01$). Moreover, patients in the cryotherapy group used significantly less analgesics.[50] A prospective study comparing cryospray ablation using LN (n = 35) with RFA (n = 59) demonstrated similar findings.[51] After cryotherapy, patients reported significantly lower post-procedural pain scores, although no significant differences were observed for dysphagia. The odds of pain after RFA were at least 5 times greater than after cryotherapy, both immediately posttreatment (OR 5.3, 95% CI 1.9–14.3) and at 48 hours posttreatment (OR 5.6, 95% CI 2.3–14.3). However, it should be noted that the comparison made in the latter study is questionable, due to the differences between the groups in terms of baseline characteristics, such as histology and length of original Barrett's segment.

Table 1 provides an overview of all data on efficacy, safety and durability of cryotherapy for eradication of dysplastic BE.

DISCUSSION

Because BE is a premalignant condition predisposing for esophageal adenocarcinoma, current guidelines recommend endoscopic treatment in case of BE-related neoplasia.[52,53] The ultimate goal of this endoscopic treatment is the complete endoscopic and histologic conversion of all Barrett's epithelium, while restoring the esophageal mucosal lining with squamous epithelium. Endoscopic treatment involves a two-step approach. First, ER is indicated for all visible, non-flat lesions. Not only for optimizing histopathological assessment, but also to make the remaining Barrett's segment susceptible for additional ablative therapy. In addition to remaining BE after

Table 1
Overview of studies on efficacy, safety and durability of cryotherapy for Barrett's esophagus

First Author, Year of Publication	Study Design	Patients, n	Baseline Histology, n (ND/ LGD/HGD/ IMC)	BE Segment Length, cm	Method	CE-D, %	CE-IM, %	BB, %	Recurrence, n (%)	Pain, n	Analgesics use, n	Stricture, n	Perforation, n
Johnston et al,[37] 2005	Prospective, single center	11	3/7/1/-	4.6	LN	100	64	0	NR	2	1	0	0
Dumot et al,[38] 2009	Prospective, single center	31	–/–/26/5	6.1	LN	33	3	NR	9 (64)	10	3	3	1
Greenwald et al,[23] 2010	Retrospective, multicenter	77	7/45/23	4.0	LN	88	53	NR	NR	57	2	3	1
Shaheen et al,[22] 2010	Retrospective, multicenter	98	–/–/98/-	5.3	LN	87	57	3	NR	NR	2	3	0
Halsey et al,[28] 2011	Retrospective, single center	36	–/–/36/-	3.0	LN	97	92	0	11 (30)	NR	NR	NR	NR
Xue et al,[21] 2011	Prospective, single center	22	-/22/–/–	2.6	CO_2	NR	91	9	3 (14)	2	0	0	0
Gosain et al,[27] 2013	Retrospective, single center	32	–/–/32/-	3.0	LN	97	81	NR	6 (19)	NR	NR	3	0
Canto et al,[16] 2015	Retrospective, single center	68	–/–/54/14	5.3	CO_2	89	55	7	20 (31)	4	2	1	0
Schölvinck et al,[43] 2015	Prospective, multicenter	39	9/10/9/11	5.0	CBF	NR	NR	NR	NR	10	3	0	0
Sengupta et al,[29] 2015	Retrospective, single center	16	-/7/7/2	7.0	LN	75	31	NR	0 (0)	NR	NR	3	1
Verbeek et al,[15] 2015	Prospective, single center	10	–/–/3/7	5.0	CO_2	44	11	0	NR	6	0	0	1
Ghorbani et al,[24] 2016	Prospective, multicenter	96	-/32/64/-	4.5	LN	81	61	NR	NR	36	0	1	0

Künzli et al,[34] 2017	Prospective, multicenter	30	-/14/7/9	0 (islands)	CBF	100	100	0	NR	8	0	0	0
Ramay et al,[26] 2017	Retrospective, single center	50 [3Y FU] 40 [5Y FU]	NR	3.5 3.0	LN	94 88	82 75	NR	15 (30) 16 (40)	NR	NR	NR	NR
Suchniak-Mussari et al,[39] 2017	Retrospective, single center	33	5/5/15/8	3.3	LN	84	49	NR	NR	2	0	5	0
Trindade et al,[30] 2017	Retrospective, multicenter	18	7/4/7/-	4.0	LN	72	50	NR	0 (0)	0	0	0	0
Canto et al,[35] 2018	Prospective, multicenter	41	-/13/23/5	3.9	CBF	95	88	NR	NR	2	2	4	0
van Munster et al,[50] 2018	Prospective, multicenter	20	-/9/11/-	2.0	CBF	NR	NR	NR	NR	14	5	0	0
Thota et al,[31] 2018	Retrospective, multicenter	81	-/11/49/21	5.2	CO_2	79	41	NR	9 (14)	NR	NR	NR	NR
Trindade et al,[33] 2018	Retrospective, multicenter	27	-/5/22/-	5.0	LN	82	70	NR	3 (11)	0	0	0	0
Solomon et al,[51] 2019	Prospective, multicenter	35	6/12/9/8	6.1	LN	NR	NR	NR	NR	10	NR	NR	NR
Spiceland et al,[32] 2019	Retrospective, single center	46	-/15/25/6	NR	LN or CBF	83	46	NR	2 [4]	NR	NR	3	NR
van Munster et al,[19] 2019	Prospective, multicenter	25	-/20/2/3	3.0	CB90	100	100	0	NR	0	0	2	0
Kaul et al,[25] 2020	Retrospective, single center	57	-/8/20/19	6.2	LN	98	75	NR	7 [21]	NR	NR	0	1

Abbreviations: BB, buried Barrett; BE, Barrett's esophagus; CBF, C2 cryoballoon focal catheter; CB90, C2 Cryoballoon 90° Catheter; CE-D, complete eradication of dysplasia; CE-IM, complete eradication of intestinal metaplasia; CO_2, carbon dioxide; FU, follow up; HGD, high-grade dysplasia; IMC, intramucosal cancer; LGD, low-grade dysplasia; LN, liquid nitrogen; ND, no dysplasia; NR, not reported; Y, year.

ER, patients should be considered for ablative therapy in case of flat type dysplastic BE.[53]

Several features are indispensable for an ideal ablation technique for BE. First of all, the ablation effect must be homogeneous and predictable without operator dependency. Other essential features include high efficacy and safety rates, and cost-effectiveness. Moreover, the tool must fit within the multimodality treatment algorithm for BE-related neoplasia. Equally important to ER of visible lesions prior to ablation, is the resection of visible abnormalities that pop-up during the ablation phase or local recurrence after prior successful eradication therapy. However, after ablation the possibility of performing ER may be impeded by submucosal fibrosis. Therefore, the ideal ablation tool should also permit post-ablation resection.

Given these essential features of an ideal ablation tool, the exact position of cryotherapy in the multimodality treatment of BE still remains unclear. Cryotherapy appears to be a safe and effective. However, evidence on the possibility of performing ER after cryotherapy is lacking. Also, the durability and cost-effectiveness of cryotherapy are largely unknown.

Currently, RFA is the most established ablative modality with high efficacy and safety rates. Any alternative ablation technique, such as cryotherapy, will be challenged to meet these high standards. Nevertheless, RFA has several disadvantages including high costs and a substantial stricture rate (6%–14%).[42,49] Another drawback is the multiple treatment endoscopies which in general are needed before reaching complete endoscopic eradication. In addition, RFA is associated with significant post-procedural pain, frequently requiring analgesics during several days.

Considering the previously mentioned, what are the potential advantages of cryotherapy over RFA? Cryotherapy theoretically allows deeper tissue ablation while preserving the esophageal wall integrity without increasing the risk of stricture formation. Studies so far, however, do not prove a significant reduction in stricture rates after cryoablation, although the reverse (higher stricture rate after cryoablation compared to RFA) also seems unlikely. Furthermore, cryotherapy is probably associated with a favorable pain course, which is shown in clinical studies and is also the general perception of endoscopists.[50,51]

To date, the exact position of cryoablation in the treatment algorithm of BE remains uncertain. Clearly, appropriately powered non-inferiority randomized controlled trials directly comparing RFA with cryotherapy are needed to determine the latter technology's role in primary endoscopic eradication therapy. Cryotherapy might become a worthy alternative to RFA if future studies further document equal effectiveness and safety. If so, patient tolerability might become a guiding element in the choice for one ablation technique over the other.

In addition, cryotherapy might find some niche indications where it might prove to be a valuable complementary, instead of a competing technology. One potential niche for cryotherapy might be the treatment of RFA-refractory cases. Increased mucosal thickness of Barrett's epithelium might be a factor contributing to the decreased susceptibility for RFA in these cases. Considering cryotherapy enabling deeper tissue ablation, it might be an appealing treatment option for patients in whom RFA previously failed. Future studies, ideally randomizing RFA-refractory patients to additional RFA ablations or cryoablation are needed. Finally, the possibility of deeper tissue ablation also suggests a possible role of cryotherapy in patients with persisting or recurrent lesions that are not amendable for ER, in inoperable patients with a positive deep resection margin after endoscopic resection, or even in patients deemed inoperable with local cancer recurrences after definitive chemoradiotherapy for advanced esophageal cancer. These potential purposes of cryotherapy warrant further investigation in order to determine the specific role of cryotherapy in the management of BE.

DISCLOSURE

For C.N. Frederiks no conflict of interest was declared. M.I. Canto has received research grants for IRB-approved studies from Pentax Medical Corporation (America). B.L.A.M. Weusten has received financial support for IRB-approved studies from Pentax Medical Corporation (America).

REFERENCES

1. Korpan NN. A history of cryosurgery: its development and future. J Am Coll Surg 2007;204(2):314–24.
2. Cooper SM, Dawber RP. The history of cryosurgery. J R Soc Med 2001;94(4): 196–201.
3. Arnott J. Practical Illustrations of the Remedial Efficacy of a Very Low Or Anaesthetic Temperature.-I. in Cancer. Lancet 1850;56(1411):316–8.
4. Rodgers BM, Pappelis P. Profound endoesophageal cryotherapy. Cryobiology 1985;22(1):86–92.
5. Johnston CM, Schoenfeld LP, Mysore JV, et al. Endoscopic spray cryotherapy: a new technique for mucosal ablation in the esophagus. Gastrointest Endosc 1999; 50(1):86–92.
6. Baust JG, Gage AA, Bjerklund Johansen TE, et al. Mechanisms of cryoablation: clinical consequences on malignant tumors. Cryobiology 2014;68(1):1–11.
7. Gage AA, Baust J. Mechanisms of Tissue Injury in Cryosurgery. Cryobiology 1998;37(3):171–86.
8. Gage AA, Baust JM, Baust JG. Experimental cryosurgery investigations in vivo. Cryobiology 2009;59(3):229–43.
9. Shin EJ, Amateau SK, Kim Y, et al. Dose-dependent depth of tissue injury with carbon dioxide cryotherapy in porcine GI tract. Gastrointest Endosc 2012; 75(5):1062–7.
10. Allaf ME, Varkarakis IM, Bhayani SB, et al. Pain control requirements for percutaneous ablation of renal tumors: cryoablation versus radiofrequency ablation–initial observations. Radiology 2005;237(1):366–70.
11. Truesdale CM, Soulen MC, Clark TWI, et al. Percutaneous computed tomography-guided renal mass radiofrequency ablation versus cryoablation: doses of sedation medication used. J Vasc Interv Radiol 2013;24(3):347–50.
12. Chan NY, Choy CC, Lau CL, et al. Cryoablation versus radiofrequency ablation for atrioventricular nodal reentrant tachycardia: patient pain perception and operator stress. Pacing Clin Electrophysiol 2011;34(1):2–7.
13. Erinjeri JP, Clark TWI. Cryoablation: mechanism of action and devices. J Vasc Interv Radiol 2010;21(8 Suppl):S187–91.
14. Sreenarasimhaiah J. Endoscopic applications of cryospray ablation therapy-from Barrett's esophagus and beyond. World J Gastrointest Endosc 2016;8(16):546.
15. Verbeek R, Vleggaar F, ten Kate F, et al. Cryospray ablation using pressurized CO2 for ablation of Barrett's esophagus with early neoplasia: early termination of a prospective series. Endosc Int Open 2015;03(02):E107–12.
16. Canto MI, Shin EJ, Khashab MA, et al. Safety and efficacy of carbon dioxide cryotherapy for treatment of neoplastic Barrett's esophagus. Endoscopy 2015; 47(7):591.

17. Lal P, Thota PN. Cryotherapy in the management of premalignant and malignant conditions of the esophagus. World J Gastroenterol 2018;24(43):4862–9.
18. Schölvinck D, Künzli H, Kestens C, et al. Treatment of Barrett's esophagus with a novel focal cryoablation device: a safety and feasibility study. Endoscopy 2015; 47(12):1106–12.
19. van Munster SN, Overwater A, Raicu MGM, et al. A novel cryoballoon ablation system for eradication of dysplastic Barrett's esophagus: a first-in-human feasibility study. Endoscopy 2019;193–201. https://doi.org/10.1055/a-1024-3967.
20. Louie BE, Hofstetter W, Triadafilopoulos G, et al. Evaluation of a novel cryoballoon swipe ablation system in bench, porcine, and human esophagus models. Dis Esophagus 2018;31(8):69–70.
21. Xue HB, Tan HH, Liu WZ, et al. A pilot study of endoscopic spray cryotherapy by pressurized carbon dioxide gas for Barrett's esophagus. Endoscopy 2011;43(5): 379–85.
22. Shaheen NJ, Greenwald BD, Peery AF, et al. Safety and efficacy of endoscopic spray cryotherapy for Barrett's esophagus with high-grade dysplasia. Gastrointest Endosc 2010;71(4):680–5.
23. Greenwald BD, Dumot JA, Horwhat JD, et al. Safety, tolerability, and efficacy of endoscopic low-pressure liquid nitrogen spray cryotherapy in the esophagus. Dis Esophagus 2010;23(1):13–9.
24. Ghorbani S, Tsai FC, Greenwald BD, et al. Safety and efficacy of endoscopic spray cryotherapy for Barrett's dysplasia: Results of the National Cryospray Registry. Dis Esophagus 2016;29(3):241–7.
25. Kaul V, Bittner K, Ullah A, et al. Liquid nitrogen spray cryotherapy-based multimodal endoscopic management of dysplastic Barrett's esophagus and early esophageal neoplasia: retrospective review and long-term follow-up at an academic tertiary care referral center. Dis Esophagus 2020;1–6. https://doi.org/10.1093/dote/doz095.
26. Ramay FH, Cui Q, Greenwald BD. Outcomes after liquid nitrogen spray cryotherapy in Barrett's esophagus-associated high-grade dysplasia and intramucosal adenocarcinoma: 5-year follow-up. Gastrointest Endosc 2017;86(4): 626–32.
27. Gosain S, Mercer K, Twaddell WS, et al. Liquid nitrogen spray cryotherapy in Barrett's esophagus with high-grade dysplasia: Long-term results. Gastrointest Endosc 2013;78(2):260–5.
28. Halsey KD, Chang JW, Waldt A, et al. Recurrent disease following endoscopic ablation of Barretts high-grade dysplasia with spray cryotherapy. Endoscopy 2011;43(10):844–8.
29. Sengupta N, Ketwaroo GA, Bak DM, et al. Salvage cryotherapy after failed radiofrequency ablation for Barrett's esophagus-related dysplasia is safe and effective. Gastrointest Endosc 2015;82(3):443–8.
30. Trindade AJ, Inamdar S, Kothari S, et al. Feasibility of liquid nitrogen cryotherapy after failed radiofrequency ablation for Barrett's esophagus. Dig Endosc 2017; 29(6):680–5.
31. Thota PN, Arora Z, Dumot JA, et al. Cryotherapy and radiofrequency ablation for eradication of Barrett's esophagus with dysplasia or intramucosal cancer. Dig Dis Sci 2018;63(5):1311–9.
32. Spiceland CM, Elmunzer BJ, Paros S, et al. Salvage cryotherapy in patients undergoing endoscopic eradication therapy for complicated Barrett's esophagus. Endosc Int Open 2019;07(07):E904–11.

33. Trindade AJ, Pleskow DK, Sengupta N, et al. Efficacy of liquid nitrogen cryotherapy for Barrett's esophagus after endoscopic resection of intramucosal cancer: A multicenter study. J Gastroenterol Hepatol 2018;33(2):461–5.
34. Künzli HT, Schölvinck DW, Meijer SL, et al. Efficacy of the CryoBalloon Focal Ablation System for the eradication of dysplastic Barrett's esophagus islands. Endoscopy 2017;49(2):169–75.
35. Canto MI, Shaheen NJ, Almario JA, et al. Multifocal nitrous oxide cryoballoon ablation with or without EMR for treatment of neoplastic Barrett's esophagus (with video). Gastrointest Endosc 2018;88(3):438–46.e2.
36. Canto MI, Trindade AJ, Abrams J, et al. Safety and Efficacy of Multifocal Cryoballoon Ablation for Eradication of Previously Untreated Barrett'S Neoplasia: Preliminary Results of a Large Multicenter American Trial. Gastrointest Endosc 2019; 89(6):AB98.
37. Johnston MH, Eastone JA, Horwhat JD, et al. Cryoablation of Barrett's esophagus: A pilot study. Gastrointest Endosc 2005;62(6):842–8.
38. Dumot JA, Vargo JJ, Falk GW, et al. An open-label, prospective trial of cryospray ablation for Barrett's esophagus high-grade dysplasia and early esophageal cancer in high-risk patients. Gastrointest Endosc 2009;70(4):635–44.
39. Suchniak-Mussari K, Dye CE, Moyer MT, et al. Efficacy and safety of liquid nitrogen cryotherapy for treatment of Barrett's esophagus. World J Gastrointest Endosc 2017;9(9):480.
40. Phoa KN, van Vilsteren FGI, Weusten BLAM, et al. Radiofrequency Ablation vs Endoscopic Surveillance for Patients With Barrett Esophagus and Low-Grade Dysplasia. JAMA 2014;311(12):1209.
41. Shaheen NJ, Sharma P, Overholt BF, et al. Radiofrequency Ablation in Barrett's Esophagus with Dysplasia. N Engl J Med 2009;360(22):2277–88.
42. van Vilsteren FGI, Pouw RE, Seewald S, et al. Stepwise radical endoscopic resection versus radiofrequency ablation for Barrett's oesophagus with high-grade dysplasia or early cancer: a multicentre randomised trial. Gut 2011;60(6):765–73.
43. Schölvinck DW, Friedland S, Triadafilopoulos G, et al. Balloon-based esophageal cryoablation with a novel focal ablation device: Dose-finding and safety in porcine and human models. Dis Esophagus 2017;30(11):1–8.
44. Van Laethem JL, Peny MO, Salmon I, et al. Intramucosal adenocarcinoma arising under squamous re-epithelialisation of Barrett's oesophagus. Gut 2000;46(4): 574–7.
45. Gray NA, Odze RD, Spechler SJ. Buried metaplasia after endoscopic ablation of Barrett's esophagus: a systematic review. Am J Gastroenterol 2011;106(11): 1899–908 [quiz: 1909].
46. Pouw RE, Visser M, Odze RD, et al. Pseudo-buried Barrett's post radiofrequency ablation for Barrett's esophagus, with or without prior endoscopic resection. Endoscopy 2014;46(2):105–9.
47. Weusten BLAM, Bergman JJGHM. Cryoablation for managing Barrett's esophagus refractory to radiofrequency ablation? Don't embrace the cold too soon! Gastrointest Endosc 2015;82(3):449–51.
48. Haidry RJ, Butt Ma, Dunn JM, et al. Improvement over time in outcomes for patients undergoing endoscopic therapy for Barrett's oesophagus-related neoplasia: 6-year experience from the first 500 patients treated in the UK patient registry. Gut 2015;64(8):1192–9.
49. Phoa KN, Pouw RE, Bisschops R, et al. Multimodality endoscopic eradication for neoplastic Barrett oesophagus: results of an European multicentre study (EURO-II). Gut 2016;65(4):555–62.

50. van Munster SN, Overwater A, Haidry R, et al. Focal cryoballoon versus radiofrequency ablation of dysplastic Barrett's esophagus: impact on treatment response and postprocedural pain. Gastrointest Endosc 2018;88(5):795–803.e2.
51. Solomon SS, Kothari S, Smallfield GB, et al. Liquid Nitrogen Spray Cryotherapy is Associated With Less Postprocedural Pain Than Radiofrequency Ablation in Barrett's Esophagus: A Multicenter Prospective Study. J Clin Gastroenterol 2019;53(2):e84–90.
52. Shaheen NJ, Falk GW, Iyer PG, et al. ACG clinical guideline: diagnosis and management of Barrett's esophagus. Am J Gastroenterol 2016;111(1):30–50 [quiz: 51].
53. Weusten B, Bisschops R, Coron E, et al. Endoscopic management of Barrett's esophagus: European Society of Gastrointestinal Endoscopy (ESGE) Position Statement. Endoscopy 2017;49(2):191–8.

Role of Endoscopic Mucosal Resection and Endoscopic Submucosal Dissection in the Management of Barrett's Related Neoplasia

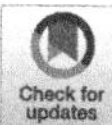

Esther A. Nieuwenhuis, MD[a], Oliver Pech, MD, PhD[b],
Jacques J.G.H.M. Bergman, MD, PhD[a], Roos E. Pouw, MD, PhD[a,*]

KEYWORDS

- Barrett's esophagus • Barrett's neoplasia • High-grade dysplasia
- Early esophageal adenocarcinoma • Endoscopic resection
- Endoscopic mucosal resection • Endoscopic submucosal dissection

KEY POINTS

- Endoscopic resection provides accurate histopathological assessment of neoplastic lesions in Barrett's esophagus.
- Endoscopic resection is among the key steps in the endoscopic work-up of early Barrett's cancer in terms of diagnosis and treatment.
- Multiband mucosectomy is the most commonly used technique for endoscopic resection in the Western world.
- Endoscopic submucosal dissection is preferred for lesions with suspicion for submucosal invasion, or bulky lesions, to ensure en bloc and radical resection of the lesion.

 **Video content accompanies this article at http://www.giendo.theclinics.com.**

INTRODUCTION

Barrett's esophagus (BE) is defined as a metaplastic change of the normal squamous lining of the distal esophagus, with replacement of squamous epithelium by an intestinal-type epithelium caused by longstanding gastroesophageal reflux

[a] Department of Gastroenterology and Hepatology, Amsterdam University Medical Centers, Location VUmc, De Boelelaan 1118, Amsterdam 1081 HV, the Netherlands; [b] Department of Gastroenterology and Hepatology, Krankenhaus Barmherzige Brüder Regensburg, Prüfeninger Str. 86, Regensburg 93049, Germany
* Corresponding author.
E-mail address: r.e.pouw@amsterdamumc.nl

Gastrointest Endoscopy Clin N Am 31 (2021) 171–182
https://doi.org/10.1016/j.giec.2020.09.001 giendo.theclinics.com

disease. BE has malignant potential through the sequence of no dysplasia to low-grade dysplasia (LGD), high-grade dysplasia (HGD), and eventually early esophageal adenocarcinoma (EAC).[1,2] BE patients have a 30- to 40-fold higher risk of EAC compared with the general population.[3] Therefore, endoscopic surveillance is recommended to detect dysplasia before it progresses to EAC, and to detect EAC at a curable stage.

Surgical esophagectomy has traditionally been recommended for patients found to have early neoplasia arising in BE. However, esophagectomy is associated with high morbidity (up to 65%) and significant mortality rates even in high-volume centers (2%–4%).[4] For the past 2 decades, much research has focused on development of endoscopic imaging techniques to detect EAC at an early stage, and on endoscopic treatment techniques to create less-invasive treatment modalities for early BE-related neoplasia.

The endoscopic resection (ER) technique for the treatment of neoplastic lesions was first developed in Japan for the treatment of early gastric cancer.[5] The technique has been adapted by Western endoscopists in subsequent years for various indications, including Barrett's neoplasia. ER has proven to be a safe, effective, and minimally invasive alternative to surgery for treatment of early neoplastic lesions in BE, and is considered to be the cornerstone of endoscopic treatment. ER is an endoscopic approach in which the neoplastic epithelium is excised, providing adequate tissue specimens, enabling accurate histologic staging of a lesion while also potentially being curative. Staging consists of assessing invasion depth, differentiation grade, presence of lympho-vascular invasion, and radicality of the resection, and is important to determine further management.[6–9] There are 2 common methods to perform ER: cap-based ER and endoscopic submucosal dissection (ESD). Both methods will be discussed in this article.

INDICATIONS FOR ENDOSCOPIC RESECTION

Because ER only allows for local therapy of suspicious visible lesions arising from BE, it is essential to adequately select patients for whom the risk of lymph node involvement or hematogenous dissemination is low enough to justify performing local ER instead of esophagectomy with lymph node dissection. This risk should also be balanced against the high morbidity and mortality rates of esophagectomy, and the clinician should take the patient's wish and performance status into account.

Mucosal Cancer

ER for the treatment of BE with HGD or EAC limited to the mucosa (ie, T1m1-m3) has been established as first-choice treatment, with excellent efficacy and safety, also in long-term analyses. In one of the largest published studies in which data from 1000 patients with endoscopically resected mucosal EAC were collected, 96.3% of patients had achieved a complete response shortly after ER. After 5 years of follow-up, the long-term complete remission rate was 93.8%, and only 2 patients died of BE-associated cancer.[10] Furthermore, several studies have shown that the risk of lymph node involvement is minimal (1%) in patients with mucosal EAC.[10,11] Therefore, ER is considered the treatment of choice for this indication. Nevertheless, data for patients with a mucosal EAC containing high-risk features (ie, poor differentiation and/or lymphovascular invasion) are not available in the current literature. Therefore, the risk of lymph node metastases in these specific patients is currently unknown.

Submucosal Cancer

In the last few years, the indication for endoscopic therapy has extended to tumors invading the submucosa superficially (ie, invasion depth ≤500 μm) without any other histopathological risk factors for lymph node metastasis (ie, good-to-moderate differentiation [G1-G2], no presence of lymphovascular invasion [LVI], and negative vertical resection margins [R0]), since the risk to develop lymph node metastasis appears to be less than 2%.[12,13] This is lower than the mortality risk of esophagectomy. Therefore, endoscopic treatment and follow-up seem to be valid alternatives to surgical resection for this indication.

Patients with high risk submucosal cancer (ie, deep submucosal infiltration >500 μm, and/or poor differentiation [G3], and/or presence of LVI, and/or R1 resection) are considered surgical candidates, as the risk of lymph node metastasis is thought to be much higher (16%–44%).[14,15] However, these numbers are mainly based on old surgical series. These numbers may also be overestimated, as these studies often did not differentiate between various submucosal infiltration depths, and this was not required for patient management. Furthermore, surgical resection specimens are cut in larger slices than ER specimens, which may lead to underestimation of the presence of histologic risk factors associated with higher risk of lymph node metastasis, and the deepest infiltrating part of a tumor, poor differentiation, or presence of LVI may have been missed.

Recently, several studies, which only included patients who underwent ER for high-risk submucosal cancer, were published indicating that the risk of metastases may be lower than generally assumed (0%–30%).[13,16,17] Nevertheless, it does exceed the mortality rate of surgical resection. Therefore, endoscopic management after ER of high-risk submucosal cancer is not advised by current guidelines. However, in selected patients, a strict endoscopic follow-up protocol with regular endoscopic and endosonographic follow-up to detect lymph node metastases at a curable stage can be considered.

ENDOSCOPIC WORK-UP

Patients with HGD or cancer found on biopsies, and all patients with a visible abnormality, regardless of the pathology outcome, should be referred to a center with high expertise in endoscopic evaluation and treatment of BE-related neoplasia to confirm these findings. Repeating endoscopy at an expert center with experienced endoscopists and pathologists provides a more reliable final diagnosis. More importantly, patients referred with flat HGD or cancer in random biopsies are likely to actually have a visible abnormality that was missed during the first endoscopy. A study comparing the detection rate of neoplastic BE lesions between community and expert endoscopists showed that 76% of patients who were referred for evaluation of HGD or cancer in random biopsies without a visible abnormality reported, did have a visible abnormality detected by an expert endoscopist.[18] Furthermore, repeat endoscopy assures the detection of other abnormalities elsewhere in the BE segment that otherwise might be left untreated. Contrarily, if a visible abnormality is detected but biopsies do not show dysplasia or cancer, one should keep the possibility of a false-negative histopathological diagnosis in mind with a low threshold to refer for a diagnostic ER or at least perform repeat endoscopy with biopsies. Moreover, high-quality documentation during endoscopy by taking multiple photos and recording videos can be used while consulting an expert center.

Detection of Early Neoplasia

Thorough endoscopic inspection of the entire BE segment is necessary to detect early neoplastic lesions, as they often present as subtle mucosal irregularities. It is preferred to use high-resolution endoscopy, complemented with virtual chromoendoscopy (ie, narrow-band imaging, blue-laser imaging, i-scan) to delineate the extent of a lesion.

Other than using the best available equipment and having familiarity with the endoscopic appearance of BE-related early neoplasia, it is also important to perform a systematic procedure, such as cleaning, pull back, inspection of the gastroesophageal junction in the inverted position, endoscopic classification by macroscopic appearance of visible lesions, and biopsies.

Cleaning

After inflation of the esophagus, adequate cleaning of the esophageal wall by rinsing with water to remove all mucus contributes to better sight and therefore less chance of missing subtle abnormalities. Suctioning of fluids should be done in the stomach and hernia to avoid suction lesions within the Barrett's segment.

Pull back

Using white light, the endoscope should be carefully withdrawn in a continuous way to examine the BE segment for mucosal abnormalities and to describe the extent of the BE according to the validated Prague C & M criteria.[19] Special attention to the area between 12 o'clock and 6 o'clock in the endoscopic view is recommended. Several studies have shown that early cancer in BE is most commonly found in the right hemisphere of the esophagus, with the highest rate in the 12 o'clock to 3 o'clock quadrant.[20,21]

Inspection of the gastroesophageal junction in the inverted position

Lesions in this area are easily missed when only looking antegrade.

Endoscopic classification by macroscopic appearance of visible lesions

The macroscopic appearance of a lesion in BE should be classified according to the Paris classification, a classification based on earlier Japanese classifications, which was developed to allow morphologic classification of early and/or superficial lesions in the gastrointestinal (GI) tract.[22,23] The classification divides lesions into 3 major types: protruded, flat, and excavated. Protruded lesions (Paris type 0-Ip and 0-Is) are defined as having more than double the amount of mucosal thickness in a histologic specimen.[24] In clinical practice, a biopsy forceps placed longitudinally next to the lesion is a helpful reference value, where the height of protruded lesions is defined as being higher than a closed biopsy forceps (2.5 mm). Flat lesions are divided into 3 subtypes: slightly elevated lesions (Paris type 0-IIa), which are defined as less than double the amount of mucosal thickness in a histologic specimen or as less high than a closed biopsy forceps; completely flat lesions (Paris type 0-IIb); and slightly depressed lesions (Paris type 0-IIc), which are defined as less deep than 1 cup of an open biopsy forceps. Excavated lesions (Paris type 0-III) are predominantly ulcerative and are defined as deeper than half the cup of an open biopsy forceps.

The macroscopic appearance of a lesion is associated with infiltration depth and therefore indirectly with the risk of metastatic lymph nodes. A retrospective study evaluating the histopathology of specimens obtained from 296 ER procedures in correlation with endoscopic characteristics showed that Paris type 0-I and 0-IIc lesions were more likely to infiltrate into the submucosa (26% and 25%) compared with types 0-IIa, 0-IIa-IIb, and 0-IIa-IIc (9%, 8% and 10%, respectively) (P=.009). None of the type 0-IIb lesions showed submucosal invasion. However, a limitation to this study was that not all resection specimens were reassessed in this retrospective setting.25 Pech and colleagues21 did overcome this limitation by prospectively assessing macroscopic types of 380 early neoplastic lesions in BE and their histopathological outcomes. The study showed that slightly depressed lesions (Paris type 0-IIc) infiltrated into the submucosa more often (25%) than elevated (11%) and slightly elevated lesions (Paris type 0-I and 0-IIa) (14%) or flat lesions (Paris type 0-IIb) (4%). Type 0-IIb neoplasia was significantly more frequently associated with early local tumor stage and a good differentiation grade than all other types. However, none of the Paris type 0-I or type 0-II lesions were associated with a very high risk of submucosal invasion. Diagnostic ER therefore is considered indicated and safe for these lesions. No sufficient data are available on the rate of submucosal invasion in excavated lesions, but these types of lesions tend to include invasive tumors and are also less suitable for treatment with ER given the ulceration.

Biopsies

Targeted biopsies can be obtained from visible abnormalities. However, when the lesion is evidently present and diagnostic ER already planned, targeted biopsies of the lesion are optional. Nevertheless, whether visible lesions are found or not, tissue sampling is still required for mapping the (residual) BE. In inexperienced hands, 10% to 20% of lesions are missed with targeted biopsies alone.[26] The Seattle biopsy protocol is recommended for mapping the whole BE segment by randomly taking 4-quadrant biopsies. This biopsy protocol starts from the top of the gastric folds moving upwards up to the most proximal extent of the BE segment, while sampling at 2 cm intervals.[27] The reason for working in the proximal direction is to minimize bleeding obscuring the endoscopic view.

Diagnostic Endoscopic Resection for Visible Lesions as a Staging Procedure

When a visible lesion is first identified upon endoscopic inspection, it needs to be accurately evaluated by classifying the lesion using the previously described Paris classification to determine whether it is suitable for ER. When the appearance does not raise suspicion for deep submucosal infiltration, which is most important for determining the chances of radicality and lymph node metastases, the lesion may be removed by ER. This is a valuable diagnostic step, because the pathologist will be able to accurately assess risk factors for lymph node metastases such as infiltration depth, differentiation grade, and lymphovascular invasion. As described earlier, mucosal cancer and low-risk submucosal cancers are indications for further endoscopic management.

Other Staging Procedures

Because the risk of LNM is considered low among patients diagnosed with mucosal or low-risk submucosal tumors (1% and <2%, respectively), additional staging procedures such as endoscopic ultrasound (EUS) and positron emission tomography (PET) computed tomography (CT) scan are not necessarily required. For patients with suspicion on a deeper submucosal invading lesion, or presence of poor differentiation of LVI in biopsies, baseline staging may be helpful before deciding on performing ER. EUS is the most accurate technique for locoregional staging of esophageal cancer and has a high negative predictive value (>95%) for the absence of local lymph nodes. However, EUS is more reliable in patients with more advanced cancer than in patients with early EAC. Moreover, accuracy is affected by the experience of the endosonographer.[28,29] Just as for EUS, PET-CT is only advised for baseline staging in patients with a high-risk EAC, as the value mainly lies in the detection of distant metastasis.

There is no evidence in the literature that PET-CT is better for detection of distant metastasis in submucosal EAC compared with CT.[30–32]

PERFORMING ENDOSCOPIC RESECTION

Expertise and experience are required to resect esophageal lesions in a safe and effective way.

First of all, the endoscopist needs to decide whether a lesion will be removed by en bloc or piecemeal resection, depending on the size and the macroscopic appearance of the lesion. The most commonly used ER technique in the Western world is a cap-based technique named multiband mucosectomy (MBM), which allows for en bloc resection of lesions up to 20 mm in diameter. Larger lesions require multiple resections in the same endoscopic treatment session, a so-called piecemeal procedure, or ESD. Different established techniques will be described. One of the disadvantages of the piecemeal procedure is that the radicality of the resection at the lateral margins is impossible to assess for the evaluating pathologist. Endoscopic assessment of the radicality of a resection is therefore important. Other downsides of piecemeal resections are that they tend to be more technically demanding to perform, have a higher complication risk, and are more time consuming.[10]

After detection of the visible lesion, it is essential to mark the lesion by delineating the lateral borders by placing coagulation marks. Without these markings, it may be difficult to recognize the lateral margins of the lesion during the endoscopic resection because of reduced visibility due to bleeding or coagulation effects. By placing markers beforehand, one ensures the macroscopic lateral radicality when all coagulation markers are removed after the resection.

Different Endoscopic Resection Techniques

There are currently 2 common methods to perform an endoscopic resection: cap-based endoscopic resection and ESD.

Cap-based endoscopic resection techniques

These techniques include the MBM technique (**Fig. 1**, Video 1) and the endoscopic resection-cap technique.

Multiband mucosectomy technique The most commonly used ER technique nowadays is the MBM technique, which uses a modified variceal band ligator with a transparent cap and a polypectomy snare. First, the neoplastic lesion is sucked into the cap. Subsequently, by triggering the releasing handle, a rubber band is released, which only captures the mucosa. The rubber band is not strong enough to hold on to the deeper layers of the esophageal wall. Therefore, the target mucosa can be resected by using the polypectomy snare with a minimal risk of damaging the deeper muscle layer, even without prior submucosal lifting. The MBM technique can be performed by using the Duette System (Cook, Limerick, Ireland), or the Captivator device (Boston Scientific).

Endoscopic resection-cap technique Another technique for ER of BE lesions is the ER-cap technique, which involves the use of a specifically designed transparent oblique cap with a distal ridge, which allows for the placement of an asymmetrical crescent-shaped electrocoagulation snare. This technique is performed by lifting the lesion with fluid that is injected into the submucosal layer. Subsequently, the snare is prelooped in the ridge of the cap, whereafter the lesion is sucked into the cap, and the snare is tightened. The created pseudopolyp can then be resected.

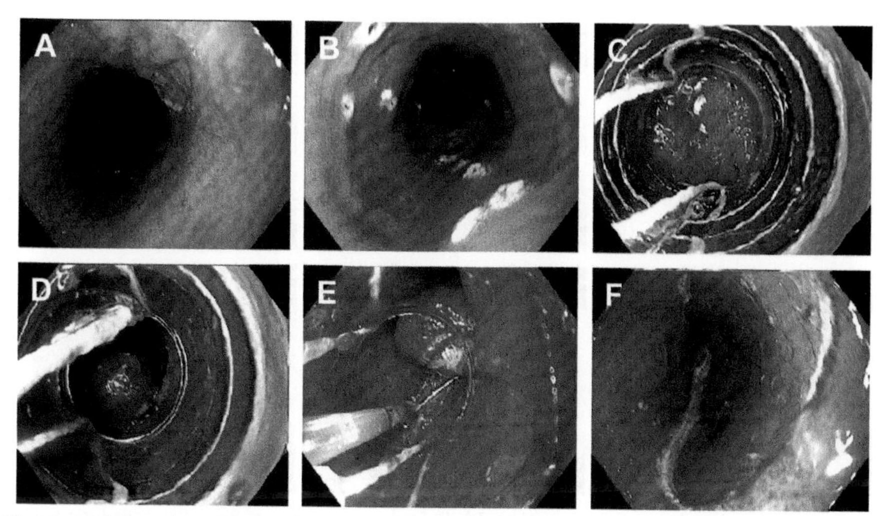

Fig. 1. Multiband mucosectomy using the Duette system (Cook, Limerick, Ireland). (*A, B*) Endoscopic view of Barrett's neoplasia, which is delineated with electrocoagulation markers before starting the endoscopic resection procedure. (*C, D*) Endoscopic view through the Duette cap. A pseudopolyp is created by suctioning the mucosa into the ligation cap and releasing a rubber band. (*E*) Pseudopolyp resection by hexagonal snare. (*F*) View on the resection wound after removal of the cap.

Several studies have shown that both cap-based techniques are safe and effective for the removal of visible lesions in a BE segment.[33–35] The overall complication rate mentioned in a large trial including 1000 BE patients with mucosal EAC was 1.5% (n = 15). Major complications were bleeding (n = 14) and perforation (n = 1), but these could all be managed conservatively. The complete eradication rate of neoplasia was 96%.[10]

As already mentioned, the MBM technique is currently the most commonly used in all Barrett's expert centers. A randomized-controlled trial comparing both techniques for piecemeal ER showed that MBM and ER-cap achieve comparable success and safety rates. However, MBM was cheaper and quicker compared to ER-cap, and most endoscopists consider MBM easier to learn.[36] Furthermore, the indication to perform an ER-cap resection is mostly replaced by ESD (**Fig. 2**, Videos 2 and 3).

Endoscopic submucosal dissection

ESD allows for en bloc resection of early neoplasia irrespective of the lesion's size and therefore overcomes the problem of piecemeal ER, which is required for lesions larger than 2 cm. The procedure starts with delineation of the lateral margins and lifting of the submucosal layer with injection fluid. The mucosal incision alongside the coagulation markers is performed using an electrosurgical knife. After completing the incision, the submucosa is dissected step by step, while repeating submucosal lesion to ensure a safety margin toward the muscle layer. Indications for ESD are strong suspicion of submucosal invasion and the resection of lesions with a large intraluminal component (ie, very bulky lesions). Because ESD appears to be a technically demanding procedure and is time consuming, ESD is, in the Western world, still only applied in selected cases by experienced endoscopists. Furthermore, ESD has not been shown to be superior to ER for excision of mucosal cancer. A trial directly comparing cap-based ER and ESD in patients with early Barrett's neoplasia randomized 40 patients (cap-based

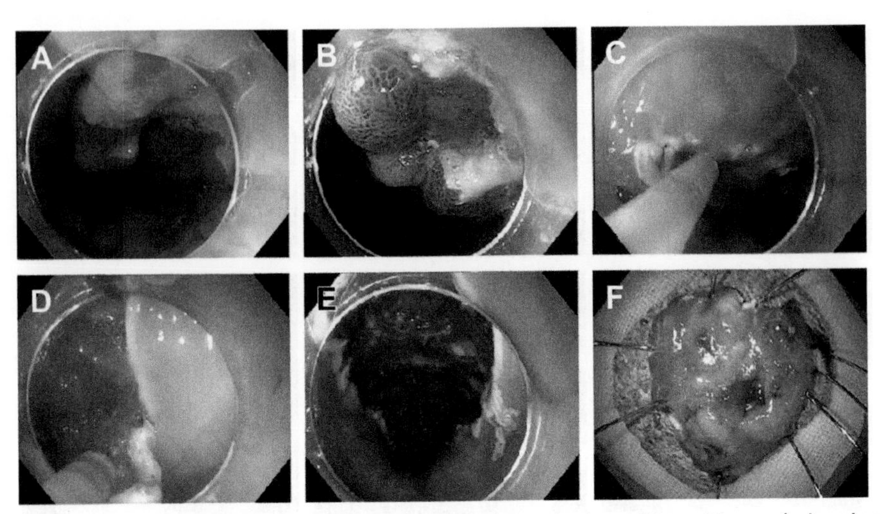

Fig. 2. Endoscopic submucosal dissection. (*A, B*) Endoscopic view of Barrett's neoplasia using white-light and narrow-band imaging. (*C*) View on the delineated lesion that is being lifted by submucosal fluid injection. (*D*) Dissection of the submucosal layer using the Dual knife, (*E*) View on the resection wound through the cap. (*F*) Resection specimen pinned on a corkboard.

ER technique, n = 20 vs ESD, n = 20). The study did not show any difference in complete remission of neoplasia at 3 months (cap-based ER 16 of 17 vs ESD 15 of 16, *P*=1.0). During a mean follow-up of 23 months, cancer recurrence was observed in 1 patient treated with ESD. Two adverse events were seen, both perforations during ESD. Although the study was underpowered, this may confirm that there is only little clinical relevance to perform ESD in most BE patients with early neoplasia.[37–39] Nevertheless, larger studies on ESD for Barrett's neoplasia in the Western world are yet to be performed.

Post-Treatment Management

Maintenance therapy with high-dose proton pump inhibitors (PPIs) is recommended for all patients with BE containing neoplasia. Besides PPIs, extra acid suppression during 2 weeks directly after ER is advisable to allow the ER wound to heal adequately with neosquamous epithelium (eg, with sucralfate suspension). Adherence to a liquid diet until 24 hours after ER is advisable, after which the diet can gradually be advanced to a soft and then a normal diet guided by the patients' symptoms. Most common symptoms after ER are chest discomfort, sore throat, and pain when swallowing. If necessary, patients can use painkillers such as acetaminophen or if necessary nonsteroidal anti-inflammatory drug suppositories. The wound generally is healed in 3 to 6 weeks after the procedure, depending on the extent of resection.

HISTOPATHOLOGICAL EVALUATION ENDOSCOPIC RESECTION SPECIMENS

Esophageal neoplasia is classified according to the Vienna classification, which divides neoplasia into 5 categories[40]: 1: no dysplasia; 2: indefinite for dysplasia; 3: low-grade dysplasia; 4: high-grade dysplasia; 5: invasive carcinoma. Category 5 is subdivided based upon whether there is invasion into the lamina propria or muscularis mucosae (category 5.1, also referred to as intramucosal cancer) or into the submucosa (category 5.2, also referred to as submucosal cancer). In case invasive carcinoma is found, the infiltration depth, differentiation grade (good, moderate, poor, or undifferentiated), presence of LVI, and radicality of the resection should be assessed. Infiltration depth is divided into mucosal and submucosal invasion. T1m2: infiltration into the lamina propria; T1m3: infiltration into the muscularis mucosae. For submucosal infiltration, measuring and reporting the depth in μm are preferred over subdividing the submucosa in 3 equal parts, because not the entire submucosal layer is present in the ER specimen. T1sm1: infiltration of no more than 500 μm, T1sm2: infiltration greater than 500 to no more than 1000 μm, T1sm3: infiltration greater than 1000 μm. Radicality is assessed at the vertical (deep) resection margin. In case of en bloc resection, the radicality of the lateral margins is assessed also. There exists interobserver reliability among pathologists. As a result, it may be helpful to achieve a consensus among more than 1 pathologist in categorizing such specimens.

EFFICACY OF ENDOSCOPIC RESECTION IN MANAGEMENT OF BARRETT'S-RELATED NEOPLASIA

Available evidence shows that ER is a successful diagnostic tool and treatment modality in patients with mucosal or low-risk submucosal Barrett's cancer. ER provides accurate histopathological assessment of the tumor and is therefore considered as the key step in the work-up of early Barrett's neoplasia. Several large prospective studies analyzing the efficacy and safety of ER have been performed in the past 10 to 15 years. Studies have consistently demonstrated ER success rates between 91% and 99%, with major complication rates (ie, bleeding, perforation, or stricture after ER) ranging from only 1.5% to 4%.[33,41,42] One of these series contains an international, single-arm, prospective international, multicenter registry primarily examining the success rate of ER using MBM. Successful ER was reached in 322 of 332 lesions (97%; 95% confidence interval [CI], 94.6%-98.4%). A perforation occurred in 3 patients (0.9%); all could be managed endoscopically, and patients were admitted for several days with intravenous antibiotics. Late bleeding requiring intervention occurred in 5 patients (1.5%), and dysphagia requiring dilatation occurred in 11 patients (3.8%).[42] In one of the largest retrospective studies analyzing the long-term follow-up results of 1000 BE patients treated with ER for HGD or mucosal EAC, 96% achieved complete remission of neoplasia. Recurrent or metachronous lesions developed in 15% of patients and were successfully endoscopically re-treated in 82% of patients. Only 0.2% died because of metastatic EAC during follow-up. The overall long-term complete remission rate was 94%.[10] Therefore, ER is considered as the cornerstone of endoscopic therapy in BE-related neoplasia. Nevertheless, the optimal strategy for patients with a high-risk submucosal lesion is yet to be defined and should therefore be discussed during a multidisciplinary team meeting, including a gastroenterologist, oncologist, and surgeon.

SUMMARY

ER is a safe and effective diagnostic tool and treatment modality in patients with early Barrett's neoplasia. ER offers multiple advantages, such as enabling accurate histopathological assessment, high success rates, and low complication rates. Multiple techniques have been reviewed in this article. In summary, MBM is the most commonly used ER technique; however, ESD is currently upcoming in the Western world. Evidence shows that ER for low risk-lesions is justifiable; however, future studies should assess whether ER is also justified in selected patients with high-risk submucosal lesions.

CLINICS CARE POINTS

- ER is justified in mucosal and low-risk submucosal cancer because of the low risk of lymph node metastasis.
- In selected patients a strict endoscopic follow-up protocol can be considered after radical removal of a high-risk submucosal lesion.

DISCLOSURE

E.A. Nieuwenhuis; no disclosures. O. Pech; disclosures: speaker fees from Medtronic, Olympus, Fujifilm, Boston Scientific, Falk, AbbVie, Bristol Myers Squibb, and Creo Medical. J.J.G.H.M. Bergman; disclosures: financial support for research from Covidien/Medtronic, Olympus Endoscopy, Cook Medical, Boston scientific, Erbe Medical, C2Therapeutic, Ninepoint Medical. Consultancy: Boston Scientific, Cook Medical, Covidien/Medtronic. R.E. Pouw; no disclosures.

SUPPLEMENTARY DATA

Supplementary data to this article can be found online at https://doi.org/10.1016/j.giec.2020.09.001.

REFERENCES

1. Shaheen NJ, Richter JE. Barrett's oesophagus. Lancet 2009;373(9666):850–61.
2. Spechler SJ, Souza RF. Barrett's esophagus. N Engl J Med 2014;371(8):36–45.
3. Solanky D, Krishnamoorthi R, Crews N, Johnson M, Wang K, Wolfsen H, Fleischer D, Ramirez FC, Katzka D, Buttar N, Iyer PG. Barrett Esophagus Length, Nodularity, and Low-grade Dysplasia are Predictive of Progression to Esophageal Adenocarcinoma. J Clin Gastroenterol 2019 May/Jun;53(5):361–5. https://doi.org/10.1097/MCG.0000000000001027. PMID: 29608452.
4. Markar SR, Karthikesalingam A, Thrumurthy S, et al. Volume-outcome relationship in surgery for esophageal malignancy: systematic review and meta-analysis 2000-2011. J Gastrointest Surg 2012;16(5):1055–63.
5. Inoue H, Endo M. Endoscopic esophageal mucosal resection using a transparent tube. Surg Endosc 1990;4(4):198–201.
6. Ell C, May A, Gossner L, et al. Endoscopic mucosal resection of early cancer and high-grade dysplasia in Barrett's esophagus. Gastroenterology 2000;118(4):670–7.
7. Nijhawan PK, Wang KK. Endoscopic mucosal resection for lesions with endoscopic features suggestive of malignancy and high-grade dysplasia within Barrett's esophagus. Gastrointest Endosc 2000;52(3):328–32.
8. Vieth M, Ell C, Gossner L, et al. Histological analysis of endoscopic resection specimens from 326 patients with Barrett's esophagus and early neoplasia. Endoscopy 2004;36(9):776–81.
9. Pech O, Behrens A, May A, et al. Long-term results and risk factor analysis for recurrence after curative endoscopic therapy in 349 patients with high-grade intraepithelial neoplasia and mucosal adenocarcinoma in Barrett's oesophagus. Gut 2008;57(9):1200–6.

10. Pech O, May A, Manner H, et al. Long-term efficacy and safety of endoscopic resection for patients with mucosal adenocarcinoma of the esophagus. Gastroenterology 2014;146(3):652–60.e1.
11. Alvarez Herrero L, Pouw RE, van Vilsteren FG, et al. Risk of lymph node metastasis associated with deeper invasion by early adenocarcinoma of the esophagus and cardia: study based on endoscopic resection specimens. Endoscopy 2010; 42(12):1030–6.
12. Manner H, May A, Pech O, et al. Early Barrett's carcinoma with "low-risk" submucosal invasion: long-term results of endoscopic resection with a curative intent. Am J Gastroenterol 2008;103(10):2589–97.
13. Schölvinck D, Künzli H, Meijer S, et al. Management of patients with T1b esophageal adenocarcinoma: a retrospective cohort study on patient management and risk of metastatic disease. Surg Endosc 2016;30(9):4102–13.
14. Buskens CJ, Westerterp M, Lagarde SM, et al. Prediction of appropriateness of local endoscopic treatment for high-grade dysplasia and early adenocarcinoma by EUS and histopathologic features. Gastrointest Endosc 2004;60(5):703–10.
15. Westerterp M, Koppert LB, Buskens CJ, et al. Outcome of surgical treatment for early adenocarcinoma of the esophagus or gastro-esophageal junction. Virchows Arch 2005;446(5):497–504.
16. Manner H, Pech O, Heldmann Y, et al. The frequency of lymph node metastasis in early-stage adenocarcinoma of the esophagus with incipient submucosal invasion (pT1b sm1) depending on histological risk patterns. Surg Endosc 2015; 29(7):1888–96.
17. Künzli HT, Belghazi K, Pouw RE, et al. Endoscopic management and follow-up of patients with a submucosal esophageal adenocarcinoma. United European Gastroenterol J 2018;6(5):669–77.
18. Schölvinck DW, van der Meulen K, Bergman JJGHM, et al. Detection of lesions in dysplastic Barrett's esophagus by community and expert endoscopists. Endoscopy 2017;49(2):113–20.
19. Sharma P, Dent J, Armstrong D, et al. The development and validation of an endoscopic grading system for Barrett's esophagus: The Prague C & M criteria. Gastroenterology 2006;131(5):1392–9.
20. Enestvedt BK, Lugo R, Guarner-Argente C, et al. Location, location, location: does early cancer in Barrett's esophagus have a preference? Gastrointest Endosc 2013;78(3):462–7.
21. Pech O, Gossner L, Manner H, et al. Prospective evaluation of the macroscopic types and location of early Barrett's neoplasia in 380 lesions. Endoscopy 2007; 39(7):588–93.
22. The Paris endoscopic classification of superficial neoplastic lesions: esophagus, stomach, and colon. Available at: https://www.worldendo.org/wp-content/uploads/2016/03/ParisClassification2000.pdf.
23. Endoscopic Classification Review Group. Update on the Paris classification of superficial neoplastic lesions in the digestive tract. Endoscopy 2005;37(6):570–8.
24. Japanese Gastric Cancer Association. Japanese gastric cancer treatment guidelines 2014 (ver. 4). Gastric Cancer 2017;20(1):1–19.
25. Peters FP, Brakenhoff KPM, Curvers WL, et al. Histologic evaluation of resection specimens obtained at 293 endoscopic resections in Barrett's esophagus. Gastrointest Endosc 2008;67(4):604–9.
26. Curvers WL, Bergman JJGHM. Multimodality imaging in Barrett's esophagus: looking longer, seeing better, and recognizing more. Gastroenterology 2008; 135(1):297–9.

27. Levine DS, Blount PL, Rudolph RE, et al. Safety of a systematic endoscopic biopsy protocol in patients with Barrett's esophagus. Am J Gastroenterol 2000; 95(5):1152–7.
28. Bergman JJ, Fockens P. Endoscopic ultrasonography in patients with gastro-esophageal cancer. Eur J Ultrasound 1999;10(2–3):127–38.
29. Fockens P, Van den Brande JH, van Dullemen HM, et al. Endosonographic T-staging of esophageal carcinoma: a learning curve. Gastrointest Endosc 1996;44(1):58–62.
30. van Westreenen HL, Westerterp M, Sloof GW, et al. Limited additional value of positron emission tomography in staging oesophageal cancer. Br J Surg 2007; 94(12):1515–20.
31. Noble F, Bailey D, SWCIS Upper Gastrointestinal Tumour Panel, et al. Impact of integrated PET/CT in the staging of oesophageal cancer: a UK population-based cohort study. Clin Radiol 2009 Jul;64(7):699–705.
32. Cuellar SLB, Carter BW, Macapinlac HA, et al. Clinical staging of patients with early esophageal adenocarcinoma: does FDG-PET/CT have a role? J Thorac Oncol 2014;9(8):1202–6.
33. Ell C, May A, Pech O, et al. Curative endoscopic resection of early esophageal adenocarcinomas (Barrett's cancer). Gastrointest Endosc 2007;65(1):3–10.
34. Behrens A, May A, Gossner L, et al. Curative treatment for high-grade intraepithelial neoplasia in Barrett's esophagus. Endoscopy 2005;37(10):999–1005.
35. Larghi A, Lightdale CJ, Ross AS, et al. Long-term follow-up of complete Barrett's eradication endoscopic mucosal resection (CBE-EMR) for the treatment of high grade dysplasia and intramucosal carcinoma. Endoscopy 2007;39(12):1086–91.
36. Pouw RE, van Vilsteren FGI, Peters FP, et al. Randomized trial on endoscopic resection-cap versus multiband mucosectomy for piecemeal endoscopic resection of early Barrett's neoplasia. Gastrointest Endosc 2011;74(1):35–43.
37. Terheggen G, Horn EM, Vieth M, et al. A randomised trial of endoscopic submucosal dissection versus endoscopic mucosal resection for early Barrett's neoplasia. Gut 2017;66(5):783–93.
38. Pimentel-Nunes P, Dinis-Ribeiro M, Ponchon T, et al. Endoscopic submucosal dissection: European Society of Gastrointestinal Endoscopy (ESGE) Guideline. Endoscopy 2015;47(9):829–54.
39. Bourke MJ, Neuhaus H, Bergman JJ. Endoscopic submucosal dissection: indications and application in Western endoscopy practice. Gastroenterology 2018; 154(7):1887–900.e5.
40. Schlemper RJ, Riddell RH, Kato Y, et al. The Vienna classification of gastrointestinal epithelial neoplasia. Gut 2000;47(2):251–5.
41. Alvarez Herrero L, Pouw RE, van Vilsteren FGI, et al. Safety and efficacy of multiband mucosectomy in 1060 resections in Barrett's esophagus. Endoscopy 2011; 43(3):177–83.
42. Pouw RE, Beyna T, Belghazi K, et al. A prospective multicenter study using a new multiband mucosectomy device for endoscopic resection of early neoplasia in Barrett's esophagus. Gastrointest Endosc 2018;88(4):647–54.

A Practical Approach to Refractory and Recurrent Barrett's Esophagus

Domenico A. Farina, MD[a,1], Ashwinee Condon, MD[b,1], Srinadh Komanduri, MD, MS[a], V. Raman Muthusamy, MD, MAS[b,*]

KEYWORDS

- Barrett's esophagus • Dysplasia • Ablation • Refractory disease
- Recurrent disease • Endoscopic eradication therapy

KEY POINTS

- Barrett's esophagus (BE) that is refractory to standard endoscopic eradication therapy (EET) is defined as inability to achieve complete eradication of intestinal metaplasia after up to 3 sessions of EET and occurs in about 4% to 14% of patients with BE.
- Recurrent BE following EET occurs in up to 7% to 13% of patients and should be treated with repeat EET.
- Validated risk factors for both refractory and recurrent BE include lack of long-term reflux control, presence of a hiatal hernia, and BE segment length greater than 5 cm.
- Aggressive antireflux therapy and monitoring is crucial in preventing refractory and recurrent BE.
- In patients who fail standard EET despite optimization of reflux control, salvage cryotherapy with liquid nitrogen, endoscopic mucosal resection, or argon plasma coagulation may be safe and effective alternative treatments.

INTRODUCTION

Barrett's esophagus (BE) affects 5% to 15% of all patients with gastroesophageal reflux disease (GERD) and approximately 1% to 2% of the entire population.[1] It is a condition of the esophagus characterized by the replacement of normal squamous cell epithelium with intestinal columnar cells through intestinal metaplasia (IM).[1–4] This process can lead to dysplasia and eventual stepwise progression to esophageal

[a] Department of Gastroenterology and Hepatology, Northwestern University, 676 North St. Clair Street, Arkes Pavilion Suite 1400, Chicago, IL 60611, USA; [b] Vatche and Tamar Manoukian Division of Digestive Diseases, David Geffen School of Medicine at UCLA, 200 UCLA Medical Plaza, Room 330-37, Los Angeles, CA 90095, USA
[1] Joint first-authors.
* Corresponding author.
E-mail address: raman@mednet.ucla.edu

Gastrointest Endoscopy Clin N Am 31 (2021) 183–203
https://doi.org/10.1016/j.giec.2020.09.002
1052-5157/21/

adenocarcinoma (EAC).[2,4–6] Those with nondysplastic BE have a low likelihood of progression to EAC, which has fueled a debate regarding the utility of ongoing endoscopic surveillance of those patients following diagnosis.[2,7–9] However, for BE-associated dysplasia and neoplasia, endoscopic eradication therapy (EET) is recommended through a combination of endoscopic mucosal resection (EMR) and ablation techniques including radiofrequency ablation (RFA) or cryotherapy.[2,3,7,9–11]

Overall, EET for dysplastic BE has been shown to be very effective in preventing progression of dysplastic BE to EAC and in achieving complete eradication of intestinal metaplasia (CE-IM).[7,8,12–15] Current guidelines support combined modality therapy using EMR for visible lesions followed by RFA of visible residual BE segments.[2,11,15,16] Complete eradication rates with RFA for low-grade dysplasia (LGD) and high-grade dysplasia (HGD) are up to 90% and 81%, respectively.[13,17] The reported efficacy of RFA for CE-IM is variable with rates ranging between 46% and 90%.[3,6,13,18,19] Given the success rate of these modalities, the primary aims of many studies in this field are focused on evaluating the efficacy and safety of combination focal EMR and RFA for the treatment of dysplastic BE and early EAC. There is a paucity of literature evaluating recurrent or refractory BE after wide-field EMR alone, argon plasma coagulation (APC), or photodynamic therapy (PDT), as these techniques are not considered to be first-line treatments. For this reason, in this article, EET refers to RFA with or without prior focal EMR.[20] EET should be performed until CE-IM is achieved regardless of pretreatment histology, as the risk of metachronous neoplasia can be as high as 30%.[6,8,20] Although there is a lack of high-quality data regarding the risk factors and management of refractory BE, studies have shown that it affects between 4% and 14% of patients.[21,22] Furthermore, despite initial high success rates in achieving CE-IM ranging from 72% to 97%,[13,17,23,24] the durability of EET has been questioned, as early studies suggested recurrence rates as high as 0% to 15% for dysplasia and 4% to 39.5% for IM following EET.[23,25–28] More recently, three large systematic reviews and meta-analyses confirmed true recurrence rates to range between 7% and 13%.[8,17,29] Despite improvements in technique and reduction in rates of recurrence, all patients should continue to undergo endoscopic surveillance after achieving CE-IM.[2,5,9,30] This review focuses on a practical approach to patients with BE that is refractory to EET and the management of recurrent BE after EET.

DEFINITION OF BARRETT'S ERADICATION, REFRACTORY BARRETT'S ESOPHAGUS, AND RECURRENCE

CE-IM has most commonly been defined as absence of IM on biopsies obtained from the entire pretreatment BE segment of the tubular esophagus, gastric cardia, and squamocolumnar junction (SCJ) (using standard protocol of 4-quadrant biopsies every 1–2 cm) after 2 consecutive surveillance endoscopies following EET.[23,30–32] CE-IM has been assessed by both 1 and 2 successive surveillance endoscopy strategies without IM. This variability in definition is seen across the multiple studies looking at rates of recurrence after EET.[6,7,9,12,13,17,18,21,24,27,28,31,33–41] Some have hypothesized that defining CE-IM after one surveillance examination may lead to an overestimation of BE recurrence, because many patients have actually experienced treatment failure rather than true recurrence.[7,17,22–41] EET protocols are also inconsistent across the literature with varied modalities of EET and differences in the number of treatments allowed in order to achieve CE-IM before being labeled treatment incomplete or refractory.[7,17,22–37]

The randomized controlled Ablation of Intestinal Metaplasia Containing Dysplasia (AIM Dysplasia) trial demonstrated that although most patients with BE and dysplasia achieved CE-IM, the number of treatments required to achieve eradication was variable and required an average of 3.5 ablations in the first year.[3,25] Currently, there is no consistent definition for refractory BE. Furthermore, differentiating between refractory and recurrent BE may be challenging if high-quality surveillance biopsies to assess for subsquamous IM following RFA are not achieved.[42,43] The US RFA Registry of more than 5000 patients, along with other large studies evaluating refractory and recurrent BE after RFA, demonstrated that most of the patients undergoing EET achieved CE-IM within 3 ablative therapy sessions.[27,30,44] Komanduri and colleagues[23] further classified patients as partial responders if CE-IM was not achieved after 3 ablative sessions and as nonresponders requiring salvage therapy if CE-IM was not achieved after 6 sessions, even after optimization of reflux control. Given that the difference in response to therapy between these 2 subsets of patients likely represents varying degrees of inadequate reflux control, it can be concluded that patients that do not achieve CE-IM (including patients with incomplete and no response) after 3 ablative sessions and optimized antireflux measures are refractory to EET.

There is also significant variation in the definition of recurrence of IM following EET.[7,17,45] Recurrence is most commonly defined as any histologic evidence of IM or dysplasia on any biopsy taken from the pretreatment tubular esophagus and/or squamocolumnar junction after CE-IM was achieved (confirmed on 2 endoscopies).[7,17,45] Variability in the reported recurrence of IM following EET can also be explained by the differences in surveillance biopsy protocols in the literature.[7,37,44] In particular, the inclusion of gastric cardia biopsies on surveillance endoscopies differs between studies.[7,13,17,25–37] Higher rates of IM are reported in the gastric cardia and may not represent true recurrence of BE.[7,17,45]

FACTORS ASSOCIATED WITH REFRACTORY BARRETT'S ESOPHAGUS

Early experience with EET found that some patients readily achieve CE-IM, whereas others require numerous ablations or fail to achieve eradication of all BE with RFA. The early identification of patients who are likely to fail EET or require prolonged therapy is of great value, as this would help providers counsel patients on what to expect in their clinical course and lead to a discussion of key factors in achieving EET, as well as possible salvage treatment modalities that may need to be used.

Multiple studies have demonstrated that severity of ongoing reflux exposure, determined by presence of esophagitis on endoscopy or pH monitoring studies, despite twice-daily proton pump inhibitor (PPI) therapy, was associated with persistent IM in patients with BE after RFA.[19,21,22,46,47] Weakly acidic reflux events, which comprise most of the reflux events in patients taking PPIs, were most strongly associated with refractory disease[19]; this may be explained by the fact that bile salts that are found in gastric contents can induce BE and EAC independently of gastric acid.[48,49] Studies have also found an association between presence and size of a hiatal hernia and response to RFA,[19,21–23] which may be explained by the fact that a hiatal hernia causes anatomic deformity of the gastroesophageal junction (GEJ) that results in the loss of the "2-sphincter mechanism" involving the alignment of the lower esophageal sphincter and diaphragmatic crus in preventing reflux events.[50] In addition, hiatal hernias compromise effective fluid clearing from the distal esophagus leading to increased acid exposure time. From a procedural standpoint, the presence of a hernia may prevent adequate tissue apposition with the ablation catheter and lead to ineffective RFA due to insufficient contact with the affected mucosa.[19] One study found that the presence of a relative narrowing of the Barrett's segment was found to be an independent predictor of poor response to RFA.[21] This is likely a reflection of a subgroup of patients with more severe reflux than others, as the narrowing may be caused by reflux-induced scarring. Narrowing may also lead to insufficient tissue apposition with the ablation catheter due to angulation of the lumen or suboptimal RFA due to selection of smaller balloon size, as it is advised to use an ablation balloon with a diameter that is 2 sizes smaller than the smallest esophageal diameter to prevent laceration during RFA.[21] This latter issue has since been resolved with the development of a single sizing and treatment balloon RFA catheter (Halo 360 Express, Medtronic, Minneapolis, MN, USA).

Van Vilsteren and colleagues[21] hypothesized that response to the index RFA treatment would predict subsequent achievement of CE-IM. They showed that patients with less than 50% regression in the endoscopically visible surface area of BE 3 months after initial RFA were less likely to achieve complete eradication, required more RFA sessions, and had a longer temporal length of treatment (median treatment period of 13 months and 4 RFA sessions for poor responders vs 7 months and 3 RFA sessions in good initial responders). This study also found that squamous regeneration within the segments previously treated by EMR was associated with complete eradication, reflecting the propensity of the tissue to regenerate as normal squamous epithelium rather than metaplastic or dysplastic epithelium. In addition, a longer duration of dysplasia or neoplasia before treatment with RFA may predict incomplete eradication. In contrast, a longer duration of IM without dysplasia seems to be protective against BE refractory to EET, possibly due to the superior regenerative capacity of metaplastic epithelium compared with dysplastic or neoplastic epithelium.[21]

Finally, the baseline length of the BE segment may also contribute to the risk for RFA refractory disease. Although there have been some conflicting reports, most studies have shown that patients with a BE segment greater than 5 to 6 cm are less likely to achieve CE-IM with RFA within 3 sessions.[3,19,21,22,51] Although the mechanism remains unclear, longer pretreatment segment length may be a marker for more severe acid exposure and injury. It may also simply be related to having a greater surface area to convert to neosquamous tissue. Additional patient-related risk factors for refractory BE that have been explored but not validated include increasing age, non-Caucasian race, increasing body mass index, and current or prior smoking history[3,19,21,46,52] (see **Box 1** for a summary of risk factors associated with refractory BE).

PHYSIOLOGIC SOLUTIONS TO REFRACTORY BARRETT'S ESOPHAGUS

It is clear that achievement of durable CE-IM requires long-term control of reflux exposure; however, the most effective strategy to eliminate reflux during EET is not well defined. Current guidelines recommend high-dose twice-daily PPI during EET. Acid suppression using PPIs has been shown to decrease symptoms of GERD, heal erosive esophagitis, and prevent peptic strictures.[48] However, despite symptom control with PPIs, abnormal acid reflux has been reported to persist in 20% to 38% of patients with BE.[47,53] In addition, there is concern that incomplete elimination of acid reflux might increase direct mucosal damage to the esophagus caused by bile salts in duodenogastroesophageal refluxate.[48,53] Given these data, antireflux surgery, specifically Nissen fundoplication, has been suggested as an alternate or adjunctive tool to achieve reflux control. Fundoplication has the benefit of being able to address physiologic abnormalities such as presence of a hiatal hernia and decreased lower esophageal sphincter tone as well as creating a physical barrier that inhibits both acid and bile reflux into the esophagus. Ferraris and colleagues[54] compared outcomes in patients treated with medical management or fundoplication for antireflux therapy before undergoing EET of BE with APC. They showed that sustained CE-IM at 5 years was

Box 1
Risk factors for Barrett's esophagus refractory to endoscopic eradication therapy (radiofrequency ablation with or without endoscopic mucosal resection)

Validated (by 2 or more studies)
- Lack of long-term reflux control
- Presence of a hiatal hernia
- Length of BE segment >5 cm

Unvalidated
- Less than 50% regression in the endoscopically visible surface area of BE 3 months after initial EET
- Asymptomatic relative narrowing of the BE segment before EET
- Squamous regeneration within EMR scar
- Longer duration of dysplasia or neoplasia before EET
- Non-Caucasian race
- Smoking history
- Obesity

Abbreviations: BE, Barrett's Esophagus; EET, endoscopic eradication therapy; EMR, endoscopic mucosal resection; RFA, radiofrequency ablation.

76% in the surgical group compared with 44% in those managed medically.[54] This was in contrast to a similar study published by Madisch and colleagues[55] that did not find any significant difference between medical and surgical antireflux therapies. The difference may be attributable to the fact that patients in the *Ferraris* study underwent optimization of antireflux therapy before, rather than after, initiation of EET. This may have aided in reducing reflux-induced damage to the newly generated neosquamous epithelium at the time of EET.[54,55] The importance of long-term reflux control was highlighted by a large prospective study by Komanduri and colleagues that aimed to assess outcomes and durability of EET (defined as RFA with or without prior focal EMR) for BE. They demonstrated that a structured reflux management protocol involving patient education, periodic medication adjustment, pH impedance and manometry testing, and antireflux surgery in select patients achieved significantly lower recurrence of CE-IM compared with patients undergoing EET without optimized reflux management (4.8% vs 10.9%, $P = .04$) (**Fig. 1**). Among patients with persistent disease after 3 sessions of RFA and proven ongoing reflux despite PPI optimization, 95% achieved sustained CE-IM at 2 years after fundoplication, again highlighting the role of reflux control after EET.[23] Lastly, O'Connell and Velanovich[56] showed that presegment length of BE correlated with persistent or recurrent BE in patients without fundoplication (median BE length in those with recurrence was 10 cm vs 3 cm in responding patients), possibly identifying a subgroup of patients who would particularly benefit from antireflux surgery. Nissen fundoplication has been the longstanding mainstay of antireflux surgery; however, over the past decade, transoral incisionless fundoplication (TIF; EsophyX® Device and SerosaFuse® Fasteners, EndoGastric Solutions, Redmond, WA, USA) and magnetic sphincter augmentation (MSA) using the LINX device (LINX®, Torax Medical Inc, Shoreview, MN, USA) have been evaluated as nonsurgical endoscopic alternatives in the treatment of chronic GERD. TIF creates a full-thickness serosa-to-serosa plication resulting in a partial fundoplication. When compared with maximum standard dose PPI therapy in patients with symptomatic GERD refractory to PPI, TIF demonstrated resolution of regurgitation and atypical GERD symptoms and improvement in health-related quality of life score at 5 years.[57] When compared with Nissen fundoplication, a network meta-

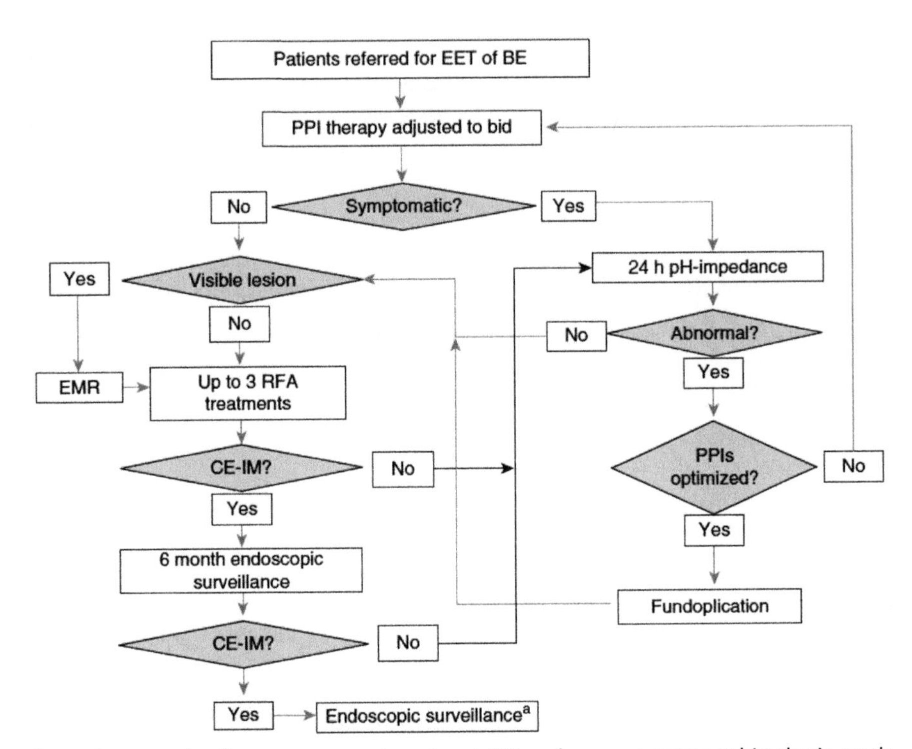

Fig. 1. Structured reflex management protocol. [a] Based on pretreatment histologic grade. (*From* Komanduri S, Kahrilas PJ, Krishnan K, et al. Recurrence of Barrett's Esophagus is Rare Following Endoscopic Eradication Therapy Coupled With Effective Reflux Control. *The American journal of gastroenterology.* 2017;112(4):556-566; with permission.)

analysis showed fundoplication was statistically superior to TIF (and PPIs) in esophageal acid control; however, given the criticisms of the validity of this study, future noninferiority randomized controlled trials comparing TIF with Nissen fundoplication are necessary.[58] The LINX Reflux Management System was approved in 2012 as a treatment of GERD and works by augmenting the lower esophageal sphincter with a ring made up of a series of rare earth magnets. Multiple meta-analyses have demonstrated comparable clinical control of reflux after MSA with LINX compared to fundoplication in both the short[59] and longer term.[60] Notably, the safety and efficacy of either TIF or LINX have not been specifically evaluated in patients with BE.[61] However, as gastroenterologists gain technical expertise and the endoscopic devices become more sophisticated, these minimally invasive procedures may play a major role in the management of chronic reflux and subsequently in patients with refractory and recurrent BE due to inadequate reflux control. Although randomized prospective data comparing CE-IM durability in patients treated with any antireflux surgery versus medical therapy in combination with EET are not available at this time, it is clear that long-term reflux control is essential for preventing disease progression and achieving and sustaining CE-IM (see **Box 2** for management principles of refractory BE).

SALVAGE ENDOSCOPIC ERADICATION THERAPY

Less than 15% of patients with dysplastic BE are refractory to EET with a combination of EMR and RFA despite an optimized antireflux regimen. However, the optimal

Box 2
Management of Barrett's esophagus refractory to endoscopic eradication therapy (radiofrequency ablation with or without endoscopic mucosal resection)

Standardized antireflux protocol (medical management)
- Patient education on appropriate use of PPI, 30 mins before meal
- Increasing PPI dose to 40 mg twice daily
- Medication reconciliation and documentation of PPI compliance at every visit
- On-treatment reflux testing (24 h pH impedence) and HRM if inability to achieve CE-IM after 3 RFA sessions

Antireflux surgery
- Optimal timing and type of surgery remains unclear
- Nissen fundoplication before EET initiation if evidence of uncontrolled reflux after PPI optimization before beginning EET
- Nissen fundoplication after initiation of EET if symptoms well controlled before beginning EET and objective evidence of ongoing reflux despite PPI optimization or inability to achieve CE-IM after 3 RFA sessions
- Consider endoscopic antireflux procedures (TIF and LINX) in select patient populations

Salvage EET
- Cryoablation
- Wide-field EMR
- Combination therapy with wide-field EMR, APC, PDT

Abbreviations: APC, argon plasma coagulation; BE, Barrett's esophagus; CE-IM, complete eradication of intestinal metaplasia; EET, endoscopic eradication therapy; EMR, endoscopic mucosal resection; HRM, high-resolution manometry; PDT, photodynamic therapy; PPI, proton-pump inhibitor; RFA, radiofrequency ablation.

management strategy in this population with a high risk of developing EAC remains undefined. Although evidence regarding the use of PDT in patients with BE and HGD shows a complete eradication of dysplasia (CE-D) rate of 77%, it remains limited by its high procedural costs, photosensitivity, and a greater than 35% chance of developing a posttreatment esophageal stricture. Most of these strictures required more than 6 dilations to achieve resolution in one prospective study.[62] In addition, the use of PDT specifically for BE refractory to RFA has not been studied. Wide-field salvage EMR of the entire Barrett's epithelium has also been shown to have a high eradication rate, up to 96% for HGD and EAC; however, this also carries a significant risk of esophageal stricture and an up to 2% risk of perforation, especially with increasing length of the affected segment.[31,63–65] The efficacy of APC has only been studied as a primary treatment of BE and reported to have a widely variable rate of eradication, an unacceptably high rate of recurrent metaplasia and dysplasia in up to one-third of patients, and a 3.3% annual risk of progression to EAC, possibly related to buried glands under the neosquamous epithelium even after complete eradication.[66] For these reasons, it is not currently recommended as a first-line treatment of dysplastic BE. However, given the availability of APC in most endoscopy units, ease of use, and endoscopists' familiarity with the device, it may be used for treating residual disease limited to the GEJ or scattered islands.[67,68]

Cryotherapy is a noncontact method of eradicating precancerous and cancerous tissue, most often liquid nitrogen or nitrous oxide, that is increasingly being studied in BE refractory to RFA. It is thought to be able to achieve a greater depth of tissue penetration via rapid freezing and thawing of affected tissue, inducing destruction followed by regeneration of healthy tissue. Cryotherapy has proved to be safe and effective as a primary treatment of dysplastic BE.[69–71] In addition, the noncontact mechanism of cryotherapy may allow treatment of patients with mucosal irregularities, hiatal hernia, and esophageal tortuosity that are technically challenging using contact therapy with RFA.[72] Multiple studies including a recent meta-analysis analyzing 11 studies (notably only 3 were full-text published studies) and 148 patients reported a CE-D with cryotherapy of 76.0% but a CE-IM of only 45.9%. Adverse effects were reported in 6.7% of patients and mostly consisted of odynophagia and esophageal strictures that were successfully treated with 1 to 2 dilations.[67,73,74] Although additional studies are warranted to better define the use of this technique, cryotherapy should be considered as a viable salvage treatment option in patients with persistent disease after RFA and EMR (see **Box 2**).

RISK OF BARRETT'S RECURRENCE FOLLOWING ENDOSCOPIC ERADICATION THERAPY

Several studies, including multiple meta-analyses, have been published on the durability of CE-IM (**Table 1**).[8,28,29] A systematic review by Orman and colleagues[17] examining 18 studies (including one randomized control trial) demonstrated a recurrence rate of 13% based on data from a combined 540 patients. In addition, they stratified studies as higher quality and lower quality studies and showed recurrence rates of 11% and 17%, respectively, which was not a statistically significant difference.[17] In terms of incidence of recurrence of BE following EET, a meta-analysis by Fujii-Lau and colleagues[8] of 39 studies showed a pooled incidence of any recurrence (either IM or dysplasia) of 7.5 per 100 patient-years. This is similar to another recent systematic review from Krishnamoorthi and colleagues[28] that included 41 studies that showed pooled incidence rates of recurrent IM at 9.5%, dysplastic BE at 2.0%, and HGD/EAC after RFA at 1.2% per patient-year.

In terms of durability of CE-IM over time, there are conflicting data regarding the timeline of recurrence of BE following EET. However, providers should be aware of which patients are at highest risk of recurrence.[21,25,29,39] A recent prospective study by Sami and colleagues[41] that required patients to have 2 negative endoscopies before achieving CE-IM showed a cumulative risk of recurrence of 19% in the first 2 years following CE-IM and an additional 49% risk over the subsequent 8.6 years. This study is notable for its particularly long follow-up time and the fact that they also showed no reduction in the annual recurrence risk with time.[41] In contrast, some literature have shown that recurrence following successful EET is likely to occur within 2 years of CE-IM/CE-D and that surveillance intervals may be lengthened 2 years after EET.[75] A meta-analysis by Sawas and colleagues[29] that looked at 22 studies to examine recurrence of BE after CE-IM found an increased risk of recurrence in the first year following EET, regardless of segment length and baseline histology. Regardless of the exact temporal occurrence, recurrence of IM after EET is significant and as such, endoscopic surveillance remains critical.[2,7,15,30]

RISK FACTORS FOR BARRETT'S ESOPHAGUS RECURRENCE

Following confirmation of CE-IM, several studies have looked at risk factors that may predispose patients to risk of recurrence of BE following EET that providers should be made aware of (**Box 3**).[32] Factors associated with an increased risk of BE recurrence include increased age, non-Caucasian race, and longer BE segment at baseline.[7,8,12,21,24] Additional studies have shown that the presence of a hiatal hernia is associated with recurrent IM following EET.[7,8,24,75] Higher grade baseline neoplasia (HGD/IMC) and a history of smoking have both independently been shown to be linked to higher rates of recurrence of BE following EET.[7,8,12,24,75] Lastly, Wani and

Table 1
Compilation of studies showing recurrence rates of Barrett's esophagus following complete eradication of intestinal metaplasia

Publication Author, Year	Study Type	Total (n)	Achieving CE-IM (n)	Surveillance CE-IM (n)	Mean Follow-up (y)	Recurrence Rate (%)	Recurrences			
							Total	IM	Dysplasia	EAC
Fleischer et al,[38] 2010	Prospective multicenter	50	46	46	5	8.7	4	4	0	0
Alvarez Herraro,[80] et al, 2011	Prospective multicenter	24	19/20	20	2.4	10.5	2	2	0	0
Shaheen et al,[26] 2011	Prospective multicenter	119	108/110	110	3	17.6	19	14	3	2
Vacarro et al,[81] 2011	Prospective single-center	47	47	47	1.1	31.9	15	11	4	0
Van Vilistren et al,[82] 2013	Prospective multicenter	22	21	20	1.8	9.5	2	2	0	0
Caillol et al,[33] 2012	Prospective single-center	34	17/30	34	1	11.8	2	0	0	2
Dulai et al,[36] 2013	Retrospective single-center	72	56/57	57	3.3	19.6	11	0	0	0
Ertan et al,[35] 2013	Prospective single-center	50	27/47	47	2.8	11.1	3	0	0	0
Haidry et al,[27] 2013	Prospective multicenter	335	208/270	256	1.6	17.8	37	17	16	4
Orman et al,[17] 2013	Retrospective single-center	262	183/188	112	1.1	4.4	8	3	2	3
Gupta et al,[37] 2013	Retrospective multicenter	448	229	229	1.1	16.2	37	29	8	0
Phoa et al,[18] 2013	Retrospective single-center	55	54	54	5	46.3	25	22	1	2
Strauss et al,[83] 2014	Retrospective multicenter	36	27/32	36	2	33.3	9	5	3	1
Anders et al,[84] 2014	Retrospective multicenter	90	81	90	5.4	45.7	37	32	2	3
Konda et al,[85] 2014	Prospective single-center	187	165	187	3.4	9.1	15	7	7	1
Lada et al,[86] 2014	Prospective single-center	57	28/49	57	3	57.1	16	4	12	0
Pasricha et al,[87] 2014	Retrospective multicenter	5521	3169	1634	2.4	10.5	334	269	52	13
Cotton et al,[34] 2015	Retrospective single-center	198	198	98	3	17.7	35	22	7	6
Phoa et al,[88] 2015	Retrospective multicenter	121	115/121	121	2.3	12.2	14	5	3	6
Le Page et al,[89] 2015	Retrospective single-center	50	35	45	1.8	5.7	2	0	0	2
Komanduri et al,[23] 2017	Prospective single-center	221	202	202	3.7	6.4	13	10	3	0
Cotton et al,[25] 2017	Prospective multicenter	119	110	110	5	31.8	35	14	19	2

(*continued on next page*)

Table 1
(continued)

Publication Author, Year	Study Type	Total (n)	Achieving CE-IM (n)	Surveillance CE-IM (n)	Mean Follow-up (y)	Recurrence Rate (%)	Recurrences			
							Total	IM	Dysplasia	EAC
Sami et al,[41] 2019	Prospective multicenter	787	787	594	2.8	19.2	151	123	19	9
Omar et al,[78] 2019	Retrospective multicenter	549	443	443	1	13.8	61	48	11	2
Wani et al,[75] 2020	Prospective multicenter	807	807	807	5	19.5	157	121	36	0

Abbreviations: IM, intestinal metaplasia; CE-IM, complete eradication-intestinal metaplasia; EAC, esophageal adenocarcinoma.

Box 3
Risk factors for Barrett's esophagus recurrence

- Longer Barrett's segment (>3 cm)
- Tobacco use
- Increased EET sessions to achieve CE-IM
- Higher grade dysplasia at baseline histology
- Presence of hiatal hernia
- Older age
- Non-Caucasian race

colleagues[75] showed that an increased number of EET sessions required for CE-IM/CE-D was an independent risk factor for BE recurrence.[76]

ASSESSMENT FOR BARRETT'S ESOPHAGUS RECURRENCE

Given the risk of recurrence following CE-IM, both the 2019 American Society for Gastrointestinal Endoscopy and 2016 American College of Gastroenterology guidelines recommend surveillance of the neosquamous epithelium following EET for recurrence.[2,7,11,15,30] The intervals between surveillance endoscopies remain controversial and continue to evolve.[2,7,15,30]

At present, patients who have completed successful EET for IMC/HGD are typically recommended to undergo endoscopy at 3-month intervals for the first year, followed by 6-month intervals in the second year and annually thereafter.[2,7,15,30] For patients with baseline LGD who achieve CE-IM, surveillance endoscopies are recommended every 6 months in the first year followed by annually thereafter.[2,7,15,30] During endoscopy, recommendations are for biopsies to be taken at the GEJ as well as every 1-2 cm in the tubular esophagus in the entire region of neosquamous epithelium.[2,7,15,30] These current surveillance guidelines are controversial, given the high cost to the health care system, the low sensitivity for detection of buried (subsquamous) IM, and the low yield of random biopsies.[2,7,15,30,34,77] As such, many endoscopists have selectively extended intervals after the first few years of surveillance or adopted a simplified post-EET surveillance biopsy protocol.[76,78]

The standard of care for posttreatment surveillance and therapy is debated, as there are several large studies where continued surveillance for primarily nondysplastic IM recurrence was done rather than retreatment that have demonstrated no progression to EAC in recurrent nondysplastic IM.[7,8,37,41,77] Recent studies have shown that recurrence of BE is most likely to occur within 2 cm of the GEJ in the first year after CE-IM, and that recurrence of IM with and without dysplasia/carcinoma is most likely to be detected on random biopsy within 1 cm of GEJ.[34,77,78] Recurrence of BE is more likely to occur at the site of visible lesions in recurrences greater than 1 year after CE-IM when compared with those occurring in the first year with low yield reported using random biopsies after 1 year.[34,77,78] A recently validated simplified biopsy protocol for post-EET surveillance advocates 4-quadrant biopsy at GEJ in addition to biopsies of the gastric cardia, 1 cm proximal to SCJ, 2 cm proximal to SCJ, and targeted biopsy of visible lesions (**Fig. 2**).[78] This would effectively eliminate the resource-intensive random 4-quadrant sampling of every centimeter of the neosquamous zone.[78]

New and emerging advanced imaging technologies for the detection of recurrent BE are being actively studied. Virtual chromoendoscopy, particularly narrow band

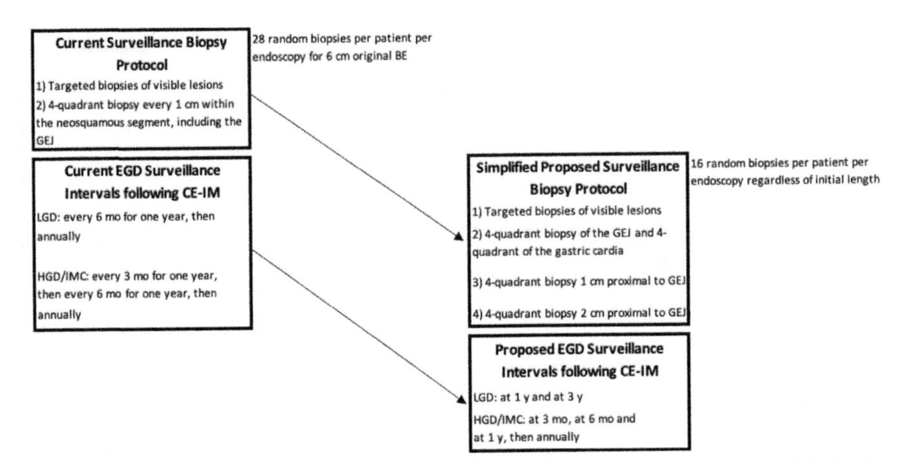

Fig. 2. Current and simplified surveillance endoscopy biopsy and interval protocol following EET. EET, endoscopic eradication therapy; EGD, esophagogastroduodenoscopy; GEJ, gastroesophageal junction; HGD, high-grade dysplasia; IMC, intramucosal cancer; LGD, low-grade dysplasia.

imaging, has been shown to improve detection of dysplasia in surveillance of BE and is recommended in post-EET surveillance.[78] Advanced endoscopic imaging techniques such as volumetric laser endomicroscopy, as well as confocal laser endomicroscopy allow for real-time assessment of esophageal mucosa for detection of IM, dysplastic BE, and IMC. However, they are not routinely recommended for post-EET surveillance due to high costs, steep learning curve, and low quality of evidence showing increased diagnostic yield.[2,7] New sampling methods, particularly wide-area transepithelial sampling (WATS-3D; CDx Diagnostics, Suffern, NY, USA), are also being studied to improve detection of recurrence after EET by limiting sampling error associated with 4-quadrant biopsies and are discussed elsewhere.[2,79]

APPROACH TO TREATMENT AND PREVENTION OF RECURRENT BARRETT'S ESOPHAGUS

The dominant approach for any recurrence following EET detected during surveillance is to pursue further EET, and this is reflected as a recommendation in the most recent Best Practice update from the American Gastroenterological Association (AGA) in 2020.[6,16,18,25,27] Despite these recommendations, there still remain questions about the natural history of recurrence of BE following EET.[5,9,28,37] Older studies show a more widely variable approach to the management of recurrent BE (**Table 2**).[8] In the Euro II study, a multicenter study with 132 patients, only those patients with recurrence of IM with HGD or intramucosal cancer (IMC) underwent retreatment.[6] Patients with LGD and IM continued with endoscopic surveillance only, although long-term follow-up of those patients was not reported at time of publication in 2016.[6] Observational data published in 2013 on 448 patients from the multicenter US RFA Registry that 37 patients had recurrence of IM.[37] Of the 37 recurrences, 25 patients underwent retreatment including one patient who underwent esophagectomy for EAC.[37] The modality of retreatment was undertaken with multiple approaches including APC or multipolar coagulation (particularly in patients who had prior strictures secondary to RFA), EMR, repeat RFA, or combination therapy.[37] At the time of publication, 19 patients had achieved repeat CE-IM and 5 were still undergoing therapy.[37] The remaining 12

Table 2
Compilation of studies showing management of recurrent Barrett's esophagus following complete eradication of intestinal metaplasia

Publication Author, Year	Study Type	Total Recurrences (n)	Treated Again (n)	Undergoing Surveillance Alone (n)	Re-CE-IM	Actively Treated	Lost to Follow-up	Retreatment Method
Fleischer et al,[38] 2010	Prospective multicenter	4	4	0	4	0	0	Not reported
Alvarez Herraro et al,[80] 2011	Prospective multicenter	2	2	0	2	0	0	Not reported
Shaheen et al,[26] 2011	Prospective multicenter	19	14	5	13	1	0	RFA
Vacarro et al,[81] 2011	Prospective single-center	15	8/12	4	3/4	0	8	RFA, EMR
Caillol et al,[33] 2012	Prospective single-center	2	2	0	0	2	0	Not reported
Dulai et al,[36] 2013	Retrospective single-center	11	5	2	5/5	0	0	RFA
Ertan et al,[35] 2013	Prospective single-center	3	3	0	0	0	0	Esophagectomy
Haidry et al,[27] 2013	Prospective multicenter	37	12	21	0	12	4	RFA
Orman et al,[17] 2013	Retrospective single-center	8	6	2	4/4	0	0	RFA, EMR, esophagectomy
Gupta et al,[37] 2013	Retrospective multicenter	37	25	12	19	5	0	RFA, EMR, and/or APC, esophagectomy
Phoa et al,[18] 2013	Retrospective single-center	25	3	22	25	0	0	APC, EMR
Strauss et al,[83] 2014	Retrospective multicenter	9	3	1	2	0	2	RFA, esophagectomy
Anders et al,[84] 2014	Retrospective multicenter	37	5	32	5	0	0	APC, EMR
Konda et al,[85] 2014	Prospective single-center	15	8	7	7	1	0	EMR
Phoa et al,[88] 2015	Retrospective multicenter	14	10	4	0	10	0	APC, EMR
Le Page et al,[89] 2016	Retrospective single-center	2	1	1	1	0	0	EMR
Komanduri et al,[23] 2017	Prospective single-center	13	13	0	13	0	0	RFA
Cotton et al,[25] 2017	Prospective multicenter	35	35	0	24	0	0	RFA, EMR; 6 referred for surgery
Sami et al,[41] 2019	Prospective multicenter	151	108	43	72	25	4	RFA, EMR, 4 surgery, 2 radiation

Abbreviation: EMR, endomucosal resection; RFA, radiofrequency ablation; APC, argon plasma coagulation; CE-IM, complete eradication-intestinal metaplasia.

patients (one of which had LGD) underwent surveillance, which the investigators attributed to differing practice patterns among the different centers.[37]

In contrast, more recent studies focus on retreatment of all recurrences of IM regardless of dysplasia status, as those areas of IM may represent incompletely treated or refractory disease with high risk for neoplastic progression (see **Table 2**).[5,8,9,28,37] Sami and colleagues[41] looked at durability of CE-IM and over the course of their study period, 151 patients had recurrence of IM on surveillance. At the time of publication, 108 had undergone retreatment and most of those patients had recurrence of only nondysplastic IM (n = 73).[41] In addition, a retrospective study published in 2017 with 306 patients who underwent EET with EMR and RFA for LGD/HGD/IMC showed 52 patients (17% of the study population) had recurrence of BE.[77] All patients underwent retreatment, with a majority (58%) achieving second CE-IM and 37% still undergoing therapy.[77] Only 4% of patients with recurrent BE reportedly failed endoscopic retreatment.[77]

Current strategies for treatment of recurrence follow the same principles of EET. All visible lesions and islands should be resected or ablated along with circumferential ablation of the squamocolumnar junction.[7,8,37,41,77] The pathogenesis of isolated IM at the GEJ is controversial and may represent a distinct nonreflux-mediated process.[8,41] In addition, some argue that recurrent IM may represent a transient process with low neoplastic potential.[8,41,77] A major limitation in replicating the results of these studies is the fact that many do not report the location of recurrence of IM in the esophagus to differentiate tubular esophageal recurrence from GEJ recurrence.[7,8,37,41,77] Given these limitations, the most recent Best Practice update from the AGA in 2020 also recommends treating the SCJ along with recurrent disease identified in the tubular esophagus with standard EET techniques.[16] IM identified within the gastric cardia (defined 1 cm distal to the GEJ, as demarcated by the top of the gastric folds) does not need to be treated.[7,8,16,37,41,77]

The hallmark of post-EET prevention of recurrent BE is aggressive reflux control to prevent the cellular changes that cause further mucosal damage and recurrence of IM with or without dysplasia/carcinoma.[7,23] Roughly 25% of patients with BE do not have normalization of their intraesophageal pH despite achieving good symptom control on PPI therapy.[7,23] Early studies have shown that poor acid suppression post-EET with CE-IM is linked to BE recurrence.[7,23] A recent study compared patients who achieved CE-IM on PPI therapy with patients who underwent antireflux surgery after CE-IM.[23] They reported an IM recurrence rate of 20% in patients maintained on PPI compared with 9.1% for those undergoing fundoplication, which was only significant in patients with baseline long-segment BE.[23] Komanduri and colleagues[23] showed improved EET durability compared with prior studies when EET is coupled with an aggressive antireflux protocol (see **Fig. 1**). In that study, patients with recurrent and refractory BE after EET who underwent optimization of acid suppression following monitoring had an IM recurrence rate of 4.8% (regardless of baseline histology) and a dysplasia recurrence rate of 1.5% with 7 years of follow-up.[23] As such, enforcing a strict antireflux regimen accompanied by early physiologic testing and modification is an effective strategy of prevention of recurrence of BE after successful EET.[7,23]

SUMMARY

Despite advances in EET and high-rates of CE-IM, BE that is refractory to EET and recurrence after successful treatment is not uncommon.[8,16,26,37] Patients who have not achieved CE-IM (including patients with incomplete or no response in disease) after EMR of nodular lesions followed by up to 3 sessions of RFA and optimized reflux control are considered refractory to EET. It is important to identify patients who are likely to be refractory to standard EET so that patients can be counseled on the potential for requiring numerous EET sessions or the need for salvage treatment strategies. Aggressive control of reflux exposure, possibly necessitating antireflux surgery including hiatal hernia repair before beginning or during EET, is likely to be the most important factor in achieving CE-IM. In patients who ultimately fail standard EET with EMR and RFA despite optimization of reflux control, salvage cryotherapy with liquid nitrogen, rescue EMR, or APC seem to be safe and effective alternative treatments. Future prospective controlled studies are warranted to identify and validate risk factors for refractory BE as well as successful management strategies including optimal methods of reflux control and salvage EET.

Because of the high rate of BE recurrence despite EET, endoscopic surveillance is recommended after achieving CE-IM.[2,15,76] Recent data have suggested that recurrence occurs early and near the GEJ. This has prompted proposed surveillance protocols to focus on visible lesions and sampling within 2 cm of the GEJ, in contrast to random sampling.[78] Although conflicting data are reported, risk factors for recurrence of BE following EET include older age, non-Caucasian race, hiatal hernia, and long-segment BE.[7,8,12,21,24] Following EET for BE, aggressive acid suppression with PPI therapy and/or antireflux surgery and early physiologic testing for incomplete responders is critical to improving durability of CE-IM/CE-D.[23] Importantly, patient-reported symptoms are not an accurate measure of appropriate acid suppression following EET.[23] Guidelines on treatment of recurrent BE are sparse, and available studies are hindered by limited data on the natural history of recurrence following EET, limited data on definition and location of IM recurrences, and heterogeneity in treatment protocols and surveillance intervals.[7,8,37,41,77] Nevertheless, current guidelines support endoscopic treatment of any recurrence.[7,8,37,41,77] Further data as to the natural history and outcomes of EET after recurrence are needed to further extend intervals and potentially discontinue endoscopic surveillance.

CLINICS CARE POINTS

- Endoscopic ablative therapy is recommended for patients with dysplastic BE and is effective in achieving CE-IM; however, refractory BE occurs in 4% to 14% of patients and recurrence occurs in 7% to 13% of patients.
- Risk factors for refractory BE include lack of long-term reflux control, presence of a hiatal hernia, and BE segment length greater than 5 cm. Risk factors for recurrence include longer segment BE, non-Caucasian race, presence of hiatal hernia, smoking history, and higher grade dysplasia at baseline.
- Recurrence of BE is most likely to occur within 2 cm of SCJ within the first year of CE-IM, and 4-quadrant biopsies every centimeter within 2 cm of SCJ is crucial during surveillance.
- All patients found to have recurrence of IM with and without dysplasia should undergo repeat EET.
- Following EET, testing and modifying antireflux strategy as needed is critical in preventing refractory and recurrent BE.
- Salvage cryotherapy with liquid nitrogen, rescue EMR, and APC seem to be safe and effective alternative treatments in patients who ultimately fail standard EET despite optimization of reflux control.

DISCLOSURE

S. Komanduri: Financial Disclosures: Consultant, Medtronic; Consultant, Boston Scientific; Consultant, Cook Medical; Consultant, Olympus Corp; Consultant, GI Supply; Educational Grant, Boston Scientific. V.R. Muthusamy: Consultant and research support: Boston Scientific and Medtronic; Consultant: Medivators and Interpace Diagnostics; Stockholder: Capsovision; Honoraria: Torax Medical/Ethicon. Drs D.A. Farina and A. Condon report no relevant disclosures.

REFERENCES

1. Runge TM, Abrams JA, Shaheen NJ. Epidemiology of Barrett's Esophagus and Esophageal Adenocarcinoma. Gastroenterol Clin North Am 2015;44(2):203–31.
2. Qumseya B, Sultan S, Bain P, et al. ASGE guideline on screening and surveillance of Barrett's esophagus. Gastrointest Endosc 2019;90(3):335–59.e2.
3. Shaheen NJ, Sharma P, Overholt BF, et al. Radiofrequency Ablation in Barrett's Esophagus with Dysplasia. N Engl J Med 2009;360(22):2277–88.
4. Yousef F, Cardwell C, Cantwell MM, et al. The Incidence of Esophageal Cancer and High-Grade Dysplasia in Barrett's Esophagus: A Systematic Review and Meta-Analysis. Am J Epidemiol 2008;168(3):237–49.
5. Reed CC, Shaheen NJ. Natural History of the Post-ablation Esophagus. Dig Dis Sci 2018;63(8):2136–45.
6. Phoa KN, Pouw RE, Bisschops R, et al. Multimodality endoscopic eradication for neoplastic Barrett oesophagus: results of an European multicentre study (EURO-II). Gut 2016;65(4):555–62.
7. Kia L, Komanduri S. Care of the Postablation Patient: Surveillance, Acid Suppression, and Treatment of Recurrence. Gastrointest Endosc Clin N Am 2017;27(3):515–29.
8. Fujii-Lau LL, Cinnor B, Shaheen N, et al. Recurrence of intestinal metaplasia and early neoplasia after endoscopic eradication therapy for Barrett's esophagus: a systematic review and meta-analysis. Endosc Int open 2017;5(6):E430–49.
9. Mansour NM, El-Serag HB, Anandasabapathy S. Barrett's esophagus: best practices for treatment and post-treatment surveillance. Ann Cardiothorac Surg 2017;6(2):75–87.
10. Sharma P, Falk GW, Weston AP, et al. Dysplasia and cancer in a large multicenter cohort of patients with Barrett's esophagus. Clin Gastroenterol Hepatol 2006;4(5):566–72.
11. Wani S, Qumseya B, Sultan S, et al. Endoscopic eradication therapy for patients with Barrett's esophagus-associated dysplasia and intramucosal cancer. Gastrointest Endosc 2018;87(4):907–31.e9.
12. Anders M, Bähr C, El-Masry MA, et al. Long-term recurrence of neoplasia and Barrett's epithelium after complete endoscopic resection. Gut 2014;63(10):1535.
13. Desai M, Saligram S, Gupta N, et al. Efficacy and safety outcomes of multimodal endoscopic eradication therapy in Barrett's esophagus-related neoplasia: a systematic review and pooled analysis. Gastrointest Endosc 2017;85(3):482–95.e4.
14. Wani S, Muthusamy VR, Shaheen NJ, et al. Development of quality indicators for endoscopic eradication therapies in Barrett's esophagus: the TREAT-BE (Treatment with Resection and Endoscopic Ablation Techniques for Barrett's Esophagus) Consortium. Gastrointest Endosc 2017;86(1):1–17.e13.
15. Shaheen NJ, Falk GW, Iyer PG, et al. ACG Clinical Guideline: Diagnosis and Management of Barrett's Esophagus. Am J Gastroenterol 2016;111(1):30–50 [quiz: 51].

16. Sharma P, Shaheen NJ, Katzka D, et al. AGA Clinical Practice Update on Endoscopic Treatment of Barrett's Esophagus With Dysplasia and/or Early Cancer: Expert Review. Gastroenterology 2020;158(3):760–9.
17. Orman ES, Li N, Shaheen NJ. Efficacy and Durability of Radiofrequency Ablation for Barrett's Esophagus: Systematic Review and Meta-analysis. Clin Gastroenterol Hepatol 2013;11(10):1245–55.
18. Phoa KN, Pouw RE, van Vilsteren FGI, et al. Remission of Barrett's esophagus with early neoplasia 5 years after radiofrequency ablation with endoscopic resection: a Netherlands cohort study. Gastroenterology 2013;145:96–104, 2013 AGA Institute. Published by Elsevier Inc.
19. Krishnan K, Pandolfino JE, Kahrilas PJ, et al. Increased risk for persistent intestinal metaplasia in patients with Barrett's esophagus and uncontrolled reflux exposure before radiofrequency ablation. Gastroenterology 2012;143(3):576–81.
20. Singh T, Sanaka MR, Thota PN. Endoscopic therapy for Barrett's esophagus and early esophageal cancer: Where do we go from here? World J Gastrointest Endosc 2018;10(9):165–74.
21. van Vilsteren FGI, Alvarez Herrero L, Pouw RE, et al. Predictive factors for initial treatment response after circumferential radiofrequency ablation for Barrett's esophagus with early neoplasia: a prospective multicenter study. Endoscopy 2013;45(07):516–25.
22. Luckett T, Allamneni C, Cowley K, et al. Length of Barrett's segment predicts failure of eradication in radiofrequency ablation for Barrett's esophagus: a retrospective cohort study. BMC Gastroenterol 2018;18(1):67.
23. Komanduri S, Kahrilas PJ, Krishnan K, et al. Recurrence of Barrett's Esophagus is Rare Following Endoscopic Eradication Therapy Coupled With Effective Reflux Control. Am J Gastroenterol 2017;112(4):556–66.
24. Pasricha S, Bulsiewicz WJ, Hathorn KE, et al. Durability and Predictors of Successful Radiofrequency Ablation for Barrett's Esophagus. Clin Gastroenterol Hepatol 2014;12(11):1840–7.e1.
25. Cotton CC, Wolf WA, Overholt BF, et al. Late Recurrence of Barrett's Esophagus After Complete Eradication of Intestinal Metaplasia is Rare: Final Report From Ablation in Intestinal Metaplasia Containing Dysplasia Trial. Gastroenterology 2017;153(3):681–8.e2.
26. Shaheen NJ, Overholt BF, Sampliner RE, et al. Durability of Radiofrequency Ablation in Barrett's Esophagus With Dysplasia. Gastroenterology 2011;141(2):460–8.
27. Haidry RJ, Dunn JM, Butt MA, et al. Radiofrequency Ablation and Endoscopic Mucosal Resection for Dysplastic Barrett's Esophagus and Early Esophageal Adenocarcinoma: Outcomes of the UK National Halo RFA Registry. Gastroenterology 2013;145(1):87–95.
28. Krishnamoorthi R, Singh S, Ragunathan K, et al. Risk of recurrence of Barrett's esophagus after successful endoscopic therapy. Gastrointest Endosc 2016; 83(6):1090–106.e3.
29. Sawas T, Iyer PG, Alsawas M, et al. Higher Rate of Barrett's Detection in the First Year After Successful Endoscopic Therapy: Meta-analysis. Am J Gastroenterol 2018;113(7):959–71.
30. Cotton CC, Haidry R, Thrift AP, et al. Development of Evidence-Based Surveillance Intervals After Radiofrequency Ablation of Barrett's Esophagus. Gastroenterology 2018;155(2):316–26.e6.
31. Konda VJA, Gonzalez Haba Ruiz M, Koons A, et al. Complete Endoscopic Mucosal Resection Is Effective and Durable Treatment for Barrett's-Associated Neoplasia. Clin Gastroenterol Hepatol 2014;12(12):2002–10.e2.

32. Tan MC, Kanthasamy KA, Yeh AG, et al. Factors Associated With Recurrence of Barrett's Esophagus After Radiofrequency Ablation. Clin Gastroenterol Hepatol 2019;17(1):65–72.e5.
33. Caillol F, Bories E, Pesenti C, et al. Radiofrequency ablation associated to mucosal resection in the oesophagus: Experience in a single centre. Clin Res Hepatol Gastroenterol 2012;36(4):371–7.
34. Cotton CC, Wolf WA, Pasricha S, et al. Recurrent intestinal metaplasia after radiofrequency ablation for Barrett's esophagus: endoscopic findings and anatomic location. Gastrointest Endosc 2015;81(6):1362–9.
35. Ertan A, Zaheer I, Correa AM, et al. Photodynamic therapy vs radiofrequency ablation for Barrett's dysplasia: efficacy, safety and cost-comparison. World J Gastroenterol 2013;19(41):7106–13.
36. Dulai PS, Pohl H, Levenick JM, et al. Radiofrequency ablation for long- and ultralong-segment Barrett's esophagus: a comparative long-term follow-up study. Gastrointest Endosc 2013;77(4):534–41.
37. Gupta M, Iyer PG, Lutzke L, et al. Recurrence of esophageal intestinal metaplasia after endoscopic mucosal resection and radiofrequency ablation of Barrett's esophagus: results from a US Multicenter Consortium. Gastroenterology 2013; 145(1):79–86.e1.
38. Fleischer DE, Overholt BF, Sharma VK, et al. Endoscopic radiofrequency ablation for Barrett's esophagus: 5-year outcomes from a prospective multicenter trial. Endoscopy 2010;42(10):781–9.
39. Korst RJ, Santana-Joseph S, Rutledge JR, et al. Patterns of recurrent and persistent intestinal metaplasia after successful radiofrequency ablation of Barrett's esophagus. J Thorac Cardiovasc Surg 2013;145(6):1529–34.
40. Lada MJ, Watson TJ, Shakoor A, et al. Eliminating a Need for Esophagectomy: Endoscopic Treatment of Barrett Esophagus With Early Esophageal Neoplasia. Semin Thorac Cardiovasc Surg 2014;26(4):274–84.
41. Sami SS, Ravindran A, Kahn A, et al. Timeline and location of recurrence following successful ablation in Barrett's oesophagus: an international multicentre study. Gut 2019;68(8):1379–85.
42. Shaheen NJ, Bronner MP, Fleischer DE, et al. Subsquamous Intestinal Metaplasia Is a Common Finding in Ablation-Naïve Patients with Dysplastic Barrett's Esophagus, and Significantly Decreases in Prevalence After Radiofrequency Ablation. Gastrointest Endosc 2008;67(5):AB176.
43. Iyer PG. A "deeper" look at subsquamous structures beneath the neosquamous epithelium after Barrett's esophagus endotherapy. Gastrointest Endosc 2016; 83:89–91.
44. Haidry RJ, Butt MA, Dunn JM, et al. Improvement over time in outcomes for patients undergoing endoscopic therapy for Barrett's oesophagus-related neoplasia: 6-year experience from the first 500 patients treated in the UK patient registry. Gut 2015;64(8):1192–9.
45. Eluri S, Earasi AG, Moist SE, et al. Prevalence and Incidence of Intestinal Metaplasia and Dysplasia of Gastric Cardia in Patients With Barrett's Esophagus After Endoscopic Therapy. Clin Gastroenterol Hepatol 2020;18(1):82–8.e1.
46. Akiyama J, Marcus SN, Triadafilopoulos G. Effective intra-esophageal acid control is associated with improved radiofrequency ablation outcomes in Barrett's esophagus. Dig Dis Sci 2012;57(10):2625–32.
47. Ouatu-Lascar R, Triadafilopoulos G. Complete elimination of reflux symptoms does not guarantee normalization of intraesophageal acid reflux in patients with Barrett's esophagus. Am J Gastroenterol 1998;93:711–6.

48. Todd JA, Basu KK, de Caestecker JS. Normalization of oesophageal pH does not guarantee control of duodenogastro-oesophageal reflux in Barrett's oesophagus. Aliment Pharmacol Ther 2005;21:969–75.
49. Vaezi MF, Richter JE. Role of acid and duodenogastroesophageal reflux in gastroesophageal reflux disease. Gastroenterology 1996;111:1192–9.
50. Kahrilas PJ, Pandolfino JE. The target of therapies: pathophysiology of gastroesophageal reflux disease. Gastrointest Endosc Clin N Am 2003;13:1–17.
51. Reed CC, Shaheen NJ. Durability of Endoscopic Treatment for Dysplastic Barrett's Esophagus. Curr Treat Options Gastroenterol 2019;17:171–86.
52. Pech O, May A, Manner H, et al. Long-term efficacy and safety of endoscopic resection for patients with mucosal adenocarcinoma of the esophagus. Gastroenterology 2014;146:652–660 e651, 2014 AGA Institute. Published by Elsevier Inc.
53. Sarela AI, Hick DG, Verbeke CS, et al. Persistent acid and bile reflux in asymptomatic patients with Barrett esophagus receiving proton pump inhibitor therapy. Arch Surg 2004;139:547–51.
54. Ferraris R, Fracchia M, Foti M, et al. Barrett's oesophagus: long-term follow-up after complete ablation with argon plasma coagulation and the factors that determine its recurrence. Aliment Pharmacol Ther 2007;25(7):835–40.
55. Madisch A, Miehlke S, Bayerdorffer E, et al. Long-term follow-up after complete ablation of Barrett's esophagus with argon plasma coagulation. World J Gastroenterol 2005;11(8):1182–6.
56. O'Connell K, Velanovich V. Effects of Nissen fundoplication on endoscopic endoluminal radiofrequency ablation of Barrett's esophagus. Surg Endosc 2011;25(3): 830–4.
57. Trad KS, Barnes WE, Simoni G, et al. Transoral incisionless fundoplication effective in eliminating GERD symptoms in partial responders to proton pump inhibitor therapy at 6 months: the TEMPO Randomized Clinical Trial. Surg Innov 2015; 22(1):26–40.
58. Abu Dayyeh B, Murad MH, Bazerbachi F, et al. Efficacy of Laparoscopic Nissen Fundoplication vs Transoral Incisionless Fundoplication or Proton Pump Inhibitors in Patients With Gastroesophageal Reflux Disease: Misleading Ranking Probabilities in Network Meta-analysis. Gastroenterology 2018;155:935–6.
59. Skubleny D, Switzer NJ, Dang J, et al. LINX((R)) magnetic esophageal sphincter augmentation versus Nissen fundoplication for gastroesophageal reflux disease: a systematic review and meta-analysis. Surg Endosc 2017;31:3078–84.
60. Aiolfi A, Asti E, Bernardi D, et al. Early results of magnetic sphincter augmentation versus fundoplication for gastroesophageal reflux disease: Systematic review and meta-analysis. Int J Surg 2018;52:82–8, 2018 IJS Publishing Group Ltd. Published by Elsevier Ltd.
61. Fass R. An Overview of Transoral Incisionless Fundoplication and Magnetic Sphincter Augmentation for GERD. Gastroenterol Hepatol (N Y) 2017;13(1):50–2.
62. Overholt BF, Lightdale CJ, Wang KK, et al. Photodynamic therapy with porfimer sodium for ablation of high-grade dysplasia in Barrett's esophagus: international, partially blinded, randomized phase III trial. Gastrointest Endosc 2005;62: 488–98.
63. Chung A, Bourke MJ, Hourigan LF, et al. Complete Barrett's excision by stepwise endoscopic resection in short-segment disease: long term outcomes and predictors of stricture. Endoscopy 2011;43(12):1025–32.
64. Larghi A, Lightdale CJ, Ross AS, et al. Long-term follow-up of complete Barrett's eradication endoscopic mucosal resection (CBE-EMR) for the treatment of high grade dysplasia and intramucosal carcinoma. Endoscopy 2007;39(12):1086–91.

65. Pouw RE, Peters FP, Sempoux C, et al. Stepwise radical endoscopic resection for Barrett's esophagus with early neoplasia: report on a Brussels' cohort. Endoscopy 2008;40(11):892–8.
66. Milashka M, Calomme A, Van Laethem JL, et al. Sixteen-year follow-up of Barrett's esophagus, endoscopically treated with argon plasma coagulation. United Eur Gastroenterol J 2014;2(5):367–73.
67. Visrodia K, Zakko L, Singh S, et al. Cryotherapy for persistent Barrett's esophagus after radiofrequency ablation: a systematic review and meta-analysis. Gastrointest Endosc 2018;87(6):1396–404.e1.
68. Dumot JA, Greenwald BD. Argon plasma coagulation, bipolar cautery, and cryotherapy: ABC's of ablative techniques. Endoscopy 2008;40(12):1026–32.
69. Shaheen NJ, Greenwald BD, Peery AF, et al. Safety and efficacy of endoscopic spray cryotherapy for Barrett's esophagus with high-grade dysplasia. Gastrointest Endosc 2010;71(4):680–5.
70. Dumot JA, Vargo JJ 2nd, Falk GW, et al. An open-label, prospective trial of cryospray ablation for Barrett's esophagus high-grade dysplasia and early esophageal cancer in high-risk patients. Gastrointest Endosc 2009;70:635–44.
71. Gosain S, Mercer K, Twaddell WS, et al. Liquid nitrogen spray cryotherapy in Barrett's esophagus with high-grade dysplasia: long-term results. Gastrointest Endosc 2013;78:260–5. United States: Inc.
72. Overwater A, Weusten B. Cryoablation in the management of Barrett's esophagus. Curr Opin Gastroenterol 2017;33(4):261–9.
73. Sengupta N, Ketwaroo GA, Bak DM, et al. Salvage cryotherapy after failed radiofrequency ablation for Barrett's esophagus-related dysplasia is safe and effective. Gastrointest Endosc 2015;82:443–8. American Society for Gastrointestinal Endoscopy. Published by Elsevier Inc.
74. Trindade AJ, Inamdar S, Kothari S, et al. Feasibility of liquid nitrogen cryotherapy after failed radiofrequency ablation for Barrett's esophagus. Dig Endosc 2017;29(6):680–5.
75. Wani S, Han S, Kushnir V, et al. Recurrence is rare following complete eradication of intestinal metaplasia in patients with barrett's esophagus and peaks at 18 months. Clin Gastroenterol Hepatol 2020. S1542-3565(20)30098-7.
76. Kahn A, Shaheen NJ, Iyer PG. Approach to the Post-Ablation Barrett's Esophagus Patient. Am J Gastroenterol 2020;115(6):823–31.
77. Guthikonda A, Cotton CC, Madanick RD, et al. Clinical Outcomes Following Recurrence of Intestinal Metaplasia After Successful Treatment of Barrett's Esophagus With Radiofrequency Ablation. Am J Gastroenterol 2017;112(1):87–94.
78. Omar M, Thaker AM, Wani S, et al. Anatomic location of Barrett's esophagus recurrence after endoscopic eradication therapy: development of a simplified surveillance biopsy strategy. Gastrointest Endosc 2019;90(3):395–403.
79. Vennalaganti PR, Kaul V, Wang KK, et al. Increased detection of Barrett's esophagus-associated neoplasia using wide-area trans-epithelial sampling: a multicenter, prospective, randomized trial. Gastrointest Endosc 2018;87(2):348–55.
80. Alvarez Herrero L, van Vilsteren FG, Pouw RE, et al. Endoscopic radiofrequency ablation combined with endoscopic resection for early neoplasia in Barrett's esophagus longer than 10 cm. Gastrointest Endosc 2011;73(4):682–90. https://doi.org/10.1016/j.gie.2010.11.016. PMID: 21292262.
81. Vaccaro BJ, Gonzalez S, Poneros JM, et al. Detection of intestinal metaplasia after successful eradication of Barrett's Esophagus with radiofrequency ablation.

Dig Dis Sci 2011;56(7):1996–2000. https://doi.org/10.1007/s10620-011-1680-4. PMID: 21468652; PMCID: PMC3144139.
82. van Vilsteren FG, Alvarez Herrero L, Pouw RE, et al. Predictive factors for initial treatment response after circumferential radiofrequency ablation for Barrett's esophagus with early neoplasia: a prospective multicenter study. Endoscopy 2013;45(7):516–25. https://doi.org/10.1055/s-0032-1326423. PMID: 23580412.
83. Strauss AC, Agoston AT, Dulai PS, et al. Radiofrequency ablation for Barrettâ™s-associated intramucosal carcinoma: a multi-center follow-up study. Surg Endosc 2014;28:3366â–3372. https://doi.org/10.1007/s00464-014-3629-0.
84. Anders M, BÃ¤hr C, El-Masry MA, et al. Long-term recurrence of neoplasia and Barrett's epithelium after complete endoscopic resection. Gut 2014;63:1535–43. https://doi.org/10.1136/gutjnl-2013-305538.
85. Konda VJ, Gonzalez Haba Ruiz M, Koons A, et al. Complete endoscopic mucosal resection is effective and durable treatment for Barrett's-associated neoplasia. Clin Gastroenterol Hepatol 2014;12(12):2002–10.e1-2. https://doi.org/10.1016/j.cgh.2014.04.010. PMID: 24732285.
86. Lada MJ, Watson TJ, Shakoor A, et al. Eliminating a need for esophagectomy: endoscopic treatment of Barrett esophagus with early esophageal neoplasia. Seminars in Thoracic and Cardiovascular Surgery 2014;26(4):274â–284. https://doi.org/10.1053/j.semtcvs.2014.12.004.
87. Pasricha S, Bulsiewicz WJ, Hathorn KE, et al. Durability and predictors of successful radiofrequency ablation for Barrett's esophagus. Clin Gastroenterol Hepatol 2014;12(11):1840–7.e1. https://doi.org/10.1016/j.cgh.2014.04.034. PMID: 24815329; PMCID: PMC4225183.
88. Phoa KN, Pouw RE, Bisschops R, et al. Multimodality endoscopic eradication for neoplastic Barrett oesophagus: results of an European multicentre study (EURO-II). Gut 2016;65(4):555–62. https://doi.org/10.1136/gutjnl-2015-309298. PMID: 25731874.
89. Le Page PA, Velu PP, Penman ID, et al. Surgical and endoscopic management of high grade dysplasia and early oesophageal adenocarcinoma. Surgeon 2015; 14(6):315–21.

Surgical Management of Barrett's-Related Neoplasia

Akshay Pratap, MD, MCh[a], Martin D. McCarter, MD[b,*], Thomas J. Watson, MD[c]

KEYWORDS

• Esophageal cancer • Esophagectomy • Barrett's esophagus • High-grade dysplasia • Intramucosal carcinoma • Minimally invasive surgery

KEY POINTS

- Accurate endoscopic and pathologic staging by an experienced team is essential for optimal care in cases of Barrett's-related neoplasia.
- Advances in endoscopic techniques have reduced the need for esophagectomy in early-stage Barrett's-related neoplasia.
- Improvements in preoperative patient evaluation and optimization, surgical techniques, and perioperative care by multidisciplinary teams, as exemplified at high-volume centers, have reduced the morbidity and mortality of esophagectomy.
- The optimal surgical approach to esophagectomy is individualized based on patient factors, tumor characteristics, and surgeon preferences.
- Minimally invasive techniques for esophagectomy have reduced pulmonary complications and quickened recovery compared with open surgery while maintaining oncologic equivalency.

INTRODUCTION

Over the past few decades, esophageal adenocarcinoma (EAC) has been increasing in incidence more rapidly than any other cancer in North America. In parallel, steadily rising incidence rates for adenocarcinoma of the cardia also have been reported.[1,2] Based on data from 2012, these rates of increase do not appear to be slowing.[3] Current estimates are that by the year 2035, 1 in 100 men in the United States will be diagnosed with EAC.[4] The only known precursor of EAC is Barrett's esophagus (BE), a metaplastic replacement of the squamous lining of the esophagus with specialized columnar epithelium. Strategies to improve survival in patients with EAC have focused

[a] Department of Surgery, University of Colorado, Aurora, CO, USA; [b] Department of Surgery, Division of Surgical Oncology, University of Colorado Denver, Academic Office One, L15-6106, 12631 East 17th Avenue, MS C325, Aurora, CO 80045, USA; [c] Department of Surgery, MedStar Georgetown University Hospital, Georgetown University School of Medicine, 3900 Reservoir Road Northwest, Washington, DC 20007, USA
* Corresponding author.
E-mail address: martin.mccarter@ucdenver.edu

Gastrointest Endoscopy Clin N Am 31 (2021) 205–218
https://doi.org/10.1016/j.giec.2020.09.003

on detection of Barrett's-related neoplasia at an early and potentially curable stage. Toward this end, screening programs have arisen for patients considered high risk for development of BE, and endoscopic surveillance of known cases of BE is now commonplace.[5]

For decades, esophagectomy has been the mainstay of treatment for patients with resectable EAC, including both early and locoregionally advanced cases. Esophageal resection, combined with a thorough lymphadenectomy, removes the primary tumor as well as sites of potential regional lymphatic spread. More recently, endoscopic resection (ER) and ablation have allowed eradication of superficial foci of esophageal neoplasia, carrying a low risk of nodal involvement, in a minimally invasive fashion. Current guidelines published by specialty medical societies and the National Comprehensive Cancer Network (NCCN) recommend endoscopic therapies for most cases of BE with high-grade dysplasia (HGD) or intramucosal carcinoma (IMC).[6] Endoscopic treatment modalities, when expertly performed in appropriately selected patients, have been shown to achieve cure rates equivalent to surgery, but with less morbidity. As a result, esophagectomy has been relegated to the minority of cases of early disease deemed inappropriate for, or having failed, endoscopic approaches. Although surgical resection reliably cures early esophageal neoplasia in a single intervention, its role has been marginalized due to a significant complication profile, the perception of high rates of perioperative mortality, particularly in low-volume centers, and the potential to impair quality of life (QOL).

Given a dramatic evolution in esophageal cancer treatment paradigms, the managing physician must remain mindful of the limitations of endoscopic therapies, as well as be knowledgeable about the indications for esophagectomy; a "one-size-fits-all" strategy does not apply. Esophagectomy remains the treatment of choice for select early neoplasms as well as for more advanced tumors, which still constitute most cases of EAC. The endoscopist must avoid being inappropriately underaggressive, following the course of endoscopic therapies when a more extensive surgical resection is indicated. On the other hand, the surgeon must avoid being overaggressive, and should perform an esophagectomy only when oncologically and medically appropriate. In addition, esophagectomy should be undertaken in experienced hands using a technique that optimizes eradication of disease while minimizing risk to the patient.

LIMITATIONS OF ENDOSCOPIC THERAPIES FOR BARRETT'S NEOPLASIA

The Risk of Nodal Metastases

A requirement for the utilization of endoscopic modalities to cure esophageal neoplasia is the absence of nodal spread; current endoscopic techniques do not allow eradication of nodal disease. The treating physician, therefore, must understand how the depth of invasion and other tumor characteristics determine the potential for lymph node metastases, which mandate surgical resection with regional lymphadenectomy should they be suspected.

The deep border of the esophageal epithelium is its basement membrane (**Fig. 1**). Neoplasia limited to the epithelium and not penetrating beyond the basement membrane is termed low-grade dysplasia (LGD) or HGD in the United States, or low-grade or high-grade intraepithelial neoplasia (LGIN or HGIN, World Health Organization terminology) in Europe.[7] The term "carcinoma in situ" is synonymous with HGD, HGIN, and Tis (American Joint Committee on Cancer Eighth Edition staging).[8] Tumors invading beyond the basement membrane to involve the lamina propria or muscularis mucosa (MM) are classified as IMC (T1a). The MM is often difficult to identify in diseased esophageal tissue and may present with 2 discrete layers in patients with

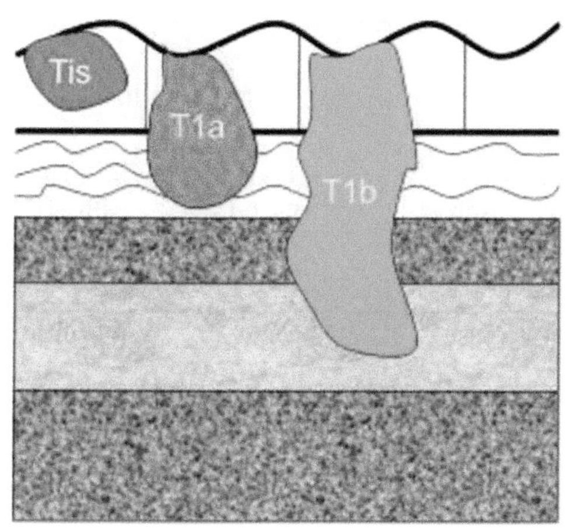

Fig. 1. Subclassification of early esophageal neoplasia based on depth of penetration. Tis is neoplasia limited to the epithelium. T1a tumors penetrate the basement membrane to involve the lamina propria and MM. T1b tumors penetrate the MM to involve the submucosa. (*From* Watson TJ. Esophagectomy for Superficial Esophageal Neoplasia. Gastrointest Endosc Clin N Am. 2017 Jul;27(3):531-546; with permission.)

BE, potentially confusing the interpretation of tumor depth, and highlighting the need for expert pathologic reveiw.[9] Tumors invading beyond the MM to involve the submucosa are considered T1b lesions (submucosal carcinoma [SMC]).

The anatomic boundaries of superficial esophageal neoplasia are relevant because multiple series assessing the prevalence of lymph node metastases in esophagectomy specimens have shown an increased risk with deeper tumor penetration (**Table 1**).[10–12] Based on these data, 3 discrete subclassifications of superficial esophageal neoplasia exist:

1. Intraepithelial neoplasia (Tis/HGD/HGIN) for which the risk of nodal spread is negligible
2. Intramucosal neoplasia (T1a, IMC) for which the risk of nodal spread is in the range of 5%
3. Submucosal neoplasia (T1b, SMC) for which the risk of nodal spread is in the range of 15% to 30%

Other factors in addition to depth of tumor invasion appear relevant in determining the potential for nodal dissemination. A multicenter study assessed esophagectomy specimens from 258 patients undergoing resection for T1 EAC in the absence of neoadjuvant treatment.[13] Nodal metastases were found in 7% (9/122) of cases of IMC (T1a), and 26% (35/136) of cases of SMC (T1b), consistent with prior reports. The analysis also determined that tumor size, differentiation, and the presence of lymphovascular invasion (LVI) were predictive of nodal spread. Based on these factors, as well as the depth of invasion, a point system was derived that stratified patients into low-risk ($\leq$2%), moderate-risk (3%–6%), and high-risk ($\geq$7%) groups.

Endoscopic therapies are considered appropriate only for cases of BE with HGD or IMC, where the risk of nodal spread is in the range of 5% or less. Once the tumor has penetrated the critical boundary of the MM to involve the submucosa, the risk of nodal disease is high enough to warrant an esophagectomy with regional lymphadenectomy in most cases. The notion of endoscopically treating select cases of SMC, with only

Table 1
Relationship between tumor depth (T-stage) and lymph node status (N-stage) for esophageal adenocarcinoma

Tumor Depth	Prevalence of Node Metastasis (%)[a]	Number of Involved Nodes Median (IQR)[b]	Number with 1–4 Involved Nodes (%)[c]	Number with >4 Involved Nodes (%)[d]
Intramucosal (T1a)	1/16 (6)	2 (n/a)	1/16 (6)	0/16 (0)
Submucosal (T1b)	5/16 (31)	1 (n/a)	4/16 (25)	1/16 (6)
Intramuscular (T2)	10/13 (77)	2 (1–4)	9/13 (69)	1/13 (8)
Transmuscular (T3)	47/55 (85)	5 (3–13.5)	22/55 (40)	25/55 (45)

Abbreviation: IQR, interquartile range.
[a] $\chi^2 = 42.0$, $P<.001$ (χ^2 for trend).
[b] $\chi^2 = 11.02$, $P \leq .0116$ (Kruskal-Wallis; includes only patients with involved nodes).
[c] $\chi^2 = 13.64$, $P = .0035$ (χ^2 for trend).
[d] $\chi^2 = 21.38$, $P<.001$ (χ^2 for trend).
Adapted from from Hagen JA, DeMeester SR, Peters JH, Chandrasoma P, DeMeester TR. Curative resection for esophageal adenocarcinoma: analysis of 100 en bloc esophagectomies. *Ann Surg* 2001;234:520-530; with permission.

very superficial submucosal invasion and a low risk of nodal dissemination, has been proposed. Such a paradigm cannot be considered standard of care until more data from larger cohorts of patients have been studied. For patients with SMC deemed high risk for undergoing an esophagectomy, however, an endoscopic treatment paradigm may be the best option, accepting the risk of untreated nodal disease.

Patient Selection

The largest experience with ER for early EAC has been reported in several publications by Ell and colleagues.[14,15] An early review of their experience assessed 100 patients who underwent ER for "low-risk" EAC, as defined by the following criteria:

- Lesion ≤20 mm
- Polypoid or flat
- Well-moderately differentiated
- Tumor limited to mucosa
- Negative deep margins
- No LVI
- No lymph node involvement or systemic metastases on staging

Of note, these cases were highly selected from 667 patients referred to their institution for consideration of endoscopic therapy over the study period. When these conservative selection criteria were observed, ER was undertaken with a high rate of success, including a 99% local remission rate, no severe complications, an 11% rate of metachronous neoplasia at a mean follow-up of 36.7 months (all cases successfully retreated by endoscopy), and a 98% 5-year survival with no cancer-related deaths. Risk factors for tumor recurrence included piecemeal resection, long-segment BE, and multifocal neoplasia.[14]

In a subsequent publication, the experience from this same center had increased to 1000 patients with IMC.[16] A complete response rate of 96.3% was noted at a mean follow-up of 56.6 months, and esophagectomy was necessary in 3.7% after failed endoscopic therapy. Only 2 patients died of Barrett's-related cancer during the follow-up period.

These excellent results were obtained in a high-volume referral center with extensive experience in ER, performed in conjunction with expert pathologists and with strict adherence to established protocols, including the assurance that the deep margins of resection were free of tumor. The regimen required commitment on the part of both the patient and the physician to remain compliant with the demands of repeat endoscopic assessments and treatments extending over the course of years. Whether similar outcomes can be achieved more broadly in nonspecialty centers awaits further study.

Based on the data attesting to the safety and efficacy of endoscopic ablation and resection for superficial esophageal neoplasia, including cases of BE with HGD and IMC, an endoscopic treatment paradigm appears appropriate for most T1a EAC cases. Esophagectomy will continue to be preferable in select circumstances, however, such as

1. When tumor characteristics (eg, large or poorly differentiated tumors, presence of LVI, positive deep margin on ER specimen, or invasion beyond the MM) impart a significant risk of lymph node metastases
2. When the patient prefers surgery, or is unwilling or unable to comply with the rigorous, often prolonged requirements of serial endoscopic treatments and subsequent surveillance
3. In cases that are difficult to eradicate with ablation, such as ultra-long segments of BE, a diffusely nodular esophagus with multifocal HGD or IMC, or long intramucosal tumors
4. When attempts at ablation have failed
5. When the esophagus is otherwise not worth salvaging (eg, recalcitrant stricture or end-stage motility disorder)

The Importance of Expert Pathologic Assessment

Of relevance to the utility of ER for treatment of superficial esophageal neoplasia is the fact that considerable interobserver variability exists in the histopathologic interpretation of ER specimens, particularly regarding the depth of tumor invasion. A recent study assessed 25 ER specimens from 4 US institutions.[17] Two expert esophageal pathologists retrospectively analyzed all the tumors and compared their findings with those of the original pathologists. The discordance rates between the original and the expert study pathologists were 44% for tumor grade, 25% for the presence of LVI, and 48% for tumor depth. Regarding tumor depth, 83% of the discordance was due to overstaging of true intramucosal (T1a) lesions.

Based on these and other reports attesting to the difficulty of interpreting biopsies in the setting of BE, the importance of expert review and consensus in the analysis of ER specimens cannot be overstated. Subtle differences in findings, particularly regarding tumor depth, can have a dramatic impact on subsequent management decisions, with obvious ramifications relative to cancer-related survival outcomes and treatment-related morbidity.

CONSIDERATIONS IN THE SURGICAL MANAGEMENT OF BARRETT'S-RELATED NEOPLASIA

Medical Operability, Performance Status, and Preoperative Risk Assessment

Before embarking on any major operation such as an esophagectomy, the surgeon must be diligent in determining whether the patient is an operative candidate. The medical history needs to be assessed for significant cardiopulmonary disease or other major comorbidities. Most patients being evaluated for esophageal resection will meet criteria for cardiac evaluation. For patients with HGD and no evidence of invasive cancer, esophageal resection may be delayed for up to 3 to 6 months until percutaneous or operative coronary revascularization has been achieved. For patients with invasive cancer, such a delay would not be recommended. Nevertheless, a pharmacologic stress test is a consideration, as it improves counseling on perioperative cardiac risk and could exclude surgery as a treatment option for some patients.

Pulmonary complications constitute the most common type of morbidity following esophagectomy. Thoracotomy causes a significant decrease in forced vital capacity (35%) and forced expiratory volume in 1 second (FEV1) (60%) in the immediate postoperative period. The performance of pulmonary function tests (PFTs) before esophagectomy may help in selecting a surgical approach and optimizing postoperative care. For example, a patient with poor lung function may not tolerate single lung ventilation and may need early bronchoscopic intervention to clear airway secretions after surgery. The results of PFTs also provide objective data to estimate the risks of postoperative pulmonary complications. In general, patients with an FEV1 or a diffusion capacity less than 40% of predicted are considered at high risk for postoperative pulmonary complications.

An assessment of functional and nutritional status is of paramount importance before considering the patient for surgery or planning neoadjuvant multimodality treatment.[18] Patients should refrain from smoking, should exercise daily by walking, and should be taught how to use an incentive spirometer. Preoperative enteral nutrition for at least 1 week is recommended to individuals with a history of significant dysphagia or anorexia with marked weight loss (>10% of ideal body weight). Patients with significant cachexia or limited mobility generally are considered high-risk for esophagectomy.

A frank discussion of perioperative risk and goals of care must be undertaken between the patient and the surgeon before embarking on a path of surgical resection. Of course, most patients are motivated to obtain the best chance of cure or long-term survival. For some with severe comorbidities and a shorter life expectancy, or for whom a major operation would severely impair their QOL, nonoperative management may be the best choice.

Volume/Outcome Relationship for Esophagectomy

Esophagectomy is a highly complex surgical procedure associated with a substantial risk of perioperative complications. The operation can be performed safely, however, with a low rate of mortality and acceptable rates of morbidity in experienced centers with a high surgical volume and a multidisciplinary team.[19] Furthermore, higher surgical volume correlates with better economic outcomes, likely due to a decreased rate of complications. Centralization of esophagectomy at dedicated centers is advocated by many experts, although an exact volume cutoff leading to improved outcomes has yet to be defined. The improved results with higher volumes of treated patients with esophageal cancer seems to be a system effect, in part due to the individual surgeon and in part to other hospital resources and expertise (Han S, Kolb JM, Hosokawa P, et al. The volume outcome effect calls for centralization of care in esophageal adenocarcinoma: results from a large cancer registry; submitted *Annals of Internal Medicine*).

Surgical Approach

The operation of choice for an adenocarcinoma of the esophagus or esophagogastric junction is dictated in part by tumor location (ie, Siewert classification) and must ensure a complete (R0) resection with adequate regional lymph node dissection (**Fig. 2**). Western investigators generally agree that the optimal procedure for Siewert type I tumors is esophagectomy, whereas for Siewert type III tumors, a total gastrectomy is preferred. No consensus has been reached on the best surgical option for Siewert type II tumors; treatment is individualized in such cases.

When considering an esophagectomy, the surgeon must choose from a multitude of esophageal resection and reconstruction options, taking into consideration not only the replacement conduit but also patient factors, the optimal incisions, the location of anastomoses, and the extent of regional lymphadenectomy. Of the incisions a surgeon might choose during the course of an esophagectomy, a thoracotomy is generally considered the most morbid given the potential for pain, both short-term and long-term, the need for single lung ventilation, and the risk of perioperative pulmonary complications.

The following are the 3 basic approaches to esophagectomy: (1) transthoracic/transabdominal with intrathoracic anastomosis (Ivor Lewis); (2) transhiatal (transabdominal with cervical anastomosis); or (3) "3-field" transthoracic/transabdominal/cervical (McKeown) with or without en bloc resection of regional lymph nodes. Each of the 3 approaches achieves the goal of resecting the primary tumor and regional nodes, albeit with varying degrees of completeness of a lymphadenectomy. Each approach can be undertaken using open, minimally invasive (including robotic) or

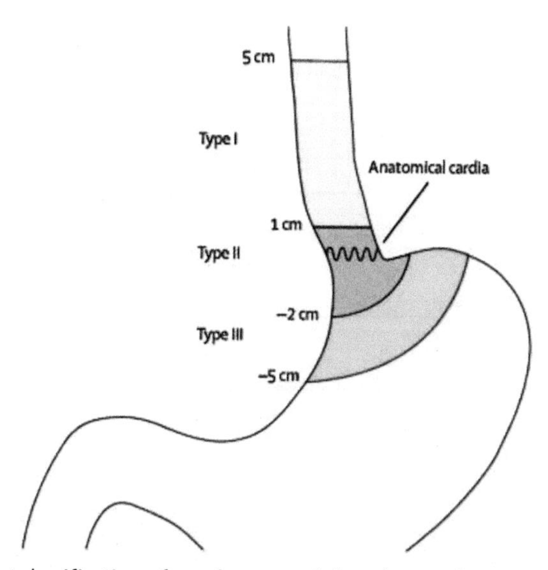

Fig. 2. The Siewert classification of esophagogastric junction carcinomas. Type I tumors have an epicenter located 1 to 5 cm proximal to the esophagogastric junction (EGJ). Type II tumors have an epicenter located between 1 cm proximal and 2 cm distal to the EGJ. Type III tumors have an epicenter 2 to 5 cm distal to the EGJ. (*From* Mariette C, Piessen G, Briez N, Gronnier C, Triboulet JP. Oesophagogastric junction adenocarcinoma: which therapeutic approach? Lancet Oncol. 2011 Mar;12(3):296-305; Reprinted with permission from Elsevier.)

hybrid techniques. The choice of approach and technique is influenced by patient factors, tumor characteristics, and the surgeon's own experiences and biases (**Table 2**).

Several studies have compared the outcomes following transhiatal versus transthoracic esophagectomy and found no differences in survival.[20,21] The transthoracic cohort, however, was associated with higher rates of respiratory complications, wound infections, and early postoperative mortality, whereas anastomotic leak, anastomotic stricture, and recurrent laryngeal nerve palsy rates were significantly higher in the group undergoing transhiatal resection.

Progress has been made in reducing the morbidity of open surgery by the introduction of minimal access procedures across many surgical specialties. Most studies have shown that minimally invasive esophagectomy (MIE) is associated with a significant reduction in pulmonary complications, blood loss, and lengths of stay in the intensive care unit, as well as quicker return to baseline function, compared with open surgery. These advantages occur without compromising oncologic effectiveness, as measured by the number of lymph nodes harvested or long-term cure.[22,23]

Robotic-assisted minimal invasive esophagectomy (RAMIE) represents the next step in the evolution of MIE, offering several potential advantages compared with other MIE approaches.[24] Current robotic technologies provide 3-dimensional optics, improved instrument articulation, and tremor filtration, all of which facilitate dissection and suturing. These advantages must be weighed against potential disadvantages of the robotic platforms, including the lack of haptics and the fact that the surgeon is situated away from the patient in a nonsterile environment. The high initial fixed costs of the systems, as well as the ongoing costs for disposables and maintenance contracts, also must be calculated into the decision regarding the use of RAMIE at a given institution. The data on RAMIE suggest that the procedure is feasible, safe, and associated with perioperative outcomes similar to other forms of MIE and open esophagectomy. Three prospective randomized trials comparing a variety of minimally invasive laparoscopic and robotic approaches to standard open esophagectomy have demonstrated consistent benefits in pulmonary complications and improved short-term QOL.[25–27]

Table 2
Comparison of surgical approaches for adenocarcinoma of the esophagus

Surgical Approach	Advantages	Disadvantages
Transhiatal	Improved pulmonary function Neck anastomosis – easier management of leak	Limited exposure Inferior nodal assessment Relatively increased anastomotic leak and stricture rate Increased risk of recurrent laryngeal nerve palsy
Transthoracic	Improved exposure Improved nodal assessment Relatively lower anastomotic leak rate	Pulmonary effects of thoracotomy More difficult management of anastomotic leak
Three field	Improved exposure Improved nodal assessment	Pulmonary effects of thoracotomy Relatively increased anastomotic leak and stricture rate Increased risk of recurrent laryngeal nerve palsy

Postoperative Management

Enhanced recovery after surgery (ERAS) programs have helped to standardize management and reduce complications following major operations across several diseases and common procedures. Post esophagectomy management is complex and several ERAS programs have been developed that show benefit.[28] Pathways focus on the key components of postoperative care, including fluid balance, pain control (via a thoracic epidural or paravertebral catheter), early mobilization, and expeditious removal of chest drains once oral fluids have recommenced. It is the authors' practice to place a feeding jejunostomy for postoperative nutritional support. There is no evidence that the routine use of contrast radiology to assess the esophageal anastomosis is of value in patients who are nonseptic in the first few days after surgery. Oral feeding is resumed based on clinical parameters at the discretion of the surgeon. A cancer nurse specialist or a dietician should counsel patients on nutritional expectations before discharge from the hospital.

Perioperative Mortality

Esophageal resection historically was associated with high rates of perioperative morbidity and mortality, especially in nonspecialty centers. In a report from 2003 describing the experience in US Veterans Administration hospitals from 1991 to 2000, 30-day postoperative mortality in 1777 esophagectomies performed in 109 facilities was 9.8%.[29] Most operations, however, were performed in low-volume institutions, as only 1.6 esophagectomies were done per year in the average facility. A later publication from 2007 used the Nationwide Inpatient Sample to assess esophagectomy outcomes in 17,395 patients over the years 1999 to 2003.[30] The overall mortality after esophagectomy was 8.7%, with high-volume centers achieving significantly lower rates compared with low-volume institutions.

A more recent analysis assessed resections for esophageal cancer between 2008 and 2011 in the Society of Thoracic Surgeons National Database, including both minimally invasive (n = 814) and open (n = 2356) procedures.[31] Mortality was 3.8% and morbidity was 62.2%; no significant differences were noted between approaches or between high-volume and low-volume centers. Contemporary data from specialty centers with the largest esophagectomy experiences reveal perioperative mortality following minimally MIE and transhiatal esophagectomy (THE) to be even lower at 1.7% and 1.0%, respectively.[22,32]

Esophagectomy for Early Barrett's-Related Esophageal Neoplasia

Rationale

The support for esophageal resection in the setting of BE with HGD, a "premalignant" condition, has been based on 2 findings: (1) occult, synchronous, invasive carcinoma has been detected in a significant proportion of esophagectomy specimens, averaging 37% in multiple surgical series[33]; and (2) invasive cancer may arise within dysplastic BE over the short to medium term. Esophagectomy, therefore, is both curative and prophylactic relative to the treatment and prevention of frank carcinoma and offers complete eradication of neoplasia and associated esophageal metaplasia in a single procedure. Of course, the desire to eliminate pathologic mucosa by surgical resection must be weighed against the invasiveness of the procedure and its risks, including pain, recovery time, perioperative morbidity, mortality, and long-term impact on QOL. Thus, esophagectomy appropriately may be considered "radical prophylaxis" for a microscopic disease process.[34]

Perioperative mortality

Of relevance to the decision regarding esophagectomy for early esophageal neoplasia are data specific to mortality in such cases rather than to the esophageal cancer population at large. A literature review published in 2007 detailed the experience with esophagectomy for HGD over the 20-year period from 1987 to 2007.[33] In 22 studies covering 530 patients, the perioperative mortality was 0.94%, roughly one-quarter to one-tenth the mortality rate reported nationally for all cases of esophagectomy for cancer. Similarly, in a single-institution case series published in 2009 of 100 patients undergoing esophagectomy for T1 esophageal cancer, the 30-day mortality was 0%.[35] Based on these analyses, and despite a possible publication bias, a perioperative mortality of $\leq$1% appears the appropriate rate to quote for the patient undergoing esophageal resection for early disease in experienced centers.

Multiple factors may explain the lower mortality in this select group compared with the population at large of patients with esophageal cancer. Individuals with BE and HGD or IMC likely represent a healthier cohort than those referred with esophageal squamous cell carcinoma, particularly when the latter present with advanced disease, given the differing risk factors and clinical manifestations of the 2 malignancies. Without esophageal obstruction and associated weight loss, patients with HGD or IMC typically do not come to surgery in a malnourished or immunocompromised state. In addition, for cases in which there is no bulky tumor, time is available for optimization of comorbidities, such as cardiovascular or pulmonary disease, smoking or alcohol use, or general deconditioning, without the urgency imposed by the physiologic and psychological manifestations of more advanced cancer. Preoperative chemotherapy or combined chemoradiation, with their deleterious effects potentially leading to increased perioperative morbidity, also are not considerations in cases of early neoplasia. Perhaps most importantly, patient selection is a major factor, as alternative management strategies, such as endoscopic surveillance, mucosal resection or ablation, can be offered to the high-risk surgical candidate. Finally, given the low risk of nodal metastasis and the fact that a regional lymphadenectomy is not a required part of the operation, the surgeon can choose from less invasive operative approaches whereby a thoracotomy, with its potential for pulmonary compromise and postoperative respiratory failure, is avoided.

Cure rates

Multiple case series have assessed cure rates when esophagectomy was undertaken for early-stage disease. The largest reported experience comes from the Worldwide Esophageal Cancer Collaboration, which assessed outcomes after esophagectomy or ER in 13,300 patients from 33 institutions spanning 6 continents.[36] Of the 7558 patients in their database with adenocarcinoma, 99.6% underwent surgical resection, none having received neoadjuvant therapy; only 32 patients underwent ER. A review of the survival curves reveals that survival decreased monotonically and distinctively with increasing depth of tumor penetration. For the 410 tumors pathologically staged Tis, the overall 5-year Kaplan-Meier actuarial survival estimates were in the range of 90%, while for the 2326 tumors pathologically staged T1, the actuarial survival was in the range of 75% to 80%. Unfortunately, data stratifying survival for T1a and T1b tumors were not reported. The results, however, were consistent with those from the smaller studies reporting outcomes from pure surgical cohorts.

The cumulative experience with esophagectomy attests to the high rate of cure for HGD and IMC, when the potential for lymph node metastases is low, and the good yet inferior results for SMC, reflecting the potential for nodal spread. The surgical cure rate is substantial even for SMC, however, underscoring the importance of appropriately aggressive treatment in this cohort.

Quality of life after esophagectomy

Given the poor prognosis associated with advanced esophageal cancer, the focus after esophagectomy traditionally has been on cure rates and perioperative morbidity. For patients undergoing esophageal resection for early neoplasia, when there is a high chance of cure and a long life expectancy, QOL becomes an important consideration, especially relative to the ability to eat and gastrointestinal side effects. A systematic review of health-related QOL published in 2011 found pooled scores for physical, role and social function after esophagectomy similar to US norms, but lower pooled scores for vitality and general health perception.[37] Symptoms of fatigue, dyspnea and diarrhea were worse at 6 months after surgery. On the other hand, emotional function had significantly improved after 6 months, perhaps attributable to the patients' perceptions that they had survived a potentially lethal experience. Of the 21 studies considered in the analysis, however, none included an average follow-up beyond 5.3 years.

A more recent study of 40 patients who underwent esophagectomy with gastric pull-up and cervical esophagogastrostomy assessed symptoms at a median follow-up of 12 years after surgery.[38] Most (88%) reported no dysphagia, 90% were able to eat ≥3 meals per day, and 93% were able to finish ≥50% of a typical meal. Dumping, diarrhea ≥3 times per day, or regurgitation occurred in 33% of patients. The median weight loss after surgery was 26 lb. Scores for QOL were at the population mean in 1 category (physical function) and above the normal mean in the remaining 7 categories. Other studies have confirmed that QOL remains normal after esophagectomy, although physical functioning and gastroesophageal reflux remain problematic.

SUMMARY

The treatment of Barrett's-related esophageal neoplasia has changed drastically in the past 10 to 15 years. With advances in endoscopic screening and surveillance programs for the detection and follow-up of BE, cases of Barrett's EAC are being detected increasingly at an early stage. The introduction, refinement, validation, and popularization of endoscopic resective and ablative techniques have allowed endoscopic treatment of early Barrett's-related esophageal neoplasia in appropriately selected cases with a high rate of cure. The need for esophagectomy, with its inherent risks, has been obviated in many cases. An endoscopic treatment paradigm, however, must be applied carefully so as not to deprive a patient with early esophageal neoplasia a chance of cure, especially when a safe and effective surgical alternative is available.

Esophagectomy with regional lymphadenectomy remains the standard of care for more advanced cases of esophageal malignancy, as well as for a subset of cases of early-stage disease unamenable to, or having failed, an endoscopic treatment paradigm. In appropriately selected and optimized individuals, and when performed at high-volume centers with specialized multidisciplinary teams and care pathways, esophagectomy can be undertaken with low mortality, acceptable morbidity, and good long-term QOL. Minimally invasive approaches to esophagectomy, including robotics, continue to advance the surgeon's ability to offer surgery with decreased morbidity and quicker recovery compared with traditional open procedures.

DISCLOSURE

A. Pratap: Financial support from Intuitive Inc for Robotic surgery fellowship grant, Consultant Medtronic Inc. M. McCarter: Medical advisory board Debbie's Dream Foundation. T.J. Watson: No disclosures.

REFERENCES

1. Eloubeidi MA, Mason AC, Desmond RA, et al. Temporal trends (1973–1997) in survival of patients with esophageal adenocarcinoma in the United States: a glimmer of hope? Am J Gastroenterol 2003;98:1627–33.
2. Kalish RJ, Clancy PE, Orringer MB, et al. Clinical, epidemiologic and morphologic comparison between adenocarcinomas arising in Barrett's esophageal mucosa and in the gastric cardia. Gastroenterology 1984;86:461–7.
3. Gupta B, Kumar N. Worldwide incidence, mortality and time trends for cancer of the oesophagus. Eur J Cancer Prev 2017;26:107–18.
4. Cook MB, Coburn SB, Lam JR, et al. Cancer incidence and mortality risks in a large US Barrett's oesophagus cohort. Gut 2018;67:418–529.
5. Shaheen NJ, Falk GW, Iyer PG, et al. ACG clinical guideline: diagnosis and management of Barrett's esophagus. Am J Gastroenterol 2016;111:30–50 [quiz: 51].
6. National Comprehensive Cancer Network (NCCN) clinical practice guidelines in oncology. Esophageal and esophagogastric junction cancers. Version 2.2016. Available at: www.NCCN.org. Accessed April 10, 2020.
7. Hamilton SR, Aaltonen LA, editors. Pathology and genetics of tumors of the digestive system (World Health Organization classification of tumors). Lyons (France): International Agency for Research on Cancer (IARC) Press; 2000.
8. Rice TW, Ishwaran H, Hofstetter WL, et al. Recommendations for pathologic staging (pTNM) of cancer of the esophagus and esophagogastric junction for the 8th edition AJCC/UICC staging manuals. Dis Esophagus 2016;29(8):897–905.
9. Lewis JT, Wang KK, Abraham SC. Muscularis mucosae duplication and the musculo-fibrous anomaly in endoscopic mucosal resections for Barrett esophagus: implications for staging of adenocarcinoma. Am J Surg Pathol 2008;32: 566–71.
10. Hagen JA, DeMeester SR, Peters JH, et al. Curative resection for esophageal adenocarcinoma: analysis of 100 en bloc esophagectomies. Ann Surg 2001; 234:520–30.
11. Sepesi B, Watson TJ, Zhou D, et al. Are endoscopic therapies appropriate for superficial submucosal adenocarcinoma? An analysis of esophagectomy specimens. J Am Coll Surg 2010;210(4):418–27.
12. Leers JM, DeMeester SR, Oezcelik A, et al. The prevalence of lymph node metastases in patients with T1 esophageal adenocarcinoma. Ann Surg 2011;253: 271–8.
13. Lee L, Ronellenfitsch U, Hofstetter WL, et al. Predicting lymph node metastases in early esophageal adenocarcinoma using a simple scoring system. J Am Coll Surg 2013;217(2):191–9.
14. Ell C, May A, Pech O, et al. Curative endoscopic resection of early esophageal adenocarcinomas (Barrett's cancer). Gastrointest Endosc 2007;65:3–10.
15. Pech O, Behrens A, May A, et al. Long-term results and risk factor analysis for recurrence after curative endoscopic therapy in 349 patients with high-grade intraepithelial neoplasia and mucosal adenocarcinoma in Barrett's oesophagus. Gut 2008;57:1200–6.

16. Pech O, May A, Manner H, et al. Long-term efficacy and safety of endoscopic resection for patients with mucosal adenocarcinoma of the esophagus. Gastroenterology 2014;146:652–60.
17. Worrell SG, Boys JA, Chandrasoma P, et al. Inter-observer variability in the interpretation of endoscopic mucosal resection specimens of esophageal adenocarcinoma; interpretation of ER specimens. J Gastrointest Surg 2016;20:140–5.
18. Bernardi D, Asti E, Aiolfi A, et al. Outcome of trimodal therapy in elderly patients with esophageal cancer: prognostic value of the Charlson comorbidity index. Anticancer Res 2018;38:1815–20.
19. Skipworth RJ, Parks RW, Stephens NA, et al. The relationship between hospital volume and post-operative mortality rates for upper gastrointestinal cancer resections: Scotland 1982-2003. Eur J Surg Oncol 2010;36:141–7.
20. Boshier PR, Anderson O, Hanna GB. Transthoracic versus transhiatal esophagectomy for the treatment of esophagogastric cancer: a meta-analysis. Ann Surg 2011;254:894–906.
21. Hulscher JB, Tijssen JG, Obertop H, et al. Transthoracic versus transhiatal resection for carcinoma of the esophagus: a meta-analysis. Ann Thorac Surg 2001;72: 306–13.
22. Luketich JD, Pennathur A, Awais O, et al. Outcomes after minimally invasive esophagectomy: review of over 1000 patients. Ann Surg 2012;256:95–103.
23. Nagpal K, Ahmed K, Vats A, et al. Is minimally invasive surgery beneficial in the management of esophageal cancer? A meta-analysis. Surg Endosc 2010;24: 1621–9.
24. Watson T. Robotic esophagectomy: is it an advance and what is the future? Ann Thorac Surg 2008;85:S757–9.
25. Biere SS, van Berge Henegouwen MI, Maas KW, et al. Minimally invasive versus open oesophagectomy for patients with oesophageal cancer: a multicentre, open-label, randomised controlled trial. Lancet 2012;379:1887–92.
26. Mariette C, Markar SR, Dabakuyo-Yonli TS, et al. Hybrid minimally invasive esophagectomy for esophageal cancer. N Engl J Med 2019;380:152–62.
27. van der Sluis PC, van der Horst S, May AM, et al. Robot-assisted minimally invasive thoracolaparoscopic esophagectomy versus open transthoracic esophagectomy for resectable esophageal cancer: a randomized controlled trial. Ann Surg 2019;269:621–30.
28. Triantafyllou T, Olson MT, Theodorou D, et al. Enhanced recovery pathways vs standard care pathways in esophageal cancer surgery: systematic review and meta-analysis. Esophagus 2020;17(2):100–12.
29. Bailey SH, Bull DA, Harpole DH, et al. Outcomes after esophagectomy: a ten-year prospective cohort. Ann Thorac Surg 2003;75:217–22.
30. Connors RC, Reuben BC, Neumayer LA, et al. Comparing outcomes after transthoracic and transhiatal esophagectomy: a 5-year prospective cohort of 17,395 patients. J Am Coll Surg 2007;205:735–40.
31. Sihag S, Kosinski AS, Gaissert HA, et al. Minimally invasive versus open esophagectomy for esophageal cancer: a comparison of early surgical outcomes from the Society of Thoracic Surgeons national database. Ann Thorac Surg 2016;101: 1281–9.
32. Orringer MB, Marshall B, Chang AC, et al. Two thousand transhiatal esophagectomies: changing trends, lessons learned. Ann Surg 2007;246:363–74.
33. Williams VA, Watson TJ, Herbella FA, et al. Esophagectomy for high grade dysplasia is safe, curative, and results in good alimentary outcome. J Gastrointest Surg 2007;11(12):1589–97.

34. Barr H. Ablative mucosectomy is the procedure of choice to prevent Barrett's cancer. Gut 2003;52(1):14–5.
35. Pennathur A, Farkas A, Krasinskas AM, et al. Esophagectomy for T1 esophageal cancer: outcomes in 100 patients and implications for endoscopic therapy. Ann Thorac Surg 2009;87:1048–55.
36. Rice TW, Chen L-Q, Hofstetter WL, et al. Worldwide esophageal cancer collaboration: pathologic staging data. Dis Esophagus 2016;29:724–33.
37. Scarpa M, Valente S, Alfieri R, et al. Systematic review of health-related quality of life after esophagectomy for cancer. World J Gastroenterol 2011;17(42):4660–74.
38. Greene CL, DeMeester SR, Worrell SG, et al. Alimentary satisfaction, gastrointestinal symptoms, and quality of life 10 or more years after esophagectomy with gastric pull-up. J Thorac Cardiovasc Surg 2014;147(3):909–14.

Measuring Quality in Barrett's Esophagus

Time to Embrace Quality Indicators

Vinay Sehgal, MBChB, MRCP, PhD[a,*],
Krish Ragunath, MBBS, MD, DNB, MPhil, FRCP[b], Rehan Haidry, MD, FRCP[a]

KEYWORDS

- Quality indicators • Barrett's esophagus • Endoscopic resection
- Endoscopic eradication therapy • Radiofrequency ablation • Dysplasia

KEY POINTS

- Endoscopic eradication therapy has revolutionized the management of patients with Barrett's neoplasia; despite numerous societal guidelines there exists significant heterogeneity in clinical practice with variable patient outcomes.
- Evidence-based, measurable quality indicators are needed to define standardized and high-quality practice for patients with Barrett's esophagus–related neoplasia.
- This article aligns recently published consensus statements from the United States and United Kingdom based on the best available evidence and expert opinion to drive improved patient outcomes.

INTRODUCTION

The evolution of minimally invasive endoscopic treatment modalities has changed the treatment paradigm for Barrett's esophagus (BE)-related neoplasia in the past decade. Endoscopic eradication therapy (EET) for BE-related neoplasia has been demonstrated to be effective, safe, and durable,[1–6] and as such, EET for BE-related neoplasia is now endorsed by all major international societal guidelines.[7–9] Despite this, there remains a significant variation in clinical practice and endoscopic management of these patients with consequent variation in outcomes. Although guidelines provide high-quality evidence-based recommendations on the management of BE-related neoplasia, these are often not measurable in daily real-life practice. It is also particularly important that medical resources and the provision of health care for

[a] Department of Gastroenterology and Endoscopy, University College London Hospitals NHS Foundation Trust, Ground Floor West, 250 Euston Road, London NW1 2PG, UK; [b] Department of Gastroenterology, Curtin University Medical School, Royal Perth Hospital, Victoria Square, Perth, Western Australia 6000, Australia
* Corresponding author.
E-mail address: vinay.sehgal@nhs.net

Gastrointest Endoscopy Clin N Am 31 (2021) 219–236
https://doi.org/10.1016/j.giec.2020.09.006
giendo.theclinics.com

BE-related neoplasia are organized and apportioned such that highest quality of care is offered in the most cost-effective manner possible. There has therefore been a driver in the past few years to develop robust, relevant, and measurable quality indicators (QIs) to define standardized clinical practice to ensure patients with BE-related neoplasia receive the highest possible quality of care.

In recent years, investigators from the United States and the United Kingdom have both published expert-led consensus statements to develop QIs for EET of BE-related neoplasia.[10,11] Both used a modified Delphi process called RAND/UCLA Appropriateness Method. In comparison with the conventional Delphi process, this method gave more than 30 experts in the field an opportunity to meet to formulate QIs in which the expected health benefits were felt to exceed the expected negative consequences by a wide margin such that it is worth performing without considering the cost. Both groups explored how current clinical evidence and experts lead opinion can develop QIs to protocolize and standardize the selection, treatment, and follow-up of patients undergoing EET for BE neoplasia.

This article has aligned the most similar statements from the Treatment with Resection and Endoscopic Ablation Techniques for Barrett's Esophagus (TREAT-BE) consortium group and UK consensus statements to provide an evidence-based summary of the most relevant QIs related to routine management of BE-related neoplasia.

PRE-PROCEDURE

EET should be Performed by Experts in High-Volume Centers

Gastroenterologists at high-volume academic centers perform significantly more EET compared with those in district general hospitals. It is important, however, to demonstrate if increased case volume correlates with improved outcomes or not. Data from the UK RFA registry has shown that increasing experience in EET is associated with significantly improved rates of complete eradication of dysplasia (CR-D: 91% vs 79.8%, $P<.05$) and intestinal metaplasia (CE-IM: 83.9% vs 71.3%, $P<.05$), a reduction in the requirement for "rescue" endoscopic mucosal resection (EMR) and faster protocol completion.[12] In light of these findings, the expert UK panel recommended that units performing more than 40 EET cases per year were suitable to perform EET for BE-related neoplasia.[11] More recently, long-term outcomes from 678 patients treated with RFA in the UK registry comparing outcomes between high-volume (more than 100), medium-volume (51–100), and low-volume (less than 50) centers were published.[13] This study did not only demonstrate significantly lower recurrence rates in high-volume versus low-volume centers but also identified a significant change-point for outcomes in CR-D (24.5% vs 10.4%, $P<.001$) and CR-IM (30.7% vs 18.6%, $P<.001$) when 12 and 18 cases of RFA were performed. This therefore suggests for the first time that a minimum of 18 supervised RFA cases should be performed before competency in RFA to treat BE dysplasia can be achieved.

All patients being considered for EET should have a formal meeting to discuss the risk, benefits and alternatives to EET alongside formal discussion in a specialist multi-disciplinary team meeting.

As with any medical or surgical intervention, it is of utmost importance that patients have all the necessary information available to them to make an informed decision regarding their care. It is important that before embarking on EET, informed consent is obtained in writing from all patients. This discussion should include the risk of progression to cancer, all treatment options (including surgery) and the risks and benefits of each and the need for long-term surveillance after treatment. This is especially relevant as although there are data reporting improved quality of life (QOL) for endoscopic treatment of early esophageal cancer versus surgery, those treated endoscopically tend to worry more about cancer recurrence than those treated surgically.[14,15]

Ideally these discussions should take place during an outpatient clinic visit; however, if this is not practical, alternative options include a telephone consultation or detailed pre-procedure discussion before the planned procedure. Patients should also have access to written information on any support groups that may be available to them and as well as a clinical nurse specialist. In addition, the guidelines from the British Society of Gastroenterology recommend that all patients being considered for EET should be discussed at specialist multi-disciplinary team (MDT) meeting, which will take into account the patients staging investigations, comorbidities and preferences for treatment.[8]

INTRA-PROCEDURE

The Prague and Paris classifications should be recorded and clearly documented in patients with BE before EET.

Accurate measurement and documentation of the circumferential and maximal extent of BE using the Prague classification (**Fig. 1**) should be recorded for all patients with BE including those having EET and is therefore advocated in all societal guidelines of BE.[7–9,16] There are data to suggest that pretreatment BE extent as measured by the Prague classification correlates with the rate of CE-IM after EET.[17] In this multicentre effectiveness study, patients with C extents of more than 2 cm were less likely to achieve CE-IM compared with those with C extents less than/equal to 2 cm (64.3% vs 73.5%, $P = .027$) thus providing validation of the Prague classification with clinically relevant outcomes in patients undergoing EET for BE-related neoplasia.

The Paris classification of endoscopically visible lesions is a uniform grading system for describing the morphology of visible lesions during endoscopy (**Fig. 2**).[18,19] The

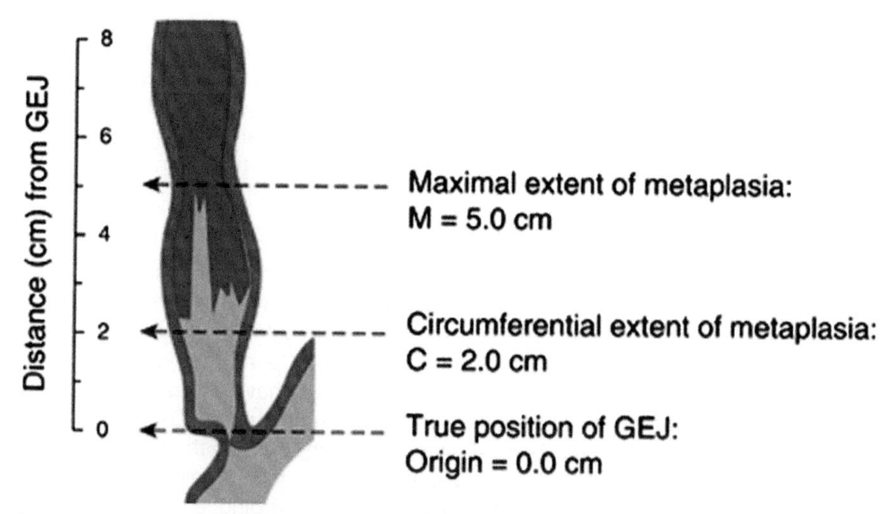

Fig. 1. Illustration of the Prague Classification for Barrett's esophagus. C indicates the circumferential extent and M indicates the maximal extent of metaplasia. This diagram demonstrates a C2M5 segment of BE. (*From* Sharma P, Dent J, Armstrong D, et al. The development and validation of an endoscopic grading system for Barrett's esophagus: the Prague C & M criteria. *Gastroenterology.* 2006;131(5):1392-1399; with permission.)

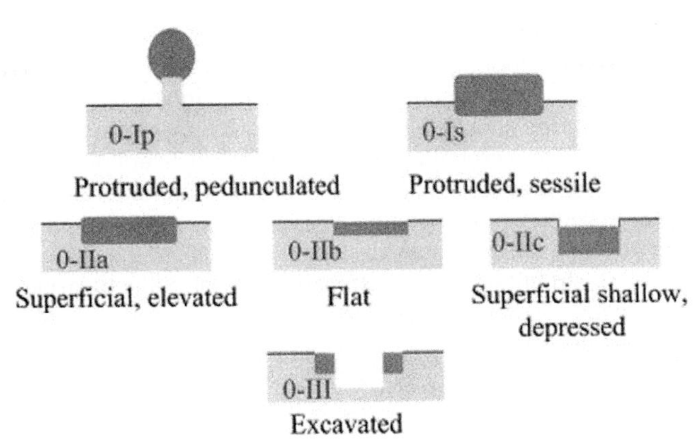

Fig. 2. Schematic representation of the Paris classification of neoplastic lesions of the digestive tracts. Protruded lesions are defined as those more than 2.5mm in height and are divided into polypoid (Ip) and sessile (Is). Flat lesions are subdivided into elevated but less than 2.5mm (IIa), flat (IIb) or depressed (IIc) and excavated lesions (III). Depressed or excavated lesions confer the highest risk of invasive malignancy. (*From* Paris Workshop Participants, The Paris endoscopic classification of superficial neoplastic lesions. Gastrointestinal Endoscopy 58 (6) (Suppl), 2003; with permission.)

Paris classification provides information on the likelihood on the invasion of cancer and helps communication between endoscopists. Whereas Paris IIa and IIb lesions are usually associated with early neoplastic disease that is confined to the mucosa in more than 83% of cases, flat or depressed lesions (0-Is, 0-IIc and 0-III) are usually associated with submucosal invasion with the attendant risk that local lymph node metastases are already present.[20] The Paris classification can therefore help endoscopists decide on the suitability of endoscopic resection and should be recorded for all patients with visible lesions and BE.

As these patients often require repeated endoscopic examinations, accurate recording of the Prague and Paris classifications serves as a useful reference point if patients are either referred onward or once therapy has begun. It is also important for audit and reimbursement purposes as well as large-scale endoscopy data collection such as the National Endoscopy Database, which has recently been introduced in the United Kingdom.

All patients undergoing EET including follow-up should have endoscopic assessment with high-definition white light endoscopy or virtual chromoendoscopy.

The primary role of endoscopic image enhancement is to improve detection of early BE neoplasia. This is vitally important, as up to 25% of patients diagnosed with esophageal cancer have had a "normal" endoscopy within the 12 months preceding their diagnosis.[21] Endoscopists at high-volume centers should have access to advanced imaging with a minimum of high-definition white light endoscopy (HD-WLE) ± virtual chromoendoscopy. HD-WLE has been shown to be more sensitive than standard definition white light endoscopy in detecting dysplasia in BE and is for all intents and purposes considered as standard of care in patients undergoing endoscopy for BE including those being considered for EET.[22–25]

Virtual chromoendoscopy uses optical filters or post-processing technologies that are built into endoscopes. Three main modalities of virtual chromoendoscopy exist: narrow band imaging (NBI; Olympus, Tokyo, Japan), i-Scan (Pentax, Tokyo, Japan), and Blue-light imaging (BLI; Fujifilm, Tokyo, Japan). All work by enhancing the mucosal and microvasculature patterns seen during endoscopy to help enhance dysplasia detection (**Fig. 3**). Data on dysplasia detection in BE surveillance using these optical enhancements has proven encouraging. i-Scan has been found to improve

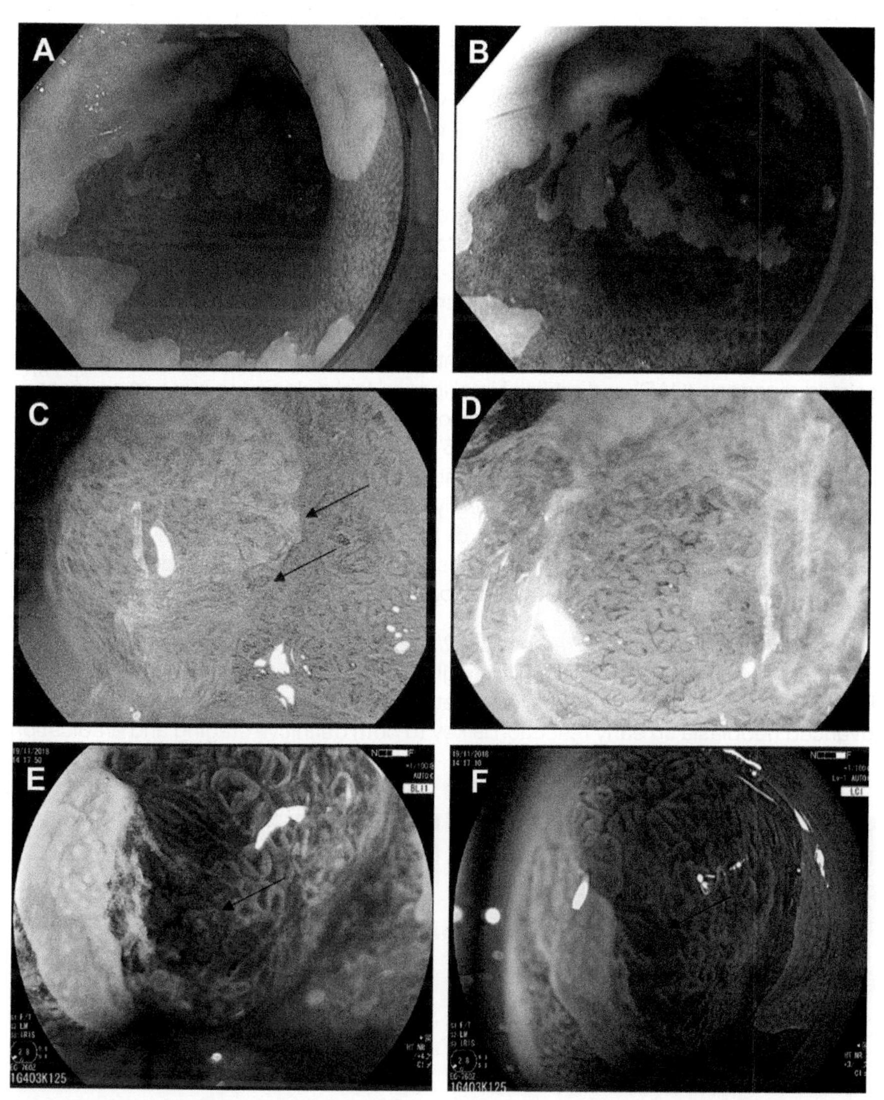

Fig. 3. Endoscopic appearances of Barrett's esophagus using different methods of virtual chromoendoscopy. Flat segment of nondysplastic BE in high definition white-light endoscopy (*A*) and corresponding appearances when using narrow-banding imaging (*B*). Appearances of BE with high-grade dysplasia using i-Scan 1 with zoom magnification revealing featureless mucosal patterns and irregular vasculature (C, *demarcation line* highlighted by *arrows*), which are further attenuated using optical filters in the optical enhancement mode (*D*). Zoom magnification blue-light imaging revealing a lack of mucosal pits (*E*) with corresponding post-processing high contrast linked color imaging demonstrating HGD (*F*).

dysplasia detection in BE compared with HD-WLE with an accuracy and sensitivity of 88%.[26] The addition of zoom magnification to i-Scan has been shown to enhance dysplasia detection even further.[27] A BE neoplasia classification system using BLI was devised and when externally validated on nonexperts after training had a sensitivity and specificity of 95.7% and 80.8%, respectively.[28] NBI has shown the most promise where it is has been reported to have an accuracy, sensitivity and specificity of 92%, 91%, and 93%, respectively.[29] The use of acetic acid (AA) has been shown to improve dysplasia detection with a sensitivity and specificity of 92% and 96%, respectively.[30] As such, only NBI and AA have surpassed the ASGE's published thresholds (sensitivity ≥90%, specificity ≥80%, and per patient negative predictive value >98%) for the preservation and incorporation of valuable endoscopic innovations (PIVI) to replace random biopsies for the detection of dysplasia.[31] All studies of virtual chromoendoscopy have, however, been performed using still images or videos in patients undergoing BE surveillance. This therefore limits the relevance that these data may have on EET for BE-related neoplasia. Given this, the expert UK panel suggested that all patients undergoing EET should have assessment with HD-WLE with chromoendoscopy or virtual chromoendoscopy.

More recently there has been growing interest in the use of endoscopic computer assisted diagnosis (CAD) and artificial intelligence technologies to support endoscopists with real-time system for the detection of early BE neoplasia. A real-time CAD system using WLI and still image analysis in 0.5 seconds per image reported an accuracy, sensitivity and specificity of 90%, 91%, and 89%, respectively.[32] More recently, a deep neural network was trained to analyze and detect neoplasia in endoscopic videos with a sensitivity and specificity of 88% and 80%, respectively.[33] This is an exciting area of endoscopic research that is likely to evolve further and in time potentially meet PIVI thresholds to replace random biopsy in BE.

All visible lesions should be removed entirely using endoscopic resection.

With advancements in endoscopic imaging, endoscopists are now able to detect visible lesions and mucosal anomalies in detail (**Fig. 4**). These are more likely to harbor advanced neoplasia so early resection is key to both definitive staging and eradication

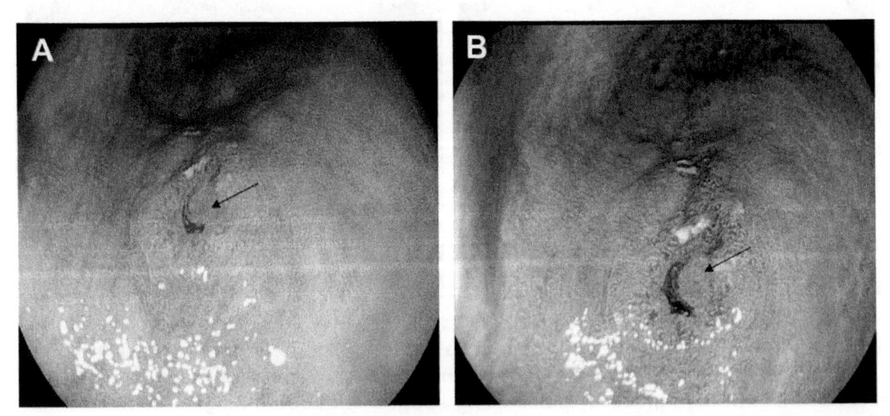

Fig. 4. Endoscopic images of a visible lesion within a segment of BE. Example of a superficially elevated lesion with a depressed center (Paris IIa/c) highlighted by the arrow using i-Scan 1 (*A*). The corresponding optical enhancement mode helps to further highlight the distorted mucosal surface pattern with featureless central depression (*arrow*) and irregular micro-vasculature suggestive of HGD at least (*B*).

before RFA. Endoscopic resection (ER) of visible lesions provides accurate histopathological staging and concomitant therapy in patients with BE-related neoplasia. Compared with biopsy, EMR results in a change of diagnosis for approximately 30% of patients with early neoplasia referred for EET (upgrade 10.1%, downgrade 21%).[34] The provision of a larger specimen has been also shown in many studies to improve interobserver agreement among pathologists compared with biopsies alone.[35] Most resection specimens also contain submucosal tissue allowing differentiation from mucosal and submucosal involvement in a more accurate manner than endoscopic ultrasound. Submucosal involvement is thought to be a poor prognostic feature for endoscopic therapy due to the risk of occult lymph node metastases. As such, ER can be used to filter out these patients to surgery, although more recently the rate of lymph node metastases was lower than those originally reported meaning more patients may be suitable for curative endoscopic therapy than originally thought possible.[36] The more widespread use of EMR is also thought to be associated with a reduction in the need for "rescue" EMR after the start of RFA treatment. Long-term outcomes from the UK RFA registry, which reported a 60% increase in EMR before RFA, found a significant reduction in the requirement for "rescue" EMR after starting RFA (13% vs 2%, $P<.0001$).[37]

EMR using a method of multiband mucosectomy has been widely studied and is safe. Numerous studies have demonstrated long-term complete remission rates of between 85% and 96% with bleeding rates of 0.7% to 7.9% and perforation rates of 0.2% to 2.3%.[38] Endoscopic submucosal dissection (ESD) is an alternative resection technique that facilitates a higher en bloc resection rate (pooled estimate 92.9%, 95% confidence interval [CI] 90.3%–95.2%) and evaluation of the lateral resection margins in a manner that is not feasible with piecemeal EMR.[39] Although complication rates are higher than EMR, they are still broadly acceptable (pooled estimates of perforation: 1.5%, bleeding 1.7%, stricture: 11.6%). ESD does however require higher operator skill and experience compared with those performing EMR alone. A randomized trial of EMR versus ESD for early BE neoplasia found no difference in complete remission (EMR 16/17 vs ESD 15/16, $P = 1.0$) and disease recurrence (EMR 0/17 vs ESD 1/16, $P = 1.0$) after 3 and 23 months, respectively.[40] Accordingly, the European Society of Gastrointestinal Endoscopy (ESGE) has recommended that EMR is acceptable for resection of lesions confined to the mucosa (regardless of size) and that ESD may be suitable for lesions larger than 15 mm, poorly lifting tumors, and those at high risk of submucosal invasion.[9] It is important to bear in mind, however, some of the unique practical and logistical challenges posed by ESD. ESD is a complex and demanding procedure that requires extensive training and expert supervision before being performed independently. ESD is also time-consuming and has a requirement for propofol or general anesthesia, which requires reorganization of therapeutic endoscopy lists and anesthetic slots that are a scarce resource in many countries including the United Kingdom.

All resected lesions should have accurate assessment and recording of histopathological prognostic features to determine if the resection is deemed curative.

Accurate histopathological assessment of all resection specimens is important for risk stratification and staging of patients undergoing EET. There is robust evidence that dysplasia is a risk factor for cancer progression although accurate diagnosis can be challenging. In contrast to high-grade dysplasia (HGD) in which there are usually strong levels of agreement among pathologists, interobserver agreement among pathologists who are diagnosing low-grade dysplasia is often weak.[41] In addition,

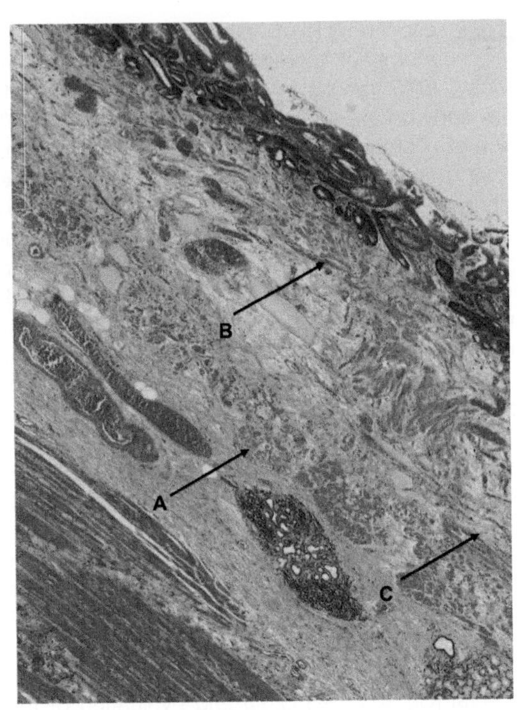

Fig. 5. Hematoxylin and eosin stain from an EMR specimen of BE. The original (A) and duplicated muscularis mucosae (B) are highlighted and converge (C) making accurate histopathological assessment challenging. (*Courtesy of* M Novelli; with permission.)

duplication of the muscularis mucosae is frequently seen in ER specimens, thus making accurate disease staging more challenging (**Fig. 5**).

Consequently, most major societal guidelines recommend that 2 expert histopathologists with a specialist interest in BE report all resection specimens particularly when dysplasia is suspected. Although the exact definition of what constitutes an "expert" histopathologist remain unclear, there is evidence to suggest that those with at least 5 years of professional experience working in a teaching hospital is protective against major diagnostic error.[42] In future, the improved performance of digital pathology reporting of whole slide imaging is expected to gain more widespread acceptance.[43] This technology will allow simultaneous assessment by multiple pathologists during a streamlined consultation using digital image analysis and opens the door to centralized histopathology reporting in BE.

There are now robust long-term data that have demonstrated that ER of neoplasia confined to the mucosa is curative in excess of 95% of patients over 5 years.[44] This study also identified adverse histopathological features that favored failure of EET including patients with a long segment of BE and poorly differentiated mucosal cancers (both $P<.0001$). The prognosis of lesions that have invaded the submucosa is also less favorable due to the significantly higher risk of occult lymph node (LN) metastases. The risk of LN metastases for mucosal neoplasia is in the range of 1% to 2%, whereas in cases of submucosal invasion the risk may be as high a 9%.[45,46] However, for those patients with low-risk submucosal lesions (submucosal invasion <500 nm, well-moderate tumor differentiation, no lymphovascular invasion), the risk of metastatic disease after a median follow-up on 5 years was lower than the mortality of esophagectomy (3%). This is in contrast to high-risk submucosal lesions with adverse histopathological features in whom the risk of LN metastases was 9%. It has therefore been recommended that only low-risk lesions with submucosal invasion should be considered for curative EET. All patients with high-risk submucosal lesions should be referred for surgery after formal discussion at the MDT and with the patient.[11]

Endoscopic ablation of all residual BE following ER and nonvisible dysplasia should be performed.

Historically ER of neoplastic BE was used as monotherapy without treatment of the residual non-neoplastic BE. It has been reported, however, that up to one-third of patients treated with ER who achieve complete resolution of the primary lesion subsequently develop recurrent HGD or EAC.[47] Pech and colleagues found that rates of metachronous neoplasia were significantly lower in patients who had ER and ablative therapies compared to ER alone (ablation 16.5% vs no ablation 29.9%, $P = .0014$). Numerous studies and meta-analyses have demonstrated that multi-modal ER combined with radiofrequency ablation (RFA) can achieve CE-D and CE-IM rates in excess of 90%.[1–3,6,12] Patients in whom dysplasia is detected without any visible lesions (in spite of careful inspection with HD-WLE and virtual chromoendoscopy) should also be offered endoscopic ablation of their BE segment. Before ablation, the histopathological diagnosis of dysplasia should again be confirmed by 2 expert BE pathologists and discussed at the MDT. An illustration of the different focal and circumferential RFA devices is shown in **Fig. 6**.

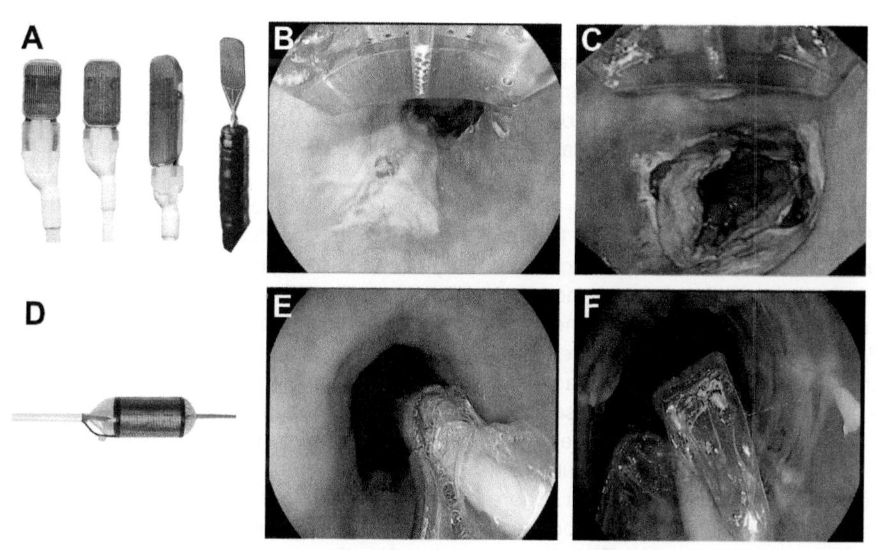

Fig. 6. Illustration of different focal and circumferential radiofrequency ablation devices used to treat patients for BE-related dysplasia. (*A*) Range of endoscope-mounted focal catheters with varying electrode lengths to help treat differing BE segments (from left to right): RFA 60 to 15 mm, RFA 90 to 20 mm, RFA Ultra Long 40 mm, RFA Endoscopic Channel Catheter 15.7 mm. Endoscopic appearances of RFA 90 catheter during (*B*) and immediately after treatment (*C*) with white visible coagulum indicating treatment coverage. (*D*) RFA 360 Express Catheter with 80 mm self-sizing balloon and 40 mm electrode length. Endoscopic appearances of RFA 360 Express Catheter with top of electrode positioned at proximal end of BE before (*E*) and after treatment (*F*). ([*A, D*] ©2020 Medtronic. All rights reserved. Used with the permission of Medtronic.)

The efficacy, safety profile, and durability of RFA has made this the ablative modality of choice. A randomized trial comparing RFA with argon plasma coagulation (APC) demonstrated similar CR-D (RFA 79% vs APC 84%; odds ratio 0.7, 95% CI 0.2–2.6) and stricture rates (RFA 8.3% vs APC 8.1%) between both treatment modalities.[48] Although RFA was more expensive per case than APC, this study was not adequately powered to detect a significant difference and thus a fully powered noninferiority trial was recommended. Other ablative strategies such as cryoablation are still in the research phase and cannot at present be recommended as first-line ablative therapy for dysplastic BE.[49]

Focal RFA dosimetry is 12 J/cm² × 3 without interval cleaning and circumferential RFA dosimetry is 10 J/cm² × 2 with interval cleaning.

Since the first circumferential RFA catheter for BE was described in 2005, a self-sizing balloon-based catheter (360 Express) and numerous focal devices have been developed to help treat different lengths of BE. This led to a number of studies with a common goal of ascertaining a standardized treatment protocol that is able to combine optimal surface regression of BE with adequate safety.

A simplified focal RFA regimen (3 × 15 J/cm², without cleaning) was shown to be as effective as the standard regimen that was first developed (2 × 15 J/cm², followed by cleaning, followed by 2 × 15 J/cm²).[50] This simplified regimen was, however, associated with a higher stenosis rate, which led to a multicenter randomized trial comparing a new simplified regimen (3 × 12 J/cm²) with the standard regimen.[51] After 2 focal RFA treatments, there was no significant difference in CE-IM rates (simplified regimen 74% vs standard regimen 83%, $P = .34$) and surface regression (simplified regimen 98% vs standard regimen 100%). There was also no difference in the adverse events in both groups such that the more recent simplified RFA regimen (3 × 12 J/cm²) is now the preferred focal ablation strategy for BE dysplasia.

The circumferential RFA balloon catheter (360 Express) is useful to treat longer segments of BE with reported surface regression of up to 85% after only 3 months.[52] This study investigated 3 different treatment regimens using the 360 Express catheter: standard (1 × 10 J/cm²-clean-1 × 10 J/cm²), simple-double (2 × 10 J/cm² with no clean) and simple-single (1 × 10 J/cm² with no clean) regimens. The simple-double arm of the study had to be terminated early because of a high stenosis rate. Despite this, the standard regimen demonstrated higher median BE regression compared with the simple-single group (standard regimen 85% vs simple-single regimen 73%, $P = .009$). Similar findings were reported by specialist centers in the United Kingdom and Ireland with a mean surface regression of 55% but stricture rate of 15% after 3 months of follow-up.[53] Consequently, the standard regimen (1 × 10 J/cm²-clean-1 × 10 J/cm²) is endorsed when using the 360 Express catheter.

The optimal endoscopic surveillance intervals for patients undergoing EET for neoplastic BE remains unclear. There is also lack of data comparing outcomes between different intervals for repeat endoscopy in those patients that have yet to complete treatment. The UK RFA registry protocol performed repeat endoscopy every 3 months after ER until all visible BE was ablated with CR-D and CR-IM rates of 92% and 83%, respectively.[12] Data from the US RFA registry showed that patients treated with RFA similarly had a repeat endoscopy every 3 months until completion of treatment.[6] In view of the lack of data and the fact that both the US and UK registries perform 3-monthly endoscopies, a 2 to 4 monthly interval would seem reasonable.

Complete eradication of dysplasia and intestinal metaplasia should be achieved by at least 80% and 70% of patients, respectively, by 18 months.

The achievement of CR-D and CR-IM are clearly defined goals for EET of BE-related neoplasia. Less well defined are the proportion of patients who should reach these thresholds after appropriate periods of treatment.

Since the landmark Ablation of Intestinal Metaplasia Containing Dysplasia (AIM Dysplasia) trial there have been a wealth of long-term observational and registry data demonstrating the effectiveness, safety, and durability of EET for the treatment of BE-related neoplasia.[1–3] The AIM Dysplasia Trial demonstrated significantly higher rates of CE-D and CE-IM in patients undergoing ablation compared with those undergoing a sham procedure (low-grade dysplasia [LGD]: CE-D 90.5% vs 22.7%, HGD: CE-D 81% vs 19%; *P*<.001).[1] Data from the UK RFA registry and the multicentre interventional EURO II study have shown that EET is capable of achieving CE-D in 92% and CE-IM in 83% to 87% of patients at 12 months. These findings have been further supported in a systematic review and meta-analysis of 18 studies (3802 patients) that reported CR-D and CR-IM rates of 91% and 78%, respectively.[2,3] Based on these data and taking into account real-world experience, including patient noncompliance or waiting list delays, the consortium of US and UK experts recommended CR-D rates of 80% and greater than 90%, respectively, and CR-IM rates of 70% and greater than 80% at 18 months after treatment.[10,11] End of treatment should be confirmed by 2 successive negative endoscopies followed by appropriate surveillance intervals that are stratified according to the risk of recurrence.

Patients with residual dysplasia after 18 months should be re-discussed at an esophagogastric MDT.

Treatment for the vast majority of patients with EET for BE-related mucosal neoplasia is effective and durable. It is important however to identify those patients who fail to respond to therapy and evaluate the appropriateness for ongoing treatment after a suitable time interval. Pech and colleagues[47] demonstrated that risk factors associated with recurrence included piecemeal resection, long-segment BE, no ablation to residual BE, time until complete response achieved of more than 10 months and multifocal neoplasia. In light of these data it has been recommended that patients with residual BE neoplasia after 18 months from the start of treatment should have their case re-discussed at a specialist esophagogastric MDT to consider further investigations and treatment options.

The symptomatic stricture rate after EET for BE neoplasia should not exceed 10% to 15%.

One of the most common side effects of EET is iatrogenic stricture formation. Although this can often be predictable (particularly for ER of lesions occupying more than 75% of the esophageal circumference) it is important these are prevented wherever possible and treated promptly to minimize the adverse effect on the patient's QOL. The symptomatic stricture rate (SSR) after EET for BE neoplasia from several major studies ranges from 2.1% to 11.6%.[39] These include research data from the UK RFA registry (SSR 6.2%), the EURO study (SSR 6%) and meta-analyses of EET with RFA/EMR (SSR 5.6%) and ESD (SSR 11.6%).[3,37,39] Wider resection of the circumference is considered to be the most important risk factor for the development of strictures independent of the technique of resection. As such, the extent of resection should be minimized to help limit the rate of stricture formation wherever possible. Endoscopic dilatation is often required repeatedly but is often inconvenient for patients and harbors a perforation rate of approximately 1%.[54] Local or system corticosteroids may reduce injury-induced inflammation leading to reduction in the formation of granulation tissue and have therefore been the subject of much research. A meta-analysis of 513 patients treated with corticosteroids post-esophageal ESD found a 60% reduction in the stricture rates and need for dilatation.[55] More recently, a randomized control trial found that a 6-week post-procedural course of Budesonide slurry twice daily after complete EMR of a short-segment BE reduced stricture formation from 37% to 14%.[56] As EMR and ESD are performed increasingly as part of EET for BE neoplasia, we would expect stricture rates to increase. Given this and the literature to date, we would suggest that centers performing EET should not have SSR which are higher than 10% to 15%.

POST-PROCEDURE

After achievement of CR-IM, patients should undergo follow-up surveillance endoscopies at appropriate time intervals that are stratified according to the risk of recurrence.

Despite the effectiveness of EET using a combination of ER and RFA, up to 15% and 40% of patients may develop recurrence of dysplasia and intestinal metaplasia respectively. This highlights the need for ongoing endoscopic surveillance after EET. The most commonly adopted surveillance intervals were based on those used in the original AIM Dysplasia Trial. Although these have been associated with low rates of recurrent untreatable BE neoplasia (CR-D 98% and CR-IM 91% at 3 years), these were not evidence-based and if anything, probably advocated too frequent endoscopic surveillance.[1] To help answer this question, Cotton and colleagues[57] published evidence-based surveillance intervals based on modeling the rates of neoplastic recurrence using data from the US and UK RFA registries. This model used the highest grade of pre-CE-IM histology to predict the risk of recurrence and performed well when validated against the UK RFA registry. Accordingly, this model divided patients into 2 groups with separate proposed surveillance intervals for each: LGD at 1 and 3 years after CE-IM and HGD/intramucosal cancer (IMC) at months 3, 6, 12 and annually after CE-IM. When compared with the original AIM Dysplasia Trial surveillance intervals, patients with LGD at baseline had a 66% reduction in endoscopic examinations and those with HGD/IMC a 22% reduction over 5 years.

At surveillance endoscopy, biopsies should be taken from the squamo-columnar junction and within the extent of the original BE. Any visible lesions should be biopsied or resected separately.

After CE-IM has been achieved, endoscopic surveillance using HD-WLE and virtual chromoendoscopy should be used to interrogate the gastro-esophageal junction (GOJ) in anterograde and retrograde views as well as the previously treated segment of BE. The GOJ is particularly important given that it is the most site for recurrence, which is often not visible. Provided no visible lesions are identified, random biopsies from the squamo-columnar junction and the original BE segment according to the Seattle protocol have been used in most long-term studies/registries to confirm CE-D and CE-IM. Although this approach seems reasonable, clinical evidence to support this is limited. In addition, this approach often requires a large number of biopsies with increased procedure time, risk of bleeding, and cost of histopathological assessment. More recently, a study has questioned the diagnostic yield of such random biopsies.[58] The highest risk of dysplasia recurrence is at the GOJ/cardia which is also more likely to be invisible. In this study, 32/198 patients developed recurrence during a mean follow-up of 3 years. The most common site for recurrence was 1 cm proximal to the GOJ (81%). Instances of recurrence more than 1 cm proximal to the GOJ was always accompanied by the presence of a visible lesion. Random biopsies more than

1 cm above the GOJ had no yield for recurrence. These data would suggest random biopsies should need only to be obtained from the OGJ (and 1 cm proximal) and from any visible lesions within the area of the previous BE segment. This study was however performed at a single center by a small group of expert endoscopists who are likely to have a better chance of detecting visible lesions than general endoscopists leading to the potential for a not insignificant rate of missed neoplasia if random biopsies were not obtained. Together with a lack of external validation, random Seattle protocol biopsies from the GOJ and from every 1 to 2 cm of the pretreatment segment of BE to exclude metachronous neoplasia remains the recommended protocol at present. A more recent study from 5 prospectively maintained databases from the United States and United Kingdom found that 82% of recurrences in the tubular esophagus were visible endoscopically. Of the 18% that were not visible, only one had LGD, meaning the yield of random biopsy sampling for dysplasia recurrence was only 0.2%.[59] Although not yet in any guidelines, these data are likely to represent future practice pertaining to surveillance biopsies moving forward (**Fig. 7**).

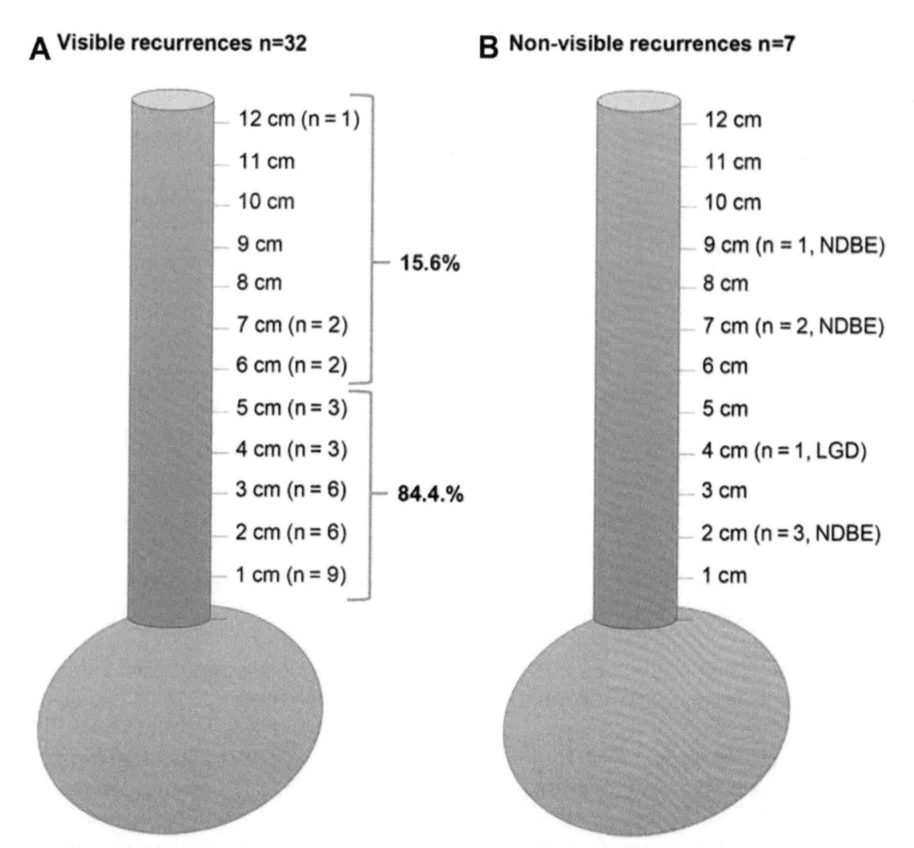

Fig. 7. Location of recurrence after completion of EET. Location of visible (*A*) and nonvisible (*B*) recurrence in the tubular esophagus (*blue cylinder*). Histology of nonvisible recurrences is also shown in (*B*). NDBE, nondysplastic BE. (*From* Sami SS, Ravindran A, Kahn A, et al. Timeline and location of recurrence following successful ablation in Barrett's oesophagus: an international multicentre study. *Gut.* 2019;68(8):1379-1385; with permission.)

DISCUSSION

The rapid evolvement of EET has drastically changed the treatment paradigm of BE-related neoplasia. Despite a breadth of published data over the past decade supporting EET, there has been a relative lack of clearly defined and measurable QIs, which this article has hopefully begun to address. It is likely that these QIs will need to be modified to take into account continued improvements in endoscopic technology and the increased uptake of ESD. Despite this, these QIs should still provide a benchmark and method of ensuring accountable delivery according to best practice for patients undergoing EET for BE-related neoplasia.

DISCLOSURE

V. Sehgal: No disclosures. K. Ragunath: Olympus: consultancy, educational grants and research grants, Pentax: educational and research grants, Boston Scientific: Consultancy, educational grants, Cook Medical: Research and educational grants, Medtronics: Educational grants, ERBE: Educational grants, CDx diagnostics: consultancy and research support. R. Haidry: Educational grants to support research: Medtronic Ltd., Cook Endoscopy (fellowship support), Pentax Europe and C2 Therapeutics, Beamline diagnostics, Fractyl Ltd.

REFERENCES

1. Shaheen NJ, Sharma P, Overholt BF, et al. Radiofrequency ablation in Barrett's esophagus with dysplasia. N Engl J Med 2009;360(22):2277–88.
2. Haidry RJ, Dunn JM, Butt MA, et al. Radiofrequency ablation and endoscopic mucosal resection for dysplastic barrett's esophagus and early esophageal adenocarcinoma: outcomes of the UK National Halo RFA Registry. Gastroenterology 2013;145(1):87–95.
3. Phoa KN, Pouw RE, Bisschops R, et al. Multimodality endoscopic eradication for neoplastic Barrett oesophagus: results of an European multicentre study (EURO-II). Gut 2016;65(4):555–62.
4. Phoa KN, van Vilsteren FG, Weusten BL, et al. Radiofrequency ablation vs endoscopic surveillance for patients with Barrett esophagus and low-grade dysplasia: a randomized clinical trial. Jama 2014;311(12):1209–17.
5. Wolf WA, Pasricha S, Cotton C, et al. Incidence of esophageal adenocarcinoma and causes of mortality after radiofrequency ablation of Barrett's esophagus. Gastroenterology 2015;149(7):1752–61.e1.
6. Orman ES, Li N, Shaheen NJ. Efficacy and durability of radiofrequency ablation for Barrett's Esophagus: systematic review and meta-analysis. Clin Gastroenterol Hepatol 2013;11(10):1245–55.
7. Shaheen NJ, Falk GW, Iyer PG, et al. ACG clinical guideline: diagnosis and management of barrett's esophagus. Am J Gastroenterol 2016;111(1):30–50 [quiz: 51].
8. Fitzgerald RC, di Pietro M, Ragunath K, et al. British Society of Gastroenterology guidelines on the diagnosis and management of Barrett's oesophagus. Gut 2014; 63(1):7–42.
9. Weusten B, Bisschops R, Coron E, et al. Endoscopic management of Barrett's esophagus: European Society of Gastrointestinal Endoscopy (ESGE) Position Statement. Endoscopy 2017;49(2):191–8.
10. Wani S, Muthusamy VR, Shaheen NJ, et al. Development of quality indicators for endoscopic eradication therapies in Barrett's esophagus: the TREAT-BE

(Treatment with Resection and Endoscopic Ablation Techniques for Barrett's Esophagus) Consortium. Gastrointest Endosc 2017;86(1):1–17.e13.
11. Alzoubaidi D, Ragunath K, Wani S, et al. Quality indicators for Barrett's endotherapy (QBET): UK consensus statements for patients undergoing endoscopic therapy for Barrett's neoplasia. Frontline Gastroenterol 2019;11(4):259–71.
12. Haidry RJ, Lipman G, Banks MR, et al. Comparing outcome of radiofrequency ablation in Barrett's with high grade dysplasia and intramucosal carcinoma: a prospective multicenter UK registry. Endoscopy 2015;47(11):980–7.
13. Lipman G, Markar S, Gupta A, et al. Learning curves and the influence of procedural volume for the treatment of dysplastic Barrett's esophagus. Gastrointest Endosc 2020;92(3):543–50.e1.
14. Rosmolen WD, Nieuwkerk PT, Pouw RE, et al. Quality of life and fear of cancer recurrence after endoscopic treatment for early Barrett's neoplasia: a prospective study. Dis Esophagus 2017;30(3):1–9.
15. Rosmolen WD, Boer KR, de Leeuw RJ, et al. Quality of life and fear of cancer recurrence after endoscopic and surgical treatment for early neoplasia in Barrett's esophagus. Endoscopy 2010;42(7):525–31.
16. Sharma P, Dent J, Armstrong D, et al. The development and validation of an endoscopic grading system for Barrett's esophagus: the Prague C & M criteria. Gastroenterology 2006;131(5):1392–9.
17. Konda VJ, Repici A, Gupta N, et al. Sa1073 the Prague criteria predict response to successful endoscopic eradication therapy for Barrett's esophagus with dysplasia or early cancer: results from an international, multi-center consortium. Gastroenterology 2015;148(4). S-214–S-215.
18. The Paris endoscopic classification of superficial neoplastic lesions: esophagus, stomach, and colon: November 30 to December 1, 2002. Gastrointest Endosc 2003;58(6 Suppl):S3–43.
19. Paris Workshop on Columnar Metaplasia in the Esophagus and the Esophagogastric Junction, Paris, France, December 11-12 2004. Endoscopy 2005;37(9): 879–920.
20. Everson MA, Ragunath K, Bhandari P, et al. How to perform a high-quality examination in patients with Barrett's esophagus. Gastroenterology 2018;154(5): 1222–6.
21. Visrodia K, Singh S, Krishnamoorthi R, et al. Magnitude of missed esophageal adenocarcinoma after Barrett's esophagus diagnosis: a systematic review and meta-analysis. Gastroenterology 2016;150(3):599–607.e7 [quiz: e514–5].
22. Wolfsen HC, Crook JE, Krishna M, et al. Prospective, controlled tandem endoscopy study of narrow band imaging for dysplasia detection in Barrett's Esophagus. Gastroenterology 2008;135(1):24–31.
23. Kara MA, Peters FP, Rosmolen WD, et al. High-resolution endoscopy plus chromoendoscopy or narrow-band imaging in Barrett's esophagus: a prospective randomized crossover study. Endoscopy 2005;37(10):929–36.
24. Curvers W, Baak L, Kiesslich R, et al. Chromoendoscopy and narrow-band imaging compared with high-resolution magnification endoscopy in Barrett's esophagus. Gastroenterology 2008;134(3):670–9.
25. Sami SS, Subramanian V, Butt WM, et al. High definition versus standard definition white light endoscopy for detecting dysplasia in patients with Barrett's esophagus. Dis Esophagus 2015;28(8):742–9.
26. Sehgal V, Rosenfeld A, Graham DG, et al. Machine learning creates a simple endoscopic classification system that improves dysplasia detection in Barrett's

oesophagus amongst non-expert endoscopists. Gastroenterol Res Pract 2018; 2018:1872437.

27. Lipman G, Bisschops R, Sehgal V, et al. Systematic assessment with I-SCAN magnification endoscopy and acetic acid improves dysplasia detection in patients with Barrett's esophagus. Endoscopy 2017;49(12):1219–28.
28. Subramaniam S, Kandiah K, Schoon E, et al. Development and validation of the international Blue Light Imaging for Barrett's Neoplasia Classification. Gastrointest Endosc 2020;91(2):310–20.
29. Sharma P, Bergman JJ, Goda K, et al. Development and validation of a classification system to identify high-grade dysplasia and esophageal adenocarcinoma in Barrett's esophagus using narrow-band imaging. Gastroenterology 2016; 150(3):591–8.
30. Coletta M, Sami SS, Nachiappan A, et al. Acetic acid chromoendoscopy for the diagnosis of early neoplasia and specialized intestinal metaplasia in Barrett's esophagus: a meta-analysis. Gastrointest Endosc 2016;83(1):57–67.e1.
31. Sharma P, Savides TJ, Canto MI, et al. The American Society for Gastrointestinal Endoscopy PIVI (Preservation and Incorporation of Valuable Endoscopic Innovations) on imaging in Barrett's Esophagus. Gastrointest Endosc 2012;76(2):252–4.
32. de Groof AJ, Struyvenberg MR, Fockens KN, et al. Deep learning algorithm detection of Barrett's neoplasia with high accuracy during live endoscopic procedures: a pilot study (with video). Gastrointest Endosc 2020;91(6):1242–50.
33. Hussein M, Gonzales J, Brandao P, et al. Deep Neural network for the detection of early neoplasia in Barrett's oesophagus. Gastrointestinal Endoscopy (Suppl), in press.
34. Wani S, Abrams J, Edmundowicz SA, et al. Endoscopic mucosal resection results in change of histologic diagnosis in Barrett's esophagus patients with visible and flat neoplasia: a multicenter cohort study. Dig Dis Sci 2013;58(6):1703–9.
35. Wani S, Mathur SC, Curvers WL, et al. Greater interobserver agreement by endoscopic mucosal resection than biopsy samples in Barrett's dysplasia. Clin Gastroenterol Hepatol 2010;8(9):783–8.
36. Künzli HT, Belghazi K, Pouw RE, et al. Endoscopic management and follow-up of patients with a submucosal esophageal adenocarcinoma. United European Gastroenterol J 2018;6(5):669–77.
37. Haidry RJ, Butt MA, Dunn JM, et al. Improvement over time in outcomes for patients undergoing endoscopic therapy for Barrett's oesophagus-related neoplasia: 6-year experience from the first 500 patients treated in the UK patient registry. Gut 2015;64(8):1192–9.
38. Tomizawa Y, Konda VJA, Coronel E, et al. Efficacy, durability, and safety of complete endoscopic mucosal resection of barrett esophagus: a systematic review and meta-analysis. J Clin Gastroenterol 2018;52(3):210–6.
39. Yang D, Zou F, Xiong S, et al. Endoscopic submucosal dissection for early Barrett's neoplasia: a meta-analysis. Gastrointest Endosc 2018;87(6):1383–93.
40. Terheggen G, Horn EM, Vieth M, et al. A randomised trial of endoscopic submucosal dissection versus endoscopic mucosal resection for early Barrett's neoplasia. Gut 2017;66(5):783–93.
41. Wani S, Falk GW, Post J, et al. Risk factors for progression of low-grade dysplasia in patients with Barrett's esophagus. Gastroenterology 2011;141(4):1179–86, 1186.e1.
42. van der Wel MJ, Coleman HG, Bergman J, et al. Histopathologist features predictive of diagnostic concordance at expert level among a large international sample

of pathologists diagnosing Barrett's dysplasia using digital pathology. Gut 2019; 69(5):811–22.
43. Mukhopadhyay S, Feldman MD, Abels E, et al. Whole slide imaging versus microscopy for primary diagnosis in surgical pathology: a multicenter blinded randomized noninferiority study of 1992 cases (pivotal study). Am J Surg Pathol 2018; 42(1):39–52.
44. Pech O, May A, Manner H, et al. Long-term efficacy and safety of endoscopic resection for patients with mucosal adenocarcinoma of the esophagus. Gastroenterology 2014;146(3):652–60.e1.
45. Dunbar KB, Spechler SJ. The risk of lymph-node metastases in patients with high-grade dysplasia or intramucosal carcinoma in Barrett's esophagus: a systematic review. Am J Gastroenterol 2012;107(6):850–62 [quiz: 863].
46. Scholvinck D, Kunzli H, Meijer S, et al. Management of patients with T1b esophageal adenocarcinoma: a retrospective cohort study on patient management and risk of metastatic disease. Surg Endosc 2016;30(9):4102–13.
47. Pech O, Behrens A, May A, et al. Long-term results and risk factor analysis for recurrence after curative endoscopic therapy in 349 patients with high-grade intraepithelial neoplasia and mucosal adenocarcinoma in Barrett's oesophagus. Gut 2008;57(9):1200–6.
48. Peerally MF, Bhandari P, Ragunath K, et al. Radiofrequency ablation compared with argon plasma coagulation after endoscopic resection of high-grade dysplasia or stage T1 adenocarcinoma in Barrett's esophagus: a randomized pilot study (BRIDE). Gastrointest Endosc 2019;89(4):680–9.
49. Canto MI, Shaheen NJ, Almario JA, et al. Multifocal nitrous oxide cryoballoon ablation with or without EMR for treatment of neoplastic Barrett's esophagus (with video). Gastrointest Endosc 2018;88(3):438–46.e2.
50. van Vilsteren FG, Phoa KN, Alvarez Herrero L, et al. A simplified regimen for focal radiofrequency ablation of Barrett's mucosa: a randomized multicenter trial comparing two ablation regimens. Gastrointest Endosc 2013;78(1):30–8.
51. Pouw RE, Kunzli HT, Bisschops R, et al. Simplified versus standard regimen for focal radiofrequency ablation of dysplastic Barrett's oesophagus: a multicentre randomised controlled trial. Lancet Gastroenterol Hepatol 2018;3(8):566–74.
52. Belghazi K, Pouw RE, Koch AD, et al. Self-sizing radiofrequency ablation balloon for eradication of Barrett's esophagus: results of an international multicenter randomized trial comparing 3 different treatment regimens. Gastrointest Endosc 2019;90(3):415–23.
53. Magee C, Gordon C, Dunn J, et al. OTU-013 Outcomes of 360 HALO express radio-frequency ablation for Barrett's oesophagus related neoplasia. Gut 2018; 67(Suppl 1):A138.
54. Uno K, Iijima K, Koike T, et al. Useful strategies to prevent severe stricture after endoscopic submucosal dissection for superficial esophageal neoplasm. World J Gastroenterol 2015;21(23):7120–33.
55. Wang W, Ma Z. Steroid administration is effective to prevent strictures after endoscopic esophageal submucosal dissection: a network meta-analysis. Medicine 2015;94(39):e1664.
56. Bahin FF, Jayanna M, Williams SJ, et al. Efficacy of viscous budesonide slurry for prevention of esophageal stricture formation after complete endoscopic mucosal resection of short-segment Barrett's neoplasia. Endoscopy 2016;48(1):71–4.
57. Cotton CC, Haidry R, Thrift AP, et al. Development of evidence-based surveillance intervals after radiofrequency ablation of Barrett's esophagus. Gastroenterology 2018;155(2):316–326 e6.

58. Cotton CC, Wolf WA, Pasricha S, et al. Recurrent intestinal metaplasia after radiofrequency ablation for Barrett's esophagus: endoscopic findings and anatomic location. Gastrointest Endosc 2015;81(6):1362–9.
59. Sami SS, Ravindran A, Kahn A, et al. Timeline and location of recurrence following successful ablation in Barrett's oesophagus: an international multicentre study. Gut 2019;68(8):1379–85.

Printed and bound by CPI Group (UK) Ltd, Croydon, CR0 4YY
08/05/2025
01864697-0003